The Medical Evaluation of Psychiatric Symptoms

Eric G. Meyer • Kelly L. Cozza
James A. Bourgeois
Editors

The Medical Evaluation of Psychiatric Symptoms

Springer

Editors
Eric G. Meyer
Department of Psychiatry
Uniformed Services University
of the Health Sciences
Bethesda, MD, USA

Kelly L. Cozza
Department of Psychiatry
Uniformed Services University
of the Health Sciences
Bethesda, MD, USA

James A. Bourgeois
Department of Psychiatry and Behavioral
Sciences
University of California, Davis
Sacramento, CA, USA

ISBN 978-3-031-14371-7 ISBN 978-3-031-14372-4 (eBook)
https://doi.org/10.1007/978-3-031-14372-4

This Springer imprint is published by the registered company Springer Nature Switzerland AG
The registered company address is: Gewerbestrasse 11, 6330 Cham, Switzerland

Dedication

To my wife and children—thank you for your ceaseless encouragement. To my amazing co-editors—without your kind mentorship this book would not have been possible. To my students, residents, and chapter authors—your questions have taught me more than you will ever know. Simon—your insatiable curiosity is missed—but not forgotten.

Eric G. Meyer

To my patients—thanks to each and every one for teaching me how to understand your symptoms and how they affect you as a person. I very much appreciate that you all have given me the honor of joining you in your health and life journey. Thanks of course to my family, Steve, Vince, and CC, for your love, support, and understanding of this night owl's work habits.

Kelly L. Cozza

To my family for their support. My wife, Kathleen M. Ayers, Psy.D., is a staff psychologist for UC Davis, specializing in psychotherapy for patients with chronic systemic illness. My son, Emile W. Ayers Bourgeois, M.B.A., is a mechanical engineer for Siemens. My daughter, Germaine A. Ayers Bourgeois, suffers from the NBIA Disorder MPAN (nbiadisorders.org). She previously worked at a remarkable facility for special needs adults, Brookwood in Georgetown (brookwoodingeorgetown.org).

James A. Bourgeois

We also dedicate this book to Dr. Robert Weick, who died prior to publication. We will miss you, Bobby.

Disclaimer

The opinions and assertions expressed herein are those of the author(s) and do not reflect the official policy or position of the Uniformed Services University of the Health Sciences or the Department of Defense.

Foreword

It is an honor to be asked to write a foreword for *The Medical Evaluation of Psychiatric Symptoms*. I have known the authors of this unique textbook for 15–30 years. The authors are all seasoned clinicians/academicians who have always worked at the interface of psychiatry and medicine. They are all highly experienced in Consultation-Liaison Psychiatry and are national and international leaders in the field. They all have strong academic credentials while retaining a love of patient care and a solidly grounded experience base in clinical medicine.

I have followed the careers of all three authors over more than three decades. Dr. Meyer's experience in psychiatry and medicine have earned him an important military medical leadership position in the Department of Defense. He is currently the Chief of Air Force Mental Health Operations and Psychiatry Consultant to the Air Force Surgeon General. He is also associate professor of Psychiatry at the F. Edward Hebert School of Medicine, Uniformed Services University of the Health Sciences, Bethesda Maryland. Dr. James A. Bourgeois, after carving out an important niche for psychiatrists who work as principal care physicians for patients needing complex medical and psychiatric care, was the Chair of Psychiatry and Baylor Scott and White Health, Central Texas Division and Clinical Professor in Medical Education at the Texas A&M University Health Science Center. He is now Vice Chair of Hospital Psychiatry Services in the Department of Psychiatry and Behavioral Sciences at the University of California, Davis Medical Center. I have known Dr. Kelly L. Cozza since she was a psychiatry resident in the early 1990s and have collaborated and worked together with her ever since, especially in the Academy of Consultation-Liaison Psychiatry. She is Professor of Psychiatry at the F. Edward Hebert School of Medicine, Uniformed Services University of the Health Sciences School of Medicine. She is a highly respected clinician, researcher, and teacher. I couldn't be more proud to see what successes these great psychiatrists have achieved, and I couldn't be happier to see them collaborate on this important textbook for our time.

At the interface between psychiatry and medicine, Consultation-Liaison Psychiatry is the American Board of Medical Specialties subspecialty uniquely positioned to provide training, expertise, and research on the important topic of the differential diagnosis of psychiatric and medical symptoms. The authors have identified an important lack of consolidated knowledge about how to approach symptoms commonly shared by psychiatry, primary care, and other medical-surgical specialty patients.

Patients present with symptoms, not diagnoses or syndromes. Yes, patients care about what their diagnosis is but what the vast majority want is relief of presenting symptoms. Approaching patients from a symptom-driven perspective assists with differential diagnosis processes and creates allies of patients by clinicians who identify with what they mostly want to address. In this respect, this textbook is long overdue. The authors have written a book that should have been in our armamentarium years and decades ago.

Readers will find a fresh approach to evaluating patients presenting with symptoms that may have psychiatric or medical etiologies and treatments. In addition to improving patient satisfaction and adherence with this approach, the structured approach to evaluating these types of symptoms is almost certain to also improve patient outcomes and patient safety. Every DSM-5-TR diagnosis includes an exclusion criterion that the disorder is not better explained by a substance or by a medical condition. Using the authors' broad and standard approach to differential diagnosis of symptoms can provide a much more confident approach to this important exclusionary criterion for psychiatric diagnoses. For psychiatrists, the authors' approach also provides a way to make certain that patients who are "medically cleared" are closer to actually being medically safe. Medical clearance does not equate to be medically ruled-out.

The Medical Evaluation of Psychiatric Symptoms is divided into chapters addressing evaluation of various symptoms commonly seen in psychiatric and medical practice, including insomnia, fatigue, decreased appetite, irritability, muscle tension, elated mood, and several others. Though each chapter has unique considerations, there is a comfortable and logical organization guiding the clinician to comprehensive evaluation of the symptoms discussed. For example, chapters typically start with clear definitions then move on to clinical evaluation. Detailed discussions of psychiatric and medical differential diagnoses are provided. As an example, for muscle tension, psychiatric differential diagnosis evaluation covers anxiety disorders, adjustment disorders, delirium, catatonia, neuroleptic malignant syndrome, and NMDA receptor encephalitis. Medical differential diagnosis for this symptom covers medication-induced etiologies, tension headaches, myositis, rhabdomyolysis, spasticity, Parkinson's disease, amyotrophic lateral sclerosis, and stiff person syndrome. For each of these conditions, there are details about incidence, prevalence and typical findings in history, physical examination, mental status examination, laboratory reports, and radiologic examinations.

This textbook will appeal to clinicians who take care of several types of patients: patients with comorbid medical and psychiatric conditions, patients with complex multi-disciplinary care needs, primary care patients with nonspecific presentations who present diagnostic dilemmas, psychiatrists who serve as patients' principal care physicians, and primary care clinicians who serve as patients' principal mental health clinicians—the latter often as a result of mental health clinician shortages, healthcare disparities, or lack of parity in healthcare coverage. I hope you are as happy as I am that this textbook has appeared at this important moment in our healthcare environment. It will truly fill a void.

James R. Rundell, MD, FACLP

Past-President,
Academy of Consultation-Liaison Psychiatry
Minneapolis, MN, USA

Preface

> What do you call the sound the wind makes? Does is merely *swoosh*? Or does it also *psithuros* which means a sort of sinister, slanderous whispering; *aeolian* for any wind that hits an object; and *rustle* for wind moving among leaves or paper? Indeed, the wind can *sigh*, *sough*, *roar*, *susurrate*, *breathe*, *zephyr*, *howl*, *chinook*, *trumpet*, and simply *blow*. To say it only *swooshes*, would rob the wind of its spirit.

Medical students are introduced to basic signs and symptoms of illness and disease within days of arriving on the doorstep of medical school. Pedantic concepts like *chest pain* quickly mature into *epigastric pain*, *cardiac pain*, and *pleuritic pain*. While students may not yet fully grasp the complete pathophysiology related to these symptoms, most beginning medical students can confidently identify and describe the different qualities of each of these symptoms, along with the etiology and even provide a cursory differential for each. Early medical students will achieve this level of competence for most symptoms—all but the symptoms of psychiatry. While this deficit may resolve with further training, medical students, residents, and even clinicians are frequently unaware of their inability to accurately describe psychiatric symptoms.

As an example, what is the difference between *anxiety* and *worry*? Are these just synonyms or are they different, like different types of chest pain? What about *stress*, *irritability*, or *being "on edge"*? Are these synonyms for anxiety? Components of anxiety? Reactions to anxiety? If all these symptoms are in fact discrete and different, do they each indicate separate differentials? If they do, what are the consequences of lumping them all together?

Lumping psychiatric symptoms together is commonplace in medicine, particularly psychiatry, and is how the Diagnostic and Statistical Manual of Mental Disorders series, the primary framework for understanding psychiatric symptoms, has been organized for over 60 years. The DSM-5-TR's A3 Criteria for major depressive disorder (MDD) combines "unexplained weight loss" with "a loss of appetite," even though a loss of appetite may not result in weight loss and unexplained weight loss may occur without a change in appetite. This lack of specificity begs the question: should these really be listed together as similar symptoms?

The DSM-5-TR lumping would be less of an issue if clinicians were more aware of what is actually listed in the DSM-5-TR. Unfortunately, too many clinicians' understanding of complicated psychiatric symptoms is limited to mnemonics or acronyms, such as SIGECAPS for major depressive disorder, or DIGFAST for bipolar disorder. While helpful recall devices, these approaches frequently disguise the complexity of the constructs they represent and leave clinicians unaware of all that they may be missing. For example, in MDD, clinicians may be unaware that the A7 criteria include "worthlessness" (not just guilt), and that the A9 criteria include morbid ideation (not just suicidal ideation).

"Short-hands" in medicine may perpetuate a lack of specificity, particularly in psychiatry. For example, "A&O" is frequently understood to simply mean *oriented*, wholly ignore whether the patient is *alert* (as if the initial "A" were just an indefinite article) and may result in a clinician missing the diagnosis of delirium entirely—which requires an alteration in *attention* and may include an alteration in *orientation*. The common shorthand "no AVH," which means "no auditory or visual hallucinations," emphasizes just two types of hallucinations (instead of including the full spectrum of auditory, visual, olfactory, tactile/kinesthetic, and gustatory hallucinations). For some clinicians, this "short-cut" combines two discrete types of hallucinating into one amorphous hallucinogenic experience. Imagine if this was acceptable in a cardiology assessment: "No rub-gallops." What about murmurs? Are gallops equal to rubs? Clearly *not*… but if this level of specificity is demanded in one field why is it not expected in another?

While lumping discrete psychiatric symptoms together affects how effectively we assess our patients, splitting diagnoses into "psychiatric" vs. "medical" or "organic" vs. "psychiatric" undermines our ability to effectively use clinical assessments to develop useful differential diagnoses and treatment plans. Dichotomous language is artificial and arbitrary at best and ignores the role of brain function and physiology. The anachronistic cartesian dualism of "brain" vs. "mind" as an "anatomic" vs. "functional" distinction between "neurologic or general medical" and "psychiatric" illness persists in common as well as medical language, despite being rendered obsolete by recent science and practice. The concept of "organic" disease in relation to psychiatric illness has been officially obsolete since the publication of the DSM-IV in 1994, yet some still refer to "neurologic" disease as "due to organic lesions," while "psychiatric" presentations are due to "functional" (implicitly non-anatomic, and, to many, purposeful or purposeful) causes.

"Psychosocial" problems, such as upbringing, distressing events, victimization/abuse, and interpersonal problems, are also considered by many clinicians as being "less real" or "less organic/physiological" than "neurologic" and "physical/organic" causes, the latter being due to "real disease." This regrettable distinction persists despite decades of research that has repeatedly demonstrated that schizophrenia, bipolar disorder, major depressive disorder, and panic disorder have substantially heritable components.[1] To further illustrate this point, the only psychiatric illnesses that *a priori* requires the experience of traumatic events are acute stress disorder and posttraumatic stress disorder.

These many cross-purposes and cross-understandings undermine our ability to diagnose important conditions effectively, and also affect how effectively we treat

[1] Kendall KM, Van Assche E, Andlauer TF, Choi KW, Luykx JJ, Schulte EC, Lu Y. The genetic basis of major depression. Psychol Med. 2021;8:1–4.

our patients. One obvious example includes the low response rate of psychiatric medications: "[O]n average a marketed psychiatric drug is efficacious in approximately half of the patients who take it. One reason for this low response rate is the artificial grouping of heterogeneous syndromes with different pathophysiological mechanisms into one disorder."[2]

Despite the groundbreaking research in connectomes, epigenetics, and biomarkers which are clearly advancing our understanding of psychiatric illnesses, these scientific advances can only be employed when clinicians are able to assess their patient's psychiatric symptoms accurately and reliably. The recent explosion of information regarding neuropsychiatric symptoms being a result of inflammation related to the body's response to SARS-CoV-2 highlights the need for specificity in describing, and ascribing, psychiatric symptoms—especially if ever hope to accurately ascribe them to their causes.

The process of developing this book has been more revealing and instructive than we ever imagined. Each of the chapter's authors have done a remarkable job of examining and developing our understanding of a singular symptom. What we thought were a collection of nine simple symptoms that have been exposed as rich, nuanced, and clinically informative. Ultimately, we hope that our symptomatic approach will enable clinicians to better hear their patients' psychiatric symptoms as important *in and of themselves*.

Department of Psychiatry
Uniformed Services University of the Health Sciences
Bethesda, MD, USA
Eric G. Meyer

Department of Psychiatry
Uniformed Services University of the Health Sciences
Bethesda, MD, USA
Kelly L. Cozza

Department of Psychiatry and Behavioral Sciences
University of California, Davis
Sacramento, CA, USA
James A. Bourgeois

[2]Wong EH, Yocca F, Smith MA, Lee CM. Challenges and opportunities for drug discovery in psychiatric disorders: the drug hunters' perspective. Int J Neuropsychopharmacol. 2010;13(9):1269–84.

Contents

Introduction

This book can be read as a complete text with each chapter exploring a different type of symptom and a new approach to appreciating that symptom. The book has also been sufficiently organized that it can be used as a reference—helping clinicians expand their thinking for a specific symptom.

Each chapter focuses on a singular symptom, with no attempt to explain that symptom as being part of a larger construct. Each symptom is treated as an independent entity. In some instances, this required being exceptionally focused. For example, a chapter on "memory loss" (Chap. 6) is too broad, so we opted to limit the chapter to a specific type of memory (recent declarative). This focus made it possible to clearly define the symptom and explore a differential of just that symptom. Conversely, for insomnia we opted to include three variants: early, middle, and late insomnia. While this resulted in a slightly longer chapter, it made it possible for the reader to compare these three variants and appreciate the different differentials for each.

Each chapter begins with a basic definition of the symptom. These definitions often involve differentiating the symptoms from other symptoms (muscle tension from muscle pain) or as a subtype of a larger symptom category (concentration as a type of attention). We also opted to include historical and literary explanations of the symptom—as these "symptoms" are frequently part of the routine human experience and their definition outside of the clinical realm is often much more revealing.

We then provide a comparison of understandings across specialties—which we hope helps consultants better understand potential misconceptions and misunderstandings of "shared concepts." As part of this, we included a general overview of how psychiatry conceptualizes the symptom to include references to the DSM-5-TR and Research Domain Criteria (RDoC). This inclusion should not be considered an endorsement or criticism of either system, but rather an effort to help readers see the multiple ways a single symptom can be organized diagnostically. Finally, we provide applicable cultural differences in understanding the symptom to further help clinicians appreciate potential questions they might ask their patients to better appreciate their cultural contexts.

Following this thorough definition, we provide a differential specific to the symptom. This section is separated by *disorders* (as described by the DSM-5-TR) and *diagnoses* as defined outside of the DSM-5-TR. For each disorder and diagnosis, we first provide the incidence. When possible, we present the incidence of a disorder presenting with the specific symptoms to assist clinicians compare their own patient panels to expected incidences. For example, given the rate of diabetes mellitus first presenting with depression, the likelihood that a clinician has no diabetic patients is highly unlikely. We also avoided prototypical diagnoses and instead focused on common diagnoses. Many clinicians are taught that depression or mania can be the result of thyroid dysfunction. While certainly true, and memorable, this is an uncommon event, certainly less likely than a patient presenting with depressive symptoms in the context of an inflammatory disorder such as diabetes mellitus. The tradition of focusing on "rare but memorable" medical diagnoses can undermine the reality that common psychiatric symptoms may be part of common systemic medical conditions. As such, we avoided rare prototypical disorders and focused on what clinicians are likely to see clinically.

Lastly, for each diagnosis we provide potential follow-up questions, physical exam maneuvers, and laboratory/radiologic tests that may help confirm or rule out a diagnosis. To further help clinicians determine the predictive value of these additional steps, we also included positive and negative predictive values as available. Psychiatric diagnoses are generally diagnoses of exclusion, so negative predictive values are especially important. For example, while conjunctival pallor does not necessary indicate anemia, a lack of conjunctival pallor is 100% specific for not having anemia—a helpful, affordable, and easy physical exam maneuver for any clinician ruling out anemia as the source of *fatigue*.

The editors hope that providing a sequenced approach to symptom ascertainment and attributions fits into the usual routine of clinical diagnosis, providing an effective supplement to the assessment and management of patients presenting with these symptoms, whether ultimately attributed to "psychiatric illness," "systemic illness" or, as oft true, *both*.

Department of Psychiatry
Uniformed Services University of the Health Sciences
Bethesda, MD, USA
Eric G. Meyer
eric.meyer@usuhs.edu

Department of Psychiatry
Uniformed Services University of the Health Sciences
Bethesda, MD, USA
Kelly L. Cozza
kelly.cozza@usuhs.edu

Department of Psychiatry and Behavioral Sciences
University of California, Davis
Sacramento, CA, USA
James A. Bourgeois
jbourgeois@ucdavis.edu

Loss of Appetite

1

Shannon C. Ford

Defining Loss of Appetite

Current Definition of Loss of Appetite

According to the Merriam-Webster dictionary, appetite is defined as "any of the instinctive desires necessary to keep up organic life," and anorexia is defined as "loss of appetite especially when prolonged" [1]. The use of anorexia in this context is separate from the DSM-5-TR diagnosis of anorexia nervosa. Appetite can also be described as a desire to eat, associated with everything that is appealing about food, or felt as the body's biological response to hunger when your stomach grumbles. One's emotional state can also influence appetite. Consuming food is a staple of social interaction; not eating is often noticed by others.

"Loss of appetite" is best described as a symptom change: a decrease from a previous appetite level as it is experienced by the patient. The underlying cause of this change can be further described as not wanting to eat, not wanting to eat more, not wanting to eat a specific food, having hunger but also nausea by the thought of food, or wanting to eat but being too weak to consume food. It could be due to not experiencing pleasure previously associated with eating due to a loss of sensation (smell, taste, texture, satiety). It could also be due to an early feeling of satiety—often coming as a surprise to the person who expects to be able or wants to eat more.

Historical Definition of Loss of Appetite

Consuming food is essential for survival, though its history is a complicated one. There is evidence of food being used as a status symbol such as in 700 BC when

S. C. Ford (✉)
Department of Psychiatry, Uniformed Services University of the Health Sciences, Bethesda, MD, USA
e-mail: shannon.c.ford.mil@health.mil

E. G. Meyer et al. (eds.), *The Medical Evaluation of Psychiatric Symptoms*,
https://doi.org/10.1007/978-3-031-14372-4_1

Romans would overindulge and then vomit so they could continue to gorge. Eating disorders are documented in Chinese scrolls. Some religions felt that starvation was necessary to deprecate or purify the body. The founder of Jainism, Vardhamana, died of voluntary starvation in the sixth century BC [2]. A Roman woman who followed the teachings of Saint Jerome starved herself in 383 AD [3]. His teachings included "Let your companions be women, pale and thin with fasting such as daily…" [2]. These cases were significantly less common following the fall of the Roman Empire [3]. During the Renaissance, fasting was used as a way to be "closer" to God, some becoming saints as a result of their faith but then the phenomenon was not well discussed until the nineteenth century [3].

The medical literature discussed one such patient in 1689, where Richard Morton's description of an 18-year-old woman is believed to be the first medical description of anorexia nervosa. In 1859, W.S. Chipley published in *American Journal of Insanity* about "sitophobia" or food refusal. Sir William Gull receives credit for first using the term "anorexia nervosa" in 1873 [2, 3]. Anorexia or sitophobia in the "insane" was considered a serious symptom. Forced feeding was often the recommended treatment of choice for severe cases with an otherwise unknown etiology, as well as removal from the patient's home environment. It is generally believed today that the description of patients with sitophobia does not completely align with how modern medicine looks at anorexia nervosa [4].

Pathophysiology of Loss of Appetite

Through a number of complex pathways, our bodies self-regulate the balance between energy requirements and expenditure. This regulatory system involves a varying combination of the availability of energy reserves, available foods, existing metabolic requirements, and individual tastes and preferences [5]. Ideally, there is a level of homeostasis that exists, but we know this is not true in nature. Foods that induce a response in the reward pathway may induce a sensation of hunger despite the lack of a need for caloric energy at the time. On the contrary, foods that are less than desirable will still be considered acceptable in times of depleted energy reserves [6]. Because this homeostasis is an integral factor in survival mechanisms, it is important to recognize and further evaluate any time it is no longer in balance.

Separating Loss of Appetite from Other Symptoms

If appetite is defined as an instinctive desire necessary to maintain life, hunger is the signal that tells the body it requires nutrition. "Loss of appetite" is the loss of this desire, contrary to the survival instinct. This loss would also presumably lead to a lack of hunger, though in the literature, "loss of appetite" is often missed as a symptom and replaced with "weight loss" (explained or unexplained) synonymously (and erroneously). This can lead to confusion and inconsistent descriptions. "Loss of appetite" does not have to correlate to decreased caloric intake and some patients will have normal nutritional intakes despite the loss of appetite.

It is also important to separate out when the patient reports having a loss of appetite despite the presence of hunger. There are many ways where patients may present with a decreased oral intake that is not necessarily related to an underlying disease process. In 1989, Robbins described the nine "d's" of geriatric weight loss: dentition, dysgeusia, dysphagia, diarrhea, disease, depression, dementia, dysfunction, and drugs [7]. Now, "Anorexia of Aging" is a loss of appetite that is seen in the elderly due to multiple factors and can have serious consequences as this population is more vulnerable to a decline or shift in food intake and other stressors. Untreated, it can lead to malnutrition and decreased survivability [8]. Especially towards the end of life, the voluntary stopping of eating and drinking (VSED) may be considered a suicidal gesture, but it is also seen as a way of keeping autonomy and control [9]. Appetite changes in VSED may or may not be present, depending upon whether there are other underlying disease processes. Another instance of poor nutritional intake is "drunkorexia," where the patient skips meals and/or induces vomiting in order to reduce weight due to the caloric load of alcohol use [10].

From the psychiatric perspective, having a loss of appetite is also not synonymous with the abnormal eating behaviors described in the differential diagnosis for an eating disorder such as anorexia nervosa or bulimia nervosa. These are diagnoses with complex underlying psychopathology and appetite may even be preserved. Also, loss of appetite is better separated from the consequences of decreased caloric intake in the A criteria for avoidant/restrictive food intake disorder. While that criterium is further described in ways that may suggest why someone would have a decreased appetite (an apparent lack of interest in eating food, avoidance based on sensory characteristics, and concern about aversive consequences), this is a pediatric diagnosis of exclusion where symptoms cannot be better described by another psychiatric or medical illness [11].

Variants of Loss of Appetite Based on Specialty

Patients who report that they are experiencing a loss of appetite may have significant variance underlying the cause of this symptom, and the differential diagnosis may be inappropriately narrowed if their is a presumption that the underlying pathology is psychiatric in nature solely due to the location (psychiatrist's office) in which the complaint is made. Just as it is important to differentiate loss of appetite as a symptom from the behavior of intentional food restriction, context is important when considering the possible etiologies.

Medicine The presumption of unexplained weight loss a may be considered secondary to underlying medical illness, psychiatric condition, or surreptitious use of substance in inappropriate dieting. Loss of interest in food may only be considered in the context of terminal illness or cases where senses may be altered and then as an expected side effect, as opposed to a symptom that requires further or independent evaluation.

Surgery A new surgical patient's presentation may be narrowed in the direction of pathology that may require surgical intervention such as an obstruction, and is often timeline-focused. Postoperatively, a lack of appetite may need to be evaluated with urgency because of the concern for intestinal blockage. In the longer postoperative time period, poor nutrition can lead to delayed healing time and prolonged recovery with excessive fatigue. It may also be a very normal response, as one study showed that it required approximately 4 weeks for patients to regain their appetite following an uncomplicated total joint arthroplasty [12].

Obstetrics Hormonal changes of pregnancy may factor in to how food is experienced, from causing nausea to changing sensitivity to smell and taste. "Morning sickness," typically associated with the first trimester of pregnancy, does neither have to occur in the morning nor only in the first trimester. Weight loss may happen and is monitored routinely. As pregnancy progresses, abdominal organs all have to share space which can constrict the stomach and cause early satiety or appetite loss. Postpartum depression may be very concerning, and appetite is closely monitored during this period especially as it relates to mood.

Pediatrics There is a difference between a child who is a "picky eater" and one who does not have a desire to eat. Sometimes their world has so many interesting things to pay attention to and explore that hunger is ignored and meals may be less of a priority. Children can choose what to eat (or not) as a way of exerting control, which is part of normal development. Many mild illnesses will present with loss of appetite as a symptoms, and as long as the behavior resolves with other symptoms and the child remains hydrated, it is generally of less concern. There are other potential underlying causes that are worthy of considering including stress response, depression, constipation, anemia, infection, or medication side effects. Eating disorders should also be considered, especially in adolescents.

Psychiatry Patients may present as referrals from primary care specialties due to their somatic complaints that do not have a yet identified medical cause or de novo to offices as a primary or secondary focus of attention. The initial differential is broad even if it excludes potential medical etiologies. In the DSM-5-TR a loss of appetite is co-located with "a significant unexpected weight loss" in the A3 criteria for major depressive disorder [11]. If this combination of appetite loss and depression is found in the geriatric population, there is an increased risk of developing dementia [13]. An underlying neurocognitive disorder may be the cause of appetite loss. But assuming the loss of appetite is secondary to psychiatric illness due to age is dangerous; less than 1/3 of these cases are attributable to psychiatric causes [14]. In some psychiatric patients, symptoms of paranoia causing fear about eating may have to be explored, even though appetite loss is not a specific criterium for a psychotic disorder. A substance use disorder may also be interfering with normal caloric intake.

Within psychiatry, the research domain criteria (RDoC) framework was designed to address the limitations seen within the way the DSM has categorized mental illnesses based upon symptoms. For eating disorders, the RDoC notes that the current DSM classification is reliant upon symptoms that have a high likelihood of being found in other disorders including weight, behaviors to affect weight control, and any associated cognitive beliefs. Eating disorders are linked to all five of the RDoC domains. The negative valence system can explore how stress can lead to the development of disordered eating behaviors. The subsystems under the positive valence system all can be associated with eating disorders, as they relate to how people interpret rewards and perpetuate habits to sustain this. Even when the reward is inconsistent with societal norms, the aberrant behavior continues to feel reinforced and allowed to perpetuate (e.g. calorie restriction in anorexia nervosa). The cognitive domain is also noted as having a strong role in eating disorders due to the pathways that lead to inhibiting behaviors related to eating disorders, as well as the ability to shift sets and reassess goals given new information (such as inadequate caloric intake). Social processes can also play a strong role in eating disorders given the importance of being a part of a group during mealtime, and that these behaviors are impaired in the case of eating disorders. Self-evaluation is more negative, attachment more insecure, and interaction with others/perception of self in relation to this are all impaired. The fifth domain, arousal and regulatory systems better categorize some of the aberrant nocturnal eating disordered behaviors. As eating disorders play a significant role in each of the five domains, it is believed that the idea of homeostatic eating is important in other psychiatric conditions [15].

Variants of Loss of Appetite Based on Culture

Cultural considerations are important when discussing food intake with patients. Calorie consumption, weight gain, weight loss, body mass index (BMI), waist size, low calorie, low fat, low sugar, high protein, and others are all words that regularly make headlines. What kinds and quantities of food people eat, how that makes them feel and look, and the "right" one for them are the constant source of advertisements for weight loss fads and special diets. Not wanting to eat may even be seen as desirable due to the constant external pressure some feel for achieving an ideal weight or successful engaging in intermittent fasting.

While once considered merely a necessity for physiological survival, the act of acquiring, preparing, and sharing food is increasingly a social construct. Some health concerns necessitate and exclude individuals from this sharing, be it allergies or special dietary requirements due to metabolic disease. Other health concerns and societal pressures may affect how people consume meals, in what quantity, and where (i.e., intermittent fasting may stop someone from participating in brunch, or someone with a binge eating disorder may eat alone and with a great deal of shame).

Sometimes a patient may prefer to attribute a loss of appetite as the underlying reason in a more socially accepted cultural context when questioned about weight loss or other symptoms consistent with poor oral intake. Eating disorders have been associated with sports such as ballet, figure skating, gymnastics, wrestling, jockeying, running, and swimming—regardless of gender [16]. Being of low socioeconomic status and financial difficulties can decrease access to food, so if asked about weight loss or another symptom suggestive of decreased caloric intake, the explanation of "I'm not hungry," can be more socially acceptable than admitting one cannot afford groceries.

A Psychiatric Differential for Loss of Appetite

In addition to the eating disorders category, psychiatric diagnoses that may present with anorexia are seen throughout DSM-5-TR.

Schizophrenia Spectrum and Other Psychotic Disorders

The disorganized behavior and/or catatonia seen in psychotic disorders including schizophrenia, could lead one to lack the planning required to eat or not recognize they are experiencing hunger. A delusional disorder with the persecutory belief that the patient is being poisoned could lead to a presentation of loss of appetite, especially if the patient is trying to minimize or normalize their paranoia.

Delusional Disorder, Persecutory Type

Incidence/Prevalence

The prevalence of delusional disorders is approximately 0.18% of the general population and between 1% and 4% of psychiatric admissions [17].

Incidence/Prevalence of Diagnosis Presenting with Loss of Appetite

Unknown.

Typical Findings of the HPI

One month of more of one or more delusion(s) without meeting the "Criterion A" for schizophrenia. Persecutory delusions may invoke anger or violent behavior [11]. There may be difficulty with occupational and social functioning.

Typical Findings on Physical and Mental Status Exam

Physical exam findings may show evidence of malnutrition.

Mental status exam will be dependent on the delusion but the patient may show dishevelment/poor grooming and hygiene, disorganized thought processes, and anger/hostility. Delusions are considered to be true by the patient.

Typical Laboratory/Radiological Findings

None are expected, but substance use will need to be ruled out.

Brief Psychotic Disorder, Schizophreniform Disorder, Schizophrenia

Incidence/Prevalence

The prevalence for brief psychotic disorder is 9%, and 0.3–0.7% for schizophreniform/schizophrenia [11].

Incidence/Prevalence of Diagnosis Presenting with Loss of Appetite

Unknown.

Typical Findings of the HPI

The timeline of illness determines the diagnosis. Onset is sudden in brief psychotic disorders, but in the case of schizophrenia prodromal symptoms tend to present in the active phase. A broad range of symptoms are seen, both positive and negative including delusions, disorganized or catatonic behavior, and avolition which may all lead to loss of appetite or food avoidance [11].

Typical Findings on Physical and Mental Status Exam

Physical exam findings may show evidence of malnutrition.

The mental status exam findings may show inappropriate effect, delusions, anxiety, occupational and social impairment, lack of insight, and disorganized thought process, but procedural memory remains intact.

Typical Laboratory/Radiological Findings

There are no notable diagnostic laboratory or radiological findings.

Substance Use Disorders

In this category, loss of appetite can be secondary to appetite suppression (nicotine, stimulant, cocaine, etc., abuse) or caloric replacement (alcohol abuse). "Drunkorexia" is a term used in both general vernacular and more academic articles that describes a person who restricts calories from nutritious foods and/or exercises excessively, in order to mitigate caloric consumption from excessive alcohol use [18].

Alcohol Use Disorders

Incidence/Prevalence

In the US, the prevalence of adults older than 18 years of age with an alcohol use disorder is 8.5%. Between 18 and 29-years old this number increases to 16.2%, with use declining with age. Americans over the age of 65-years old have a prevalence of 1.5%.

Incidence/Prevalence of Diagnosis Presenting with Loss of Appetite

Unknown.

Typical Findings of the HPI

In cases with heavy amounts of alcohol use, complaints of gastritis, stomach/duodenal ulcers, liver cirrhosis, and pancreatitis are typically seen. During alcohol withdrawal patients may exhibit nausea, vomiting, gastritis, hematemesis, dry mouth, peripheral edema, autonomic hyperactivity, tremor, auditory/visual hallucinations, and/or seizures.

Typical Findings on Physical and Mental Status Exam

Physical exam findings may show evidence of malnutrition, peripheral edema, jaundice, and/or abdominal pain.

The mental status exam findings may range from normal to signs of intoxication or withdrawal, depending on the person's substance use.

Typical Laboratory/Radiological Findings

Elevated blood alcohol level, elevated liver enzymes (2:1 AST:ALT ratio), elevated alkaline phosphatase, increased uric acid, increased gamma-glutamyl transferase (GGT), increased carbohydrate-deficient transferrin (CDT), elevated RBC MCV, decreased platelets, increased prothrombin, low albumin, low sodium, positive urine ethyl glucuronide and ethyl sulfate, positive blood alcohol level.

On imaging, there may be hepatic enlargement. Abnormal brain findings are usually seen in severe cases with associated Wernicke's-Korsakoff syndrome.

Caffeine Use Disorders

Incidence/Prevalence

The prevalence is up to 30% in small general population studies [19].

Incidence/Prevalence of Diagnosis Presenting with Loss of Appetite

Unknown.

Typical Findings of the HPI

Caffeine intoxication (usually >250 mg/2 cups of coffee) typically produces restlessness, nervousness, excitement, anxiety, insomnia, flushed face, diuresis, gastrointestinal distress, muscle twitching, and/or tachycardia or cardiac arrhythmias.

Caffeine withdrawal may cause headaches, fatigue, irritability, flu-like symptoms (nausea, vomiting, muscle pain), drowsiness, and/or depression. Withdrawal symptoms are typically seen after abrupt cessation of daily or near-daily use.

Typical Findings on Physical and Mental Status Exam

Physical exam findings may show evidence of malnutrition, tachycardia (associated with intoxication), or hypertension.

Mental status exam: In cases of caffeine intoxication, rambling flow of thought and speech, anxiety, sense of constant energy availability, and/or psychomotor agitation are seen.

For caffeine withdrawal, the patient may display dysphoric or depressed mood, irritability, and/or difficulty with concentration.

Typical Laboratory/Radiological Findings

There are no notable diagnostic laboratory or radiological findings; caffeine is not routinely used as part of a screening panel for drugs of abuse.

Cannabis Withdrawal

Incidence/Prevalence

The prevalence of cannabis use in American adults is 1.8%.

Incidence/Prevalence of Diagnosis Presenting with Loss of Appetite

Unknown.

Typical findings of the HPI

Symptoms usually present after abrupt cessation of daily or near-daily use. Patients may complain of difficulty with sleep, decreased appetite or weight loss, irritability, and/or motivation (from chronic use).

Typical Findings on Physical and Mental Status Exam

Physical exam findings are likely to be normal.

The mental status exam may show irritability, anger or aggression, anxiety, depressed mood, and/or restlessness.

Typical Laboratory/Radiological Findings

If tested for, the drug screen could be positive for cannabis.

Stimulant Use Disorder

Incidence/Prevalence

The prevalence in American adults older than 18-years old for amphetamine use is 0.2% and cocaine use is 0.3%.

Incidence/Prevalence of Diagnosis Presenting with Loss of Appetite

Unknown.

Typical Findings of the HPI

Symptoms of stimulant intoxication includes increased or decreased heart rate and blood pressure, pupillary dilation, perspiration and chills, nausea/vomiting, muscular weakness, and/or chest pain. Severe cases may lead to dyskinesias, dystonia, and coma.

Typical Findings on Physical and Mental Status Exam

Physical exam findings may show evidence of malnutrition due to the drug's tendency to suppress appetite.

Mental status exam findings may show psychomotor agitation or retardation and confusion.

Typical Laboratory/Radiological Findings

If tested for, the drug screen may be positive for amphetamines.

Tobacco Use Disorder

Incidence/Prevalence

Approximately 20% of US adults identified as current users in 2018.

Incidence/Prevalence of Diagnosis Presenting with Loss of Appetite

Unknown.

Typical Findings of the HPI

Symptoms associated with tobacco use may include tachycardia, hypertension, increased respiration, improved concentration/focus, and appetite suppression.

Patients who use tobacco regularly may have associated signs, such as clothes that smell of smoke, carrying a bottle for chew/dip spit, or having paraphernalia.

Typical Findings on Physical and Mental Status Exam

Physical exam findings may show evidence of malnutrition, stained teeth, and fingertips.

The mental status exam is likely to be most abnormal during the withdrawal phase, when the patient may have irritability, anxiety, and nicotine cravings.

Typical Laboratory/Radiological Findings

There are no notable diagnostic laboratory or radiological findings.

Depressive Disorders

Depressive and bipolar disorders that require a depressive episode as part of their diagnostic criteria can be characterized by anorexia. In the DSM-5-TR, depressive disorders are in a separate chapter from bipolar disorders. Bipolar disorder, type II requires a depressive episode, though bipolar disorder type I does not for diagnostic purposes though this is often seen. The A3 diagnostic criterion for a Major Depressive Disorder is to have weight loss or decrease or increase in appetite nearly every day. The B1 criteria for Persistent Depressive Disorder (Dysthymia) is poor appetite or overeating. Loss of appetite is not required in bereavement but can be seen as part of the associated depressive features [11]. When the depressive episode is characterized as by having melancholic features, experiencing either loss of pleasure in all or almost activities, or lack of reactivity to usually pleasurable stimuli, and meet 3 of 6 criteria where criterium 5 is "significant anorexia or weight loss" [11].

Major Depressive Disorder

Incidence/Prevalence

Per the DSM-5-TR, the annual prevalence of American adults with major depressive disorder is 7%. Women are 1.5–3 times more likely than males to have this diagnosis [11]. In patients who are hospitalized for all reasons, the prevalence is 12%, with studies reporting as high as 32% [20].

Incidence/Prevalence of Diagnosis Presenting with Loss of Appetite

Unknown.

Typical Findings of the HPI

Patients experiencing a depressive episode will demonstrate a depressed mood, anhedonia, possibly an acute stressor, difficulty with sleep, low energy, and/or changes in appetite.

Typical Findings on Physical and Mental Status Exam

Physical exam findings may show evidence of malnutrition.

Mental status exam findings may show mood and affect congruent with depression, psychomotor retardation, poor eye contact, and slowed thought processes.

Typical Laboratory/Radiological Findings

Other conditions must be ruled out to ensure that symptom presentation is not due to a medical diagnosis.

Anxiety & Obsessive-Compulsive and Related Disorders

Anxiety disorders do not require a component of appetite or food intake in their diagnostic criteria, but disordered eating can be seen in the context of anxiety. There may be fear associated with eating in public for social anxiety disorder or a preoccupation with food as part of obsessive-compulsive disorder. Personal beliefs about one's appearance in body dysmorphic disorder may lead to changes in eating behaviors, but this is not secondary to a loss of appetite as defined in this chapter.

Incidence/Prevalence

One systematic review cited the global prevalence of all anxiety disorders is 7.3%, with higher rates in conflict countries and Euro/Anglo cultures [21].

Incidence/Prevalence of Diagnosis Presenting with Loss of Appetite

Unknown.

Typical Findings of the HPI

The histories are more specific to the underlying disease that is being evaluated, with the loss of appetite not identified as a primary presenting symptom, but the eating behaviors are found to be secondary to other symptoms. Patients may report excessive worry, ruminating thoughts, obsessive or compulsive behaviors, or recent life stressors. In addition to poor appetite, they may also have insomnia, restlessness, or other somatic symptoms.

Typical Findings on Physical and Mental Status Exam

Physical exam findings should focus on any somatic complaints. Short, ragged fingernails, or restlessness may be seen.

Mental status exam findings may show psychomotor agitation or restlessness, mood and affect congruent with anxiety, but the patient demonstrates an intact sensorium without perceptual disturbances.

Typical Laboratory/Radiological Findings

There are no notable diagnostic laboratory or radiological findings.

Feeding and Eating Disorders

Feeding and eating disorders are diagnosed when there is a pathologic change in how or what a person eats. Eating nonfood items is generally not considered when working up the complaint of a loss of appetite, but eating less or not at all is a key component to many of these disorders.

Avoidant/Restrictive Food Intake Disorder

Incidence/Prevalence

The prevalence of this primarily pediatric diagnosis in children aged 8–13-years old is 3.2%. The prevalence in patients older than 15-years old is 0.3% [22].

Incidence/Prevalence of Diagnosis Presenting with Loss of Appetite

Unknown.

Typical Findings of the HPI

Avoidant or restrictive food intake disorder generally begins in childhood, but may persist to adulthood. These patients may not present for care, as they have relatively normal levels of functioning. When seen in children, the guardians or parents typically provide some of the history associated with feeding and eating behaviors. When adults are evaluated it is important to discuss the underlying cause: lack of interest in food, expressed aversion to food based on sensory characteristics, or aversive consequences of eating, all of which can help elucidate more information about the issue. Any of those behaviors may ultimately lead to a conditioned negative response associated with the intake of a specific food.

Typical Findings on Physical and Mental Status Exam

Physical exam findings of limited food intake may include symptoms or malnutrition or failure to thrive.

Mental status exam findings generally depend on the motivation for food avoidance (lack of interest, difficulty with sensory features of eating, aversive avoidance related to a previous negative event) but sensorium is typically intact without evidence of paranoia or delusions. (If present, these would suggest a different diagnosis).

Typical Laboratory/Radiological Findings

Patients with dietary deficiencies may have low iron, calcium, vitamin B12, folate, and/or vitamin D.

Anorexia Nervosa

Incidence/Prevalence

The prevalence of anorexia nervosa in young females is approximately 0.4%. The prevalence in males is believed to be approximately one tenth that of females [11].

Incidence/Prevalence of Diagnosis Presenting with Loss of Appetite

Because the diagnostic criteria for this disorder require patients to have a normal appetite but distorted body image that leads to a change in intake, the prevalence is 0%.

Typical Findings of the HPI

Typically, the presentation focuses on weight and body image. Typically, weight loss or poor growth are seen, and developmentally inappropriate concerns about body image and weight are also present. There is usually an intense fear of gaining weight, leading to a consumption of less than 500 kcal/day with a strong desire to control their environment. Other behaviors may include food refusal, rituals around mealtime, behavior that prevents/interferes with gaining weight, and inappropriate compensation mechanisms (purging, laxative abuse, excessive exercise). Patients are frequently having denial and poor insight into the severity of their disease. In females, amenorrhea or oligomenorrhea may be present. Both sexes may have diminished libido, insomnia, cold intolerance, muscular weakness, presyncope/syncope, emotional dysregulation, poor self-esteem, rigid thinking, and limited coping skills.

Typical Findings on Physical and Mental Status Exam

Physical exam findings will include low body weight and body mass index (BMI) compared to developmental norms. Findings may also include bradycardia, hypotension, orthostatic hypotension, hypothermia, loss of muscle mass and subcutaneous fat, alopecia or brittle hair, xeroderma, and/or xanthoderma.

Mental status exam findings may include depressed mood, irritability, anxiety/obsessiveness, poor stress tolerance, difficulty with concentration, and/or fatigue.

Typical Laboratory/Radiological Findings

Depending on the severity of illness, electrolyte abnormalities including low calcium, magnesium, and phosphate levels may be present. Poor protein intake may lead to hypoalbuminemia and low total protein levels. Low alkaline phosphatase, elevated amylase, and/or mild transaminitis with a normal bilirubin may also be seen. Water intoxication can lead to hyponatremia. Dehydration can cause elevated creatinine and BUN. A CBC may show normocytic-normochromic anemia. In females, central suppression of luteinizing hormone and follicle-stimulating hormone levels (subsequent decrease in estradiol and testosterone levels) may be found.

In the starvation state, on EKG there may be prolonged QT intervals.

Bulimia Nervosa

Incidence/Prevalence

The annual prevalence of bulimia nervosa in females is 1–1.5%. Similar to anorexia nervosa, less is known about the prevalence of this disorder in males but it is estimated to be one-tenth that of females [11].

Incidence/Prevalence of Diagnosis Presenting with Loss of Appetite

Unknown.

Typical Findings of the HPI

The key criteria for this diagnosis are inappropriate bingeing and subsequent compensatory behaviors. Patients may experience a lack of appetite after a binge. Generally, this diagnosis is associated with shame and an attempt to conceal behaviors so the patient may not be fully forthcoming. There is a fear of weight gain and body image dissatisfaction. Physical symptoms may include complaints of bloating, flatulence, and constipation. There may be a new onset of GERD symptoms. Despite the disordered eating behaviors, weight may be normal.

Typical Findings on Physical and Mental Status Exam

Physical exam findings may be dependent on the modality used for purging behaviors. In laxative abuse, there may be rectal prolapse. Ipecac abuse can cause cardiomyopathy that presents with left ventricular dysfunction. Vomiting can lead to enamel erosion on lingual surface of the teeth, caries, oral ulcerations, callus formation over dorsal aspects of metacorpophalangeal and interphalangeal joints, parotid swelling, or scleral hemorrhages. The patient may not be underweight.

Mental status exam findings: Bulimia nervosa has a high likelihood of psychiatric comorbidity; these patients tend to be extroverted and perfectionistic [23]. Thirty to seventy percent have a coexisting substance abuse problem, which will also affect their mental status [24].

Typical Laboratory/Radiological Findings

Electrolyte abnormalities can be seen to include: hypokalemic and hypochloremic metabolic alkalosis due to purging, hypokalemia from laxative abuse, hyponatremia secondary to water intoxication, low calcium, magnesium, and phosphate levels. There may be an elevated amylase, mild transaminitis, and low alkaline phosphatase with normal bilirubin. Malnutrition may cause hypoalbuminemia and low total protein levels. Dehydration leads to elevated creatinine and BUN levels. CBC shows normocytic-normochromic anemia.

The urinalysis may show a ratio of urine sodium to urine chloride greater than 1.16.

If nocturnal eating is occurring during periods of aberrant sleep behaviors, the patient may be less hungry during the day but will not necessarily experience weight loss. Other signs associated with nocturnal eating may be present in these instances, such as evidence of food in bed, disruption in the kitchen food storage areas, or dishes and other detritus of food preparation on the sink and counters.

A Medical Differential for Loss of Appetite

Adrenal Insufficiency (Addison's Disease)

Adrenal insufficiency is due to the inadequate secretion of corticosteroids that occurs in primary adrenal failure (partial or complete destruction of the adrenal glands) or secondary cortisol deficiency due to critical illness and pituitary insufficiency. Acute adrenal crisis is unlikely to present as a chronic condition in a psychiatry office, as it is characterized by cardiovascular collapse and hemodynamic instability. Chronic adrenal insufficiency however will present with nonspecific symptoms, especially initially. The most common cause is due to autoimmune adrenalitis [25], but malignancy, infection (tuberculosis, cytomegalovirus, HIV, candidiasis, histoplasmosis), and genetic causes can also be seen.

Incidence/Prevalence

The prevalence of chronic primary adrenal insufficiency is increasing but this disease remains rare, with a prevalence of approximately 1 in 20,000 persons in the US and Western Europe [26] and an annual incidence of approximately 4 per million in Western populations [27]. It is seen twice as often in females than males. In patients with diagnosed adrenal insufficiency, 6–8% will have an adrenal crisis annually [28].

Incidence/Prevalence of Diagnosis Presenting with Loss of Appetite

Symptoms of anorexia, weakness, tiredness, and fatigue are seen in 100% of patients diagnosed with adrenal insufficiency. Ninety-two percent complain of gastrointestinal symptoms and 86% will have nausea.

Typical Findings in the HPI

Symptoms can be subtle preceding a crisis, but most patients with this disease will present with unspecified weakness and anorexia with weight loss. Additional symptoms likely to occur include other gastrointestinal symptoms such as abdominal pain, nausea, vomiting, and changes in bowel movements (diarrhea or constipation). Eighty-eight to ninety-four percent of patients have hypotension and subsequent postural dizziness. Hyperpigmentation is common and vitiligo is less common (10–20%).

Typical Physical Exam Findings

Physical exam is significant for these skin and mucosal membrane pigmentation changes, which is more prominent in palmar creases, buccal mucosa, pressure points, perianal mucosa, and around areolas of nipples.

Typical Laboratory/Radiological Findings

Laboratory findings will include electrolyte disturbances including hyponatremia, hyperkalemia, hypercalcemia, azotemia (increased BUN/Cr ratio), anemia (less than half), and eosinophilia (less than 1 in 5). Hypercalcemia and hypoglycemia may also be present. A low early morning serum cortisol (<3 μg/dL) is diagnostic, and if the cortisol is between 3 and 15 μg/dL, a rapid adrenocorticotropic hormone (ACTH) test can be used for confirmation.

Radiological studies are not necessary for diagnosis but may be helpful to identify underlying causes.

Screening Tools

To diagnose, obtain either a short 250 μg ACTH stimulation test or an early morning salivary cortisol concentration. Cortisol levels greater than 16 nmol/L will exclude adrenal insufficiency [27].

Positive Predictive Values

Early morning salivary cortisol concentration has 33% sensitivity and 20% specificity [29].

Pitfalls/Differential Diagnoses

- Depressive disorders
- Anorexia nervosa
- GI malignancy
- Chronic infection
- Salt-losing nephritis
- Hemochromatosis

Alcoholic Hepatitis

Alcohol-induced hepatitis is a spectrum of liver disease caused by chronic, excessive alcohol use. In the early stages of alcoholic fatty liver, the damage is reversible with abstinence in 90–95% of patients and the patients generally appear healthy. Five to ten percent of cases progress to fibrosis and cirrhosis. In the later stages, symptoms can appear abruptly with jaundice a predominant feature.

Incidence/Prevalence

Approximately 1% of the population in the United States are affected, typically presenting in their fourth or fifth decade. Males are twice as likely as females to abuse alcohol however females develop alcoholic hepatitis with a shorter duration of abuse and smaller amounts compared to males.

Incidence/Prevalence of Diagnosis Presenting with Loss of Appetite

Unknown.

Typical Findings in the HPI

Symptoms frequently seen are malaise, nausea/vomiting, anorexia (accompanied by weight loss due to poor caloric intake), right upper quadrant pain, jaundice, fever, proximal muscle wasting, weakness, and complications of liver impairment.

Typical Physical Exam Findings

Physical exam findings are minimal in alcoholic fatty liver. The patient generally appears healthy and may have mild hepatomegaly and splenomegaly. In cases of alcoholic hepatitis, exam findings include jaundice and ascites, hepatomegaly (tender to palpitation), asterixis, tachycardia, hypotension, peripheral edema, abdominal distention with ascites, and a hepatic bruit.

Typical Laboratory/Radiological Findings

Laboratory findings include elevated aspartate aminotransferase (AST) and alanine aminotransferase (ALT) (not always in the early stages), elevated gamma-glutamyl transferase (GGT), elevated carbohydrate-deficient transferrin (CDT), elevated C-reactive protein (CRP), hypokalemia, hypomagnesemia, low zinc, hypophosphatemia, hypoalbuminemia, hyperferritinemia, and elevated mean corpuscular volume seen in CBC. Liver biopsy is rarely needed, though can be used to confirm the diagnosis, rule out cirrhosis, and exclude other diagnoses.

Ultrasonography is the preferred radiographic study and can be used to evaluate size, parenchyma, vasculature, and bile ducts of the liver. It cannot determine if alcohol consumption is the cause of the disease however.

Screening Tools

AUDIT-C or AUDIT questionnaires or similar.

Positive Predictive Values

One study identified total bilirubin and CRP as independent factors to predict alcoholic hepatitis. Positive predictive value was 92% and negative predictive value was 81% [30].

Pitfalls/Differential Diagnoses

- Hepatitis
- Failing to make the diagnosis secondary to premature closure focusing only on the substance use

Gastric Cancer

Gastric cancer is an adenocarcinoma arising from the stomach. Classifications are made depending on location and histological subdivision (intestinal and diffuse). The diffuse form is more common in women and young patients, and the intestinal type is predominantly related to environmental factors and ethnicity.

Incidence/Prevalence

Gastric cancer is the fourth most common cancer in the world, with 70% occurring in developing countries. In the United States, the incidence is 6.7 per 100,000 people. It is more common in males than females (3:2 ratio) and 70% of cases are in patients over 50-years old.

Incidence/Prevalence of Diagnosis Presenting with Loss of Appetite

Unknown.

Typical Findings in the HPI

Symptoms include early satiety with postprandial fullness, significant weight loss (70–80%), nausea/emesis (20–40%), dysphagia (20%), and dyspepsia that is unresponsive to treatment.

Typical Physical Exam Findings

Physical exam can be significant for epigastric or abdominal mass (30–50%). A palpable, firm liver may indicate metastatic disease, as would ascites, lymphadenopathy, or pleural effusions.

Typical Laboratory/Radiological Findings

Laboratory findings may include microcytic anemia, hemoccult-positive stools, hypoalbuminemia, and abnormal liver enzymes if there are metastases to the liver. There are a number of genetic abnormalities that are seen and further evaluation is recommended in familial cases.

Screening Tools

Endoscopy is recommended in persons of high risk (family history or from regions with a high risk of cancer) [31].

Positive Predictive Values

H. pylori serology is not useful but endoscopy allows for biopsy and definitive diagnosis.

Pitfalls/Differential Diagnoses

- Somatic symptom disorder

Gastroesophageal Reflux Disease (GERD)

GERD is classified as a motility disorder, where the primary symptom is typically heartburn and regurgitation caused by a reflux of gastric contents into the esophagus [32]. The severity of reflux varies from annoyance to damage to the esophageal mucosa [33].

Incidence/Prevalence

GERD is probably the most prevalent GI disorder, with a prevalence of 10–20% and an annual incidence of 0.38–0.45% [32]. Almost 7% of adults in the US complain of daily symptoms, 20% report experiencing symptoms monthly, and almost 2/3 (60%) have intermittent symptoms. In pregnancy, the incidence pushes 80%.

Incidence/Prevalence of Diagnosis Presenting with Loss of Appetite

Unknown.

Typical Findings in the HPI

Loss of appetite is typically described as early satiety, accompanied by a sensation of abdominal fullness and bloating. Additional symptoms include heartburn, dysphagia, sour taste in one's mouth, laryngitis, and regurgitation of gastric contents. Sometimes there is chronic cough, bronchospasm, or noncardiac chest pain.

Typical Physical Exam Findings

Physical exam is generally unremarkable.

Typical Laboratory/Radiological Findings

Laboratory tests include endoscopy for diagnostic confirmation. If treatment is initiated without endoscopy, endoscopy is recommended if symptoms recur after an 8-week trial of a proton-pump inhibitor (PPI) [33]. Ambulatory pH monitoring is sometimes completed when there is a failure to respond to therapy and an absence of endoscopic evidence to confirm diagnosis [34].

Screening Tools

None, but empiric therapy with a proton pump inhibitor (PPI) for 8 weeks can be considered.

Positive Predictive Values

Not applicable.

Pitfalls/Differential Diagnoses

- Somatic symptom disorder
- Anxiety disorder

Hyperthyroidism

Hyperthyroidism is the result of excessive production and secretion of thyroid hormone. While less common than hypothyroidism, it can be seen in patients on long-term lithium therapy, usually presenting as thyrotoxicosis earlier in therapy. The majority of these patients will go on to develop hypothyroidism however [35].

Incidence/Prevalence

The incidence of hyperthyroidism is 2% in females and 0.2% in males across their lifetimes. Eighty to ninety percent of all cases of hyperthyroidism are due to Graves' disease (diffuse toxic goiter). Hyperthyroidism can also be due to toxic multinodular goiter (more common than Graves' disease in women >55-years old), toxic adenoma, factitious (abuse of synthetic thyroid hormone), iatrogenic, or transient (in the cases of subacute thyroiditis or Hashimoto thyroiditis). Rarer causes are secondary to neoplasms that are secreting TSH, carcinoma of the thyroid, side effect of amiodarone, or hydatidiform mole.

Incidence/Prevalence of Diagnosis Presenting with Loss of Appetite

Unknown.

Typical Findings in the HPI

In addition to anorexia, patients will complain of tachycardia, tremor, anxiety, irritability, emotional lability, panic attacks, heat intolerance, increased or decreased appetite, diarrhea, weight loss, and menstrual dysfunction. In the case of Graves' ophthalmopathy the patient may have blurring of vision, photophobia, increased lacrimation, double vision, and deep orbital pressure. Elderly patients may develop apathetic hyperthyroidism, where they will present with lethargy, weight loss, tachycardia, brittle nails, and fine skin. The patients maintain insight about weight loss and do not intentionally restrict calorie intake.

Typical Physical Exam Findings

Physical exam may show tachycardia, tremor, hyperreflexia, or pretibial myxedema. In the case of Graves' disease, exophthalmos, lid retraction, and lid lag may be present. Periosteal new bone formation (Graves' acropachy) may lead to clubbing of fingers.

Typical Laboratory/Radiological Findings

Laboratory testing will show elevated T4 (free thyroxine), elevated T3 (free triiodothyronine), and low TSH (except in rare cases of TSH hypersecretion from a pituitary adenoma).

Radiography can be used to differentiate the cause of hyperthyroidism. An overactive thyroid gland will have increased uptake of radioactive iodine, whereas a normal thyroid (in cases of iatrogenic or factitious thyroid ingestion or subacute thyroiditis) will have normal or decreased uptake.

Screening Tools
TSH (low), T_4 (high).

Positive Predictive Values
TSH has a sensitivity of 98% and specificity of 92%. It is recommended to do multiple tests over a 3–6 month interval to confirm or rule out abnormal findings [36].

Pitfalls/Differential Diagnoses
- Panic disorder
- Other anxiety disorder

Hypothyroidism

Hypothyroidism is insufficient thyroid hormone due to inadequate synthesis and secretion. Subclinical hypothyroidism is defined as an elevated thyroid stimulating hormone (TSH) level with a normal free thyroxine (T4) level. In psychiatric patients, Lithium is a common suspected culprit, as it can inhibit synthesis and secretion of thyroid hormones. Goiter can be found in over half of patients prescribed Lithium, and hypothyroidism or subclinical hypothyroidism is also reported in up to 52% of patients [35]. Multiple psychiatric medications can cause hypothyroidism including carbamazepine, oxcarbazepine, and phenytoin [37].

Incidence/Prevalence
Overall, approximately 1 in 300 patients in the US has hypothyroidism. Patients over 60 years old are more likely to develop this disease, and up to 20% of the elderly may have subclinical hypothyroidism.

Incidence/Prevalence of Diagnosis Presenting with Loss of Appetite
Unknown.

Typical Findings in the HPI
In addition to anorexia, common presenting symptoms include fatigue, weakness, constipation, weight gain (modest 2–5 kg, despite decreased appetite), cold intolerance, and difficulty with thinking clearly.

Typical Physical Exam Findings
Physical exam may show brittle, coarse hair, thickened tongue, possibly palpable thyroid gland, bradycardia, muscle stiffness, delayed relaxation phase of deep tendon reflexes, cerebellar ataxia, and peripheral neuropathies with paresthesia. Mental status exam may show poor memory and slowed thought processes.

Typical Laboratory/Radiological Findings
Laboratory testing will show an increased TSH in primary hypothyroidism. It may be normal in secondary or tertiary hypothyroidism if the patient is on dopamine or

corticosteroids, or after a severe illness. Free T4 will also be decreased (but may be normal in subclinical cases). Additionally, hyperlipidemia, hyponatremia, and anemia may also be found.

Screening Tools

TSH (high), T_4 (low).

Positive Predictive Values

Elevated TSH has a sensitivity of 98% and specificity of 92%. It is recommended to complete multiple tests over a 3–6 month interval to confirm or rule out abnormal findings [36].

Pitfalls/Differential Diagnoses

- Depressive disorder
- Major neurocognitive disorder
- Another systemic disorder dependent on presenting symptoms

Human Immunodeficiency Virus (HIV)

HIV is a transmissible retrovirus that attacks the CD4 subset of lymphocytes, causing progressive immunodeficiency in nearly all infected individuals without adequate antiretroviral therapy. Most patients are asymptomatic. A few weeks after the initial infection, patients may experience a mononucleosis-like illness with fever, headache, sore throat, myalgias, arthralgias, and lymphadenopathy. Later stages of the disease may present with opportunistic infections and/or constitutional symptoms.

Incidence/Prevalence

In the United States in 2016, the CDC estimated 1.1 million people aged 13 and older were infected, and 14% of them had not been diagnosed [38]. Of those who know their status, 20% may not be connected to care [39]. In populations that fall outside of the CDC recommended guidelines for screening (13–64-years old) a level of suspicion should be maintained.

Incidence/Prevalence of Diagnosis Presenting with Loss of Appetite

Unknown.

Typical Findings in the HPI

Initial history of present illness would be significant for the potential of exposure to the virus.

In the acute phase, 50–80% of patients experience a mononucleosis-like illness, which could present with decreased appetite, fever, sore throat lymphadenopathy, headache, and roseola-like rash. Symptoms of chronic HIV infection, in addition to opportunistic infection, can include weight loss, diarrhea, lymphadenopathy, fatigue, and skin changes. HIV-related encephalopathy can be mistaken for chronic dementia.

Typical Physical Exam Findings

Physical exam will be significant for lymphadenopathy in the initial stage. Later stages will present depending on the presenting opportunistic infection and stage of disease—wasting symptoms are increasingly predominant with disease progression.

Typical Laboratory/Radiological Findings

A sensitive screening test is an enzyme-linked immunosorbent assay (ELISA) for HIV antibodies, for which a Western Blot is used for confirmation. Depending on the severity of illness, the CD4 T cell count may be relatively normal to nonexistent.

Screening Tools

FDA-approved antigen/antibody immunoassay that detects HIV-1 and HIV-2 antibodies and the HIV-1 p24 antigen [40].

Positive Predictive Values

The immunoassay has 99.76–100% sensitivity and 99.5–100% specificity [40].

Pitfalls/Differential Diagnoses

- Common flu-like illness
- Failure to take appropriate history looking for risk factors

Pancreatic Cancer

Pancreatic exocrine cancer is an adenocarcinoma derived from pancreatic duct epithelium. Initial symptoms are often nonspecific (anorexia, malaise, nausea, fatigue), which can be attributed to many other illnesses but then delays diagnosis. Despite being the tenth most common cancer in men and ninth in women, it is responsible for 8% of all cancer deaths [41].

Incidence/Prevalence

The number of annual cases differs by gender. Approximately 5.5 men per 100,000 will be diagnosed and 4 women per 100,000. Most cases are not diagnosed until the patient has advanced disease; less than 20% will have potentially resectable tumors and the overall 5-year survival is less than 5%.

Incidence/Prevalence of Diagnosis Presenting with Loss of Appetite

Unknown.

Typical Findings in the HPI

Early symptoms are subtle and can include nonspecific gastrointestinal issues such as nausea, vague abdominal pain, anorexia, change in taste of food as well as pruritis, fatigue, and unexplained weight loss. While depression is classically associated with pancreatic cancer, it is an uncommon finding.

Typical Physical Exam Findings

Physical exam may be significant for jaundice and epigastric abdominal tenderness. Less common findings can include icterus, cachexia, ascites, peripheral lymphadenopathy, and excoriations (from scratching pruritic skin). Obstruction of the common bile duct can lead to a palpable gallbladder.

Typical Laboratory/Radiological Findings

Laboratory findings may include anemia on CBC, elevated serum bilirubin, alkaline phosphatase, and aminotransferase levels (seen due to ductal obstruction or metastases). Serum glucose may be elevated due to the destruction of pancreatic islet cells. CA 19-9 is a nonspecific biomarker that can be elevated in pancreatic cancer and other malignancies, though up to 10% of the population may not be able to produce a detectable level due to an inability to express Lewis blood-group antigens. Histopathology is necessary for formal diagnosis, though a needle biopsy is not recommended due to concerns for seeding.

CT (ideally multidetector CT angiography) and MRI can be used to assess metastatic disease, vascular invasion, and determining if the tumor is surgically resectable.

Screening Tools

Recommended to be limited to high-risk individuals.

CA 19-9.

Positive Predictive Values

The efficacy of checking these lab values is not well established, as in America approximately 6% of the white population and 22% of the black population do not have the necessary antigen to detect CA 19-9 [42]. CA 19-9 may also be elevated in liver cirrhosis, chronic pancreatitis, cholangitis, and other GI cancers [43]. In carcinoma cases, the sensitivity of CA 19-9 was 78.2% and in benign cases, the specificity was 82.8% [42].

Pitfalls/Differential Diagnoses

- Depression
- Mild viral illness
- Somatic symptom disorder

Viral Hepatitis

Hepatitis is an acute viral infection of the liver caused by one of five biologically unrelated hepatotropic viruses (HAV, HBV, HCV, HDV, and HEV). Other viruses that can cause hepatitis, as part of multisystemic disease, include herpes simplex virus, cytomegalovirus, Epstein-Barr virus, varicella-zoster virus, HIV, rubella, adenoviruses, enteroviruses, parvovirus B18, and arboviruses.

Incidence/Prevalence

Total numbers are dependent on the underlying virus. Viral hepatitis affects hundreds of millions of people annually. Vaccination for Hepatitis B has decreased the incidence where a vaccine is widely available.

Incidence/Prevalence of Diagnosis Presenting with Loss of Appetite

Unknown.

Typical Findings in the HPI

Symptoms are generally nonspecific and can include anorexia, fatigue, malaise, arthralgias, jaundice (frequency is dependent on the virus), and fever. Further evaluation of risk factors and potential exposures will help guide evaluation.

Typical Physical Exam Findings

Physical exam findings can include hepatomegaly with right upper quadrant tenderness and splenomegaly in 10–15% of cases.

Typical Laboratory/Radiological Findings

Elevated liver enzymes.

Positive viral hepatitis antigens.

Screening Tools

Liver function tests: Alanine aminotransferase (ALT), aspartate aminotransferase (AST), alkaline phosphatase, gamma-glutamyl transpeptidase, albumin, prothrombin time, serum bilirubin.

Serology for hepatitis B and C (HBsAg, anti-HBs, anti-HBc, anti-HCV).

Positive Predictive Values

There are multiple reasons why these tests could be abnormal, further evaluation would be guided by initial evaluation.

Weight Loss Medications

Medications, supplements, and substances can all lead to decreased appetite and weight loss. Stimulants used for treating ADHD are commonly identified as appetite suppressants and can be misused for this reason. Other medications that can suppress appetite include bupropion, topiramate, anticholinesterase inhibitors, some diabetes medications, and thyroid medications. Bupropion and topiramate are sometimes prescribed to aid in weight loss, or for this side effect when another disease is being treated primarily. It is also prudent to inquire about over-the-counter medications and herbal supplement use.

Incidence/Prevalence

Many herbals and supplements are marketed to suppress appetite and cause weight loss. In the US, approximately 15% will use a weight-loss dietary supplement in their lifetimes but less than one-third will discuss this with a healthcare professional [44]. Their safety is of ongoing study, and some are known to cause harm.

Incidence/Prevalence of Diagnosis Presenting with Loss of Appetite

Unknown, patients may have started a new supplement that has an ingredient that causes weight loss even though that was not the advertised purpose of the product purchased.

Typical Findings in the HPI

Any data or specifics will be secondary to the medication being taken, especially as individuals have varying response to the medications.

Common ingredients in weight-loss supplements that have some data with moderate effect on weight loss include African mango, Bitter orange, caffeine, capsaicinoids, carnitine, green coffee bean extract, green tea/green tea extract, and white kidney bean. Additionally, all of these supplements have their own side effect profiles that can be highly distressing for patients. In high doses, caffeine and bitter orange can cause physical symptoms that mimic anxiety, especially at higher doses.

Substances that lead to weight loss include cocaine, alcohol (usually due to nutritional deficiencies as alcohol replaces usual caloric intake), tobacco, and amphetamines. Withdrawal from marijuana can cause anorexia and weight loss (in addition to irritability and abnormal dreams).

Typical Physical Exam Findings

Findings will be dependent on the substance ingested and if there is end organ damage as a result.

Typical Laboratory/Radiological Findings

Illegal drugs would be found in a drug screen, but most supplements are not specifically tested for. Further work-up should be guided to examine when there is suspicion of organ injury.

Screening Tools

None outside of routine history.

Positive Predictive Values

Unknown.

Pitfalls/Differential Diagnoses

- Inadequate history leads to failure to recognize the cause.

References

1. Appetite. 2020. https://www.merriam-webster.com/dictionary/appetite.
2. Bemporad JR. Self-starvation through the ages: reflections on the pre-history of anorexia nervosa. Int J Eat Disord. 1996;19(3):217–37.
3. Pearce JM. Richard Morton: origins of anorexia nervosa. Eur Neurol. 2004;52(4):191–2.
4. van Deth R, Vandereycken W. Food refusal and insanity: sitophobia and anorexia nervosa in Victorian asylums. Int J Eat Disord. 2000;27(4):390–404.
5. Maclean PS, et al. Biological control of appetite: a daunting complexity. Obesity. 2017;25:S8–S16.
6. Piech RM, et al. Neural correlates of appetite and hunger-related evaluative judgments. PLoS One. 2009;4(8):e6581.
7. Robbins LJ. Evaluation of weight loss in the elderly. Geriatrics. 1989;44(4):31–4, 37.
8. Landi F, et al. Anorexia of aging: assessment and management. Clin Geriatr Med. 2017;33(3):315–23.
9. Ivanović N, Büche D, Fringer A. Voluntary stopping of eating and drinking at the end of life - a 'systematic search and review' giving insight into an option of hastening death in capacitated adults at the end of life. BMC Palliat Care. 2014;13(1):1.
10. Hunt TK, Forbush KT. Is "drunkorexia" an eating disorder, substance use disorder, or both? Eat Behav. 2016;22:40–5.
11. American Psychiatric Association. Diagnostic and statistical manual of mental disorders. 5th ed., text rev. Washington, DC: American Psychiatric Association; 2022
12. Prodger S, et al. A prospective review of appetite loss and recovery time in primary joint replacement patients. Ann R Coll Surg Engl. 2016;98(03):206–7.
13. Saha S, et al. Appetite and weight loss symptoms in late-life depression predict dementia outcomes. Am J Geriatr Psychiatry. 2016;24(10):870–8.
14. Bilbao-Garay J, et al. Assessing clinical probability of organic disease in patients with involuntary weight loss: a simple score. Eur J Intern Med. 2002;13(4):240–5.
15. Wildes JE, Marcus MD. Application of the Research Domain Criteria (RDoC) framework to eating disorders: emerging concepts and research. Curr Psychiatry Rep. 2015;17(5):30.
16. George JB, Franko DL. Cultural issues in eating pathology and body image among children and adolescents. J Pediatr Psychol. 2010;35(3):231–42.
17. Perälä J, et al. Lifetime prevalence of psychotic and bipolar I disorders in a general population. Arch Gen Psychiatry. 2007;64(1):19–28.
18. Thompson-Memmer C, Glassman T, Diehr A. Drunkorexia: a new term and diagnostic criteria. J Am Coll Heal. 2019;67(7):620–6.
19. Budney AJ, Lee DC, Juliano LM. Evaluating the validity of caffeine use disorder. Curr Psychiatry Rep. 2015;17(9):74.
20. Walker J, et al. The prevalence of depression in general hospital inpatients: a systematic review and meta-analysis of interview-based studies. Psychol Med. 2018;48(14):2285–98.
21. Baxter AJ, et al. Global prevalence of anxiety disorders: a systematic review and meta-regression. Psychol Med. 2013;43(5):897–910.
22. Katzman DK. Avoidant restrictive food intake disorder. Psychiatr Clin North Am. 2019;42(1):45–57.
23. Rushing JM, Jones LE, Carney CP. Bulimia nervosa: a primary care review. Prim Care Companion J Clin Psychiatry. 2003;5(5):217–24.
24. Vastag B. What's the connection? No easy answers for people with eating disorders and drug abuse. JAMA. 2001;285(8):1006–7.
25. Chakera AJ, Vaidya B. Addison disease in adults: diagnosis and management. Am J Med. 2010;123(5):409–13.
26. Michels A, Michels N. Addison disease: early detection and treatment principles. Am Fam Physician. 2014;89(7):563–8.

27. Charmandari E, Nicolaides NC, Chrousos GP. Adrenal insufficiency. Lancet. 2014;383(9935):2152–67.
28. Rushworth RL, Torpy DJ, Falhammar H. Adrenal crisis. N Engl J Med. 2019;381(9): 852–61.
29. Langelaan MLP, et al. Salivary cortisol in the diagnosis of adrenal insufficiency: cost efficient and patient friendly. Endocr Connect. 2018;7(4):560–6.
30. Vanbiervliet G, et al. Serum C-reactive protein: a non-invasive marker of alcoholic hepatitis. Scand J Gastroenterol. 2006;41(12):1473–9.
31. Kim GH, et al. Screening and surveillance for gastric cancer in the United States: is it needed? Gastrointest Endosc. 2016;84(1):18–28.
32. Lacy BE, et al. The diagnosis of gastroesophageal reflux disease. Am J Med. 2010;123(7): 583–92.
33. Iwakiri K, et al. Evidence-based clinical practice guidelines for gastroesophageal reflux disease 2015. J Gastroenterol. 2016;51(8):751–67.
34. Badillo R, Francis D. Diagnosis and treatment of gastroesophageal reflux disease. World J Gastrointest Pharmacol Ther. 2014;5(3):105–12.
35. Kibirige D, Luzinda K, Ssekitoleko R. Spectrum of lithium induced thyroid abnormalities: a current perspective. Thyroid Res. 2013;6(1):3.
36. LeFevre ML. Screening for thyroid dysfunction: U.S. Preventive Services Task Force recommendation statement. Ann Intern Med. 2015;162(9):641–50.
37. Burch HB. Drug effects on the thyroid. N Engl J Med. 2019;381(8):749–61.
38. HIV Surveillance CDC statistics overview.
39. Gill GS, et al. Unexpected diagnosis. Cureus. 2019;11(9):e5767.
40. Owens DK, et al. Screening for HIV infection. JAMA. 2019;321(23):2326.
41. American Cancer Society. Cancer facts & figures. Atlanta: American Cancer Society; 2020.
42. Poruk KE, et al. The clinical utility of CA 19-9 in pancreatic adenocarcinoma: diagnostic and prognostic updates. Curr Mol Med. 2013;13(3):340–51.
43. Stoffel EM, et al. Evaluating susceptibility to pancreatic cancer: ASCO provisional clinical opinion. J Clin Oncol. 2019;37(2):153–64.
44. National Institutes of Health. Dietary supplements for weight loss: fact sheet for health professionals. 2019. http://ods.od.nih.gov/factsheets/WeightLoss-HealthProfessional.

Irritability

2

Julia Jacobs and Mary C. Vance

Definition of Irritability

The classification of mental disorders has been approached from both top-down and bottom-up frameworks. The Diagnostic and Statistical Manual of Mental Disorders, Fifth Edition-Text Revision (DSM-5-TR) uses top-down diagnostic categories to identify clusters of symptoms that often occur together [1]. On the other hand, the Research Domain Criteria Initiative (RDoC) is organized by specific symptoms and seeks to understand how they manifest across mental disorders, a more bottom-up approach [2]. Irritability is an ideal symptom to examine with this bottom-up approach, as it appears in almost every chapter of the DSM-5-TR and across a variety of medical diagnoses affecting different body systems. Clinically, patients seeking treatment for irritability often leave medical clinician unsure where to begin due to its transdiagnostic nature and lack of a validated medical definition or measurement scale.

Oxford Dictionary defines irritability as "having or showing a tendency to be easily annoyed or made angry" [3]. Researchers in the fields of psychiatry and psychology have defined it as a reaction to blocked goal attainment (RDOC), interindividual differences in proneness to anger that may reach a pathological extent [4], touchiness, easy annoyance, and anger [5], and excessive reactivity to negative

J. Jacobs (✉)
Medical Corps, US Navy, Washington, DC, USA

Navy Medicine Readiness and Training Unit, Groton, CT, USA
e-mail: julia.f.jacobs2.mil@health.mil

M. C. Vance
US Public Health Service, Atlanta, GA, USA

Pacific Area, US Coast Guard, Portland, OR, USA
e-mail: mary.c.vance@uscg.mil

E. G. Meyer et al. (eds.), *The Medical Evaluation of Psychiatric Symptoms*,
https://doi.org/10.1007/978-3-031-14372-4_2

emotional stimuli [6]. Other medical specialties generally do not conceptualize irritability as a discrete symptom.

Vidal-Ribas et al. [4] addressed the relationship between irritability and the concepts of feelings, emotions, moods, and affects. In the context of irritability, they broadly define these concepts as (1) **feeling**: an individual is *consciously aware* of a set of thoughts and bodily sensations they describe as anger, (2) **emotion**: an *action tendency* toward anger that does not need to reach conscious awareness (e.g., acting "angry" without being aware of it), (3) **mood**: a valenced, *enduring irritable state* that is not in direct response to a stimulus (comparable to the sustained negative mood in depressive disorders), and (4) **affect**: the *objectively observed features* of a mood or emotion, such as an angry facial expression. "In summary, irritability is a mood, and anger is its defining emotion. When anger enters the person's awareness, it is called a feeling, and when observable to others, such as clinicians, anger is described as an affect" [4].

The DSM-5-TR describes irritability using phasic and tonic components in its definition of severe mood dysregulation (SMD). *Phasic* irritability refers to developmentally inappropriate temper outbursts, whereas *tonic* irritability refers to the negative affect that persists between outbursts [1]. For example, a 10-year old child who throws a tantrum when told to clean up after playing demonstrates the phasic component of irritability, whereas a child who consistently snaps at other children throughout the day, demonstrates the tonic component.

Irritability is also a core feature of negative emotionality in the scientific literature on temperament, which is defined by: "negative emotional reactions to thwarted goal-directed activity and anticipated distress" [7, 8]. In Psychological Trait Theory, which described personality in terms of the Big Five Personality Traits (openness to experience, conscientiousness, extraversion, agreeableness, and neuroticism) [9, 10], irritability is a core feature of trait *neuroticism* [11].

Irritability Is a Normal Response to Stressful Circumstances Surrounding Medical Conditions and Treatment

Being ill can be a frightening and vulnerable experience characterized by loss of control and having to confront one's mortality. In this context, individuals facing illnesses often act appropriately irritable when they must also navigate complex and unfamiliar social, legal, and financial systems. More practical irritants may include long wait times, complex medical bills, frustration with health insurance companies, difficult-to-find doctor's offices, and parking challenges. Additionally, factors that arise between physician and patient, such as different communication styles or a mismatch of expectations, may lead to irritability. Finally, an irritable physician, due to burnout or other causes, may *induce* irritability in their patient or perceive their patient as more irritable than they are. In a brief meeting with a patient, it may be difficult for a physician to determine whether the patient is demonstrating pathological "easy annoyance or anger" or a normal response to a stressful situation.

Historical Definition of Irritability

Throughout the nineteenth and twentieth centuries, psychoanalysts addressed irritability in discussions about depression and anxiety. In psychoanalysis, irritability is typically viewed as a means of self-directed hostility [12]. The term "irritable mood" was introduced to the *Diagnostic and Statistical Manual of Mental Disorders First Edition (DSM)* in 1952. Now, irritability appears across a range of DSM-5-TR disorders, which are outlined in detail later in this chapter. This long list demonstrates the transdiagnostic nature of irritability in psychiatry.

Pathophysiology of Irritability

Research in genetics and in structural and functional neuroimaging has examined the pathophysiology of irritability. Much of this research has focused on differentiating the pathophysiology of patients diagnosed with severe mood dysregulation (SMD) and bipolar disorder (BD), which have irritability as prominent features, from healthy volunteers.

One study examined neuroanatomical differences among youth with SMD, youth with BD, and healthy volunteers using structural magnetic resonance imaging (MRI). It revealed that, compared with healthy volunteers, youth with SMD and BD had greater gray matter volume in the presupplementary motor area, dorsolateral prefrontal cortex, and insula [13].

Various functional MRI (fMRI) studies have identified statistically significant aberrations in activity in the amygdala [14], frontal cortex [15], posterior cingulate, superior temporal gyrus [16, 17], insula, parahippocampal gyrus, and thalamus [17] during various facial emotional processing tasks in adolescents with SMD compared with healthy controls.

Twin studies demonstrate a genetic contribution to the variation of irritability of approximately 30–40% in both adults [18] and adolescents [19].

Separating Irritability from Other Symptoms

Authors seeking to define irritability, often in the context of research on oppositional defiant disorder (ODD), distinguish it from aggression, vindictiveness, and defiance [5] and from anger as a normal, healthy feeling or emotion [4].

Variants of Irritability Based on Culture

One study sought to evaluate participants' perceptions of irritability across cultures. It utilized a survey that contained qualitative questions about participants' personal causes for, experiences with, and consequences of irritability as well as how they perceived the relationship between irritability and anger. It used three quantitative questions about the frequency, intensity, and duration of their irritability. Participants were living in the US, Malaysia, Australia, New Zealand, Singapore, South Africa, the UK, India, Ireland, and China. Results revealed that residents of China, Singapore, and the US reported having a longer duration of irritability than residents of Ireland and the UK [20].

A Psychiatric Differential for Irritability

Irritability appears throughout the DSM-5-TR in three contexts (1) as a diagnostic criterion for a disorder, (2) as a feature supporting the diagnosis of a disorder, and (3) as a functional consequence of a disorder. Furthermore, it appears in many diagnostic categories, which are listed in Table 2.1. This highlights the transdiagnostic nature of irritability across diagnostic categories. The following section reviews the presence of irritability among psychiatric disorders in the DSM-5-TR.

Bipolar and Related Disorders

Irritability is a core feature of bipolar disorder (BD) and appears in criterion 1 of the diagnostic criteria for a manic episode in **bipolar I disorder** and a hypomanic episode in **bipolar II disorder**.

Bipolar I Disorder

Incidence/Prevalence

The 12-month prevalence estimate in the continental United States was 0.6% for bipolar I disorder as defined in DSM-IV [21]. Twelve-month prevalence of bipolar I disorder across 11 countries ranged from 0.0% to 0.6% [21]. The lifetime male-to-female prevalence ratio is approximately 1.1:1 [21].

Typical Findings of the HPI

Irritability is a core feature of mania. Mania is defined as a distinct period of abnormally and persistently elevated, expansive, or **irritable** mood and abnormally and persistently increased activity or energy, lasting at least 1 week and present most of the day, nearly every day (or any duration if hospitalization is necessary). **Irritability** is common in manic, mixed, and depressive episodes.

Typical Findings on Physical and Mental Status Exam

Findings on mental status exam during a manic or mixed episode may include thought content that is grandiose in the context of the individual's typical belief system including delusions of grandiosity, rapid, uninterruptible speech, flight of ideas, distractibility, psychomotor agitation, manifestations of mood lability (moving from laughing, to crying, to angry more rapidly than is normal for that individual) or hypersexual behavior or appearance that is not typical for the individual.

Table 2.1 Irritability in the DSM-5-TR

	Irritability appears as:		
Diagnosis	Diagnostic criterion	Feature supporting Dx	Functional consequence of Dx
Bipolar and related disorders			
Bipolar I disorder	X		
Bipolar II disorder	X		
Depressive disorders			
Disruptive mood dysregulation disorder	X		
Premenstrual dysphoric disorder	X		
Major depressive disorder	X (child)	X (adult)	
Anxiety disorders			
Generalized anxiety disorder	X		
Trauma- and stressor-related disorders			
Reactive attachment disorder	X		
Acute stress disorder	X		
Posttraumatic stress disorder	X		
Personality disorders			
Antisocial personality disorder	X		
Borderline personality disorder	X		
Schizophrenia spectrum and other psychotic disorders			
Delusional disorder		X	
Neurodevelopmental disorders			
ADHD		X	
Disruptive, impulse-control, and conduct disorders			
Conduct disorder		X	
Substance use disorders			
Alcohol use disorder		X	
Stimulant use disorder		X	
Alcohol withdrawal		X	
Stimulant withdrawal		X	
Cannabis withdrawal syndrome	X		
Tobacco withdrawal		X	
Alcohol withdrawal		X	
Opiate withdrawal		X	
Caffeine withdrawal	X		
Neurocognitive disorders			
Delirium		X	
Major or mild neurocognitive disorder due to Alzheimer's disease		X	
Major or mild neurocognitive disorder due to traumatic brain injury		X	
Substance/medication-induced major or mild neurocognitive disorder		X	
Sleep-wake disorders			
Insomnia disorder			X
Nightmare disorder			X

During a depressive episode, individuals with bipolar I disorder may present with the mental status exam findings described in section "Major Depressive Disorder (MDD)".

Incidence/Prevalence of Bipolar I Disorder Presenting with Irritability
100%.

Typical Laboratory/Radiological Findings
There are no notable diagnostic laboratory or radiological findings.

Bipolar II Disorder

Incidence/Prevalence
The 12-month prevalence of bipolar II disorder, internationally, is 0.3% [22]. In the United States, 12-month prevalence is 0.8% [22]. The prevalence rate of pediatric bipolar II disorder is difficult to establish.

Incidence/Prevalence of Bipolar II Disorder Presenting with Irritability
Unknown.

Typical Findings of the HPI
Individuals with bipolar II disorder are most likely to present to a physician for symptoms of depression, mood swings, or problems with interpersonal or occupational functioning, as opposed to symptoms of hypomania. **Irritability** is common in hypomanic, mixed, and depressive episodes.

Typical Findings on Physical and Mental Status Exam
Findings on mental status exam may include thought content that is grandiose in the context of the individual's typical belief system, rapid speech, flight of ideas, distractibility, psychomotor agitation, manifestations of mood lability less intense than in a manic episode (moving from laughing, to crying, to angry more rapidly than is normal for that individual) or hypersexual behavior or appearance that is not typical for the individual.

During a depressive episode, individuals with bipolar II disorder may present with the mental status exam findings described in section "Major Depressive Disorder (MDD)".

Typical Laboratory/Radiological Findings
There are no notable diagnostic laboratory or radiological findings.

Depressive Disorders

Irritability appears in three diagnoses under the DSM-5-TR diagnostic category depressive disorders: (1) disruptive mood dysregulation disorder, (2) major depressive disorder, and (3) premenstrual dysphoric disorder.

Disruptive Mood Dysregulation Disorder (DMDD)

Incidence/Prevalence

DMDD is common among children presenting to pediatric mental health clinics. Prevalence estimates of the disorder in the community are unclear. Based on rates of chronic and severe persistent irritability, which is the core feature of the disorder, the overall 6-month to 1-year period-prevalence of DMDD among children and adolescents probably falls in the 2–5% range [23]. However, rates are expected to be higher in males and school-age children than in females and adolescents.

Incidence/Prevalence of Disruptive Mood Dysregulation Disorder Presenting with Irritability

100%.

Typical Findings of the HPI

Individuals with DMDD or their caregivers report at least 12 months of severe recurrent temper outbursts that are grossly out of proportion in intensity or duration to the situation or provocation. These outbursts are inconsistent with the child's developmental level and the child is **irritable** or angry most of the day, nearly every day.

Typical Findings on Physical and Mental Status Exam

Findings on mental status exam may include verbal or behavioral outbursts out of proportion to the context that provoked them.

Typical Laboratory/Radiological Findings

There are no notable diagnostic laboratory or radiological findings.

Major Depressive Disorder (MDD)

Incidence/Prevalence

Twelve-month prevalence of MDD in the United States is approximately 7%, with marked differences by age group. The prevalence in 18–29-year-old individuals is threefold higher than the prevalence in individuals aged 60 years or older [24]. Females experience 1.5- to threefold higher rates than males beginning in early adolescence [24].

Incidence/Prevalence of Major Depressive Disorder Presenting with Irritability

Unknown.

Typical Findings of the HPI

Near daily depressed mood (or **irritable** mood in children in adolescents) is a core feature of major depressive disorder. Additional features include loss of interest or pleasure, a decrease or increase in appetite with weight change, insomnia or hypersomnia, psychomotor agitation or retardation observable by others, fatigue, or loss of energy nearly every day, feelings of worthlessness or excessive or inappropriate guilt, diminished ability to think or concentrate, or indecisiveness, recurrent thoughts of death and/or suicide.

Typical Findings on Physical and Mental Status Exam

Findings on mental status exam may include poor hygiene, speech that is slow, monotone, or characterized by increased speech latency, psychomotor slowing or restlessness, uncharacteristically poor eye contact, dysthymic mood, depressed affect, thought content that is ruminative, suicidal, or characterized by mood congruent thought distortions, and concerns about memory, concentration, or ability to pay attention.

Typical Laboratory/Radiological Findings

There are no notable diagnostic laboratory or radiological findings.

Premenstrual Dysphoric Disorder (PMDD)

Incidence/Prevalence

Twelve-month prevalence of premenstrual dysphoric disorder is between 1.8% and 5.8% of menstruating women [25, 26].

Incidence/Prevalence of Premenstrual Dysphoric Disorder Presenting with Irritability

Unknown.

Typical Findings of the HPI

Marked **irritability**, anger, or increased interpersonal conflicts is a core feature of PMDD. Additional features include affective lability, depressed mood, feelings of hopelessness, or self-deprecating thoughts, anxiety, tension, and/or feelings of being keyed up or on edge, decreased interest in usual activities, difficulty in concentration, lethargy, easy fatigability, or marked lack of energy, marked change in appetite; overeating; or specific food cravings, hypersomnia or insomnia, sense of being overwhelmed or out of control, and physical symptoms such as breast tenderness or swelling, joint or muscle pain, a sensation of "bloating," or weight gain.

Typical Findings on Physical and Mental Status Exam

Findings on physical exam may include breast tenderness or swelling, joint or muscle pain, a sensation of "bloating," or weight gain present during most menstrual cycles, in the final week before the onset of menses, and must start to improve within a few days after the onset of menses and must become minimal or absent in the week post menses.

Findings on mental status exam may include poor hygiene, tense posture, uncharacteristically poor eye contact, speech that is slow, monotone, or characterized by increased speech latency, psychomotor restlessness, dysthymic mood, depressed, **irritable**, labile, or angry affect, thought content that is uncharacteristically negative, self-deprecating, or hopeless, and concerns about memory, concentration, motivation, loss of interest, or ability to pay attention.

Typical Laboratory/Radiological Findings

There are no notable diagnostic laboratory or radiological findings.

Anxiety Disorders

Irritability appears as a diagnostic criterion for generalized anxiety disorder in the DSM-5-TR category anxiety disorders.

Generalized Anxiety Disorder

Incidence/Prevalence

The 12-month prevalence of generalized anxiety disorder is 0.9% among adolescents and 2.9% among adults in the United States [27].

Incidence/Prevalence of Generalized Anxiety Disorder Presenting with Irritability

100%.

Typical Findings of the HPI

Irritability is a core feature of generalized anxiety disorder. It occurs alongside excessive anxiety, worry, restlessness or feeling keyed up or on edge, being easily fatigued, difficulty concentrating or mind going blank, muscle tension, and sleep disturbance.

Typical Findings on Physical and Mental Status Exam

Findings on physical exam may include:

- Cardiac: tachycardia, chest pain
- Musculoskeletal: muscle tension, trembling
- Dermatologic: diaphoresis

Findings on mental status exam may include tense or restless appearance, catastrophic thought process, thought content including worry about multiple aspects of one's life out of proportion to context and functionally impairing, anxious mood, anxious or **irritable** affect.

Typical Laboratory/Radiological Findings

There are no notable diagnostic laboratory or radiological findings.

Trauma- and Stressor-Related Disorders

Irritability appears in three diagnoses under the DSM-5-TR diagnostic category trauma- and stressor-related disorders: (1) reactive attachment disorder, (2) acute stress disorder, and (3) posttraumatic stress disorder.

Reactive Attachment Disorder (RAD)

Incidence/Prevalence

The prevalence of reactive attachment disorder is unknown, but the disorder is seen relatively rarely in clinical settings. In known populations of severely neglected children, the disorder is uncommon, occurring in less than 10% of children [28].

Incidence/Prevalence of Reactive Attachment Disorder Presenting with Irritability

Unknown.

Typical Findings of the HPI

A caregiver will describe a child with a history of extreme insufficient care who presents with unexplained **irritability**, sadness, or fearfulness that are evident even during nonthreatening interactions with adult caregivers. Addition features include a consistent pattern of inhibited, emotionally withdrawn behavior toward adult caregivers manifested by rarely or minimally seeking comfort when distressed and rarely or minimally responding to comfort when distressed, social and emotional disturbance characterized by minimal social and emotional responsiveness to others, limited positive affect, and episodes of unexplained irritability, sadness, or fearfulness that are evident even during nonthreatening interactions with adult caregivers. The child's developmental age must be at least 9 months and the symptoms above must be evident before age 5. The child cannot also exhibit symptoms that meet the criteria for autism spectrum disorder.

Typical Findings on Physical and Mental Status Exam

Findings on mental status exam may include fearful behavior in non-threatening interactions with caregivers or clinicians, limited comfort-seeking, and minimal responses to reasonable attempts to comfort the child.

Typical Laboratory/Radiological Findings

There are no notable diagnostic laboratory or radiological findings.

Acute Stress Disorder (ASD)

Incidence/Prevalence

The prevalence of acute stress disorder in recently trauma-exposed populations (i.e., within 1 month of trauma exposure) varies according to the nature of the event and the context in which it is assessed. In both US and non-US populations, acute stress disorder tends to be identified in less than 20% of cases following traumatic events that do not involve interpersonal assault. Higher rates (i.e., 20–50%) are reported following interpersonal traumatic events, including assault, rape, and witnessing a mass shooting [29, 30].

Incidence/Prevalence of Acute Stress Disorder Presenting with Irritability
Unknown.

Typical Findings of the HPI
Marked alterations in arousal (**irritability**, reckless behavior, hypervigilance, exaggerated startle response, poor concentration, and sleep disturbances) are a core feature of PTSD. Other features include intrusive symptoms, persistent avoidance to stimuli associated with traumatic event, and negative alterations in thoughts and mood.

Typical Findings on Physical and Mental Status Exam
Findings on physical exam may include [LAT1]:

- Cardiovascular: elevated blood pressure, tachycardia
- Dermatologic: profuse sweating
- Musculoskeletal: twitching, psychomotor agitation

Findings on mental status exam may include tense, guarded appearance, reckless behavior, sitting in an orientation to maximize safety in the exam room, sensitive startle response, avoidance behavior relevant to the context of trauma, distorted thoughts about the cause or consequences of the event, altered perceptions including reexperiencing the event or hallucinations related to the event, altered memory of the event, detached, anxious, or depressed mood, anxious, depressed, labile, or restricted affect, limited insight into the cause or consequences of the event, and impaired judgment characterized by reckless or self-harming behavior.

Typical Laboratory/Radiological Findings
There are no notable diagnostic laboratory or radiological findings.

Posttraumatic Stress Disorder

Incidence/Prevalence
In the United States, projected lifetime risk for PTSD using DSM-IV criteria at the age of 75 years is 8.7% [31].

Incidence/Prevalence of Diagnosis Presenting with Irritability
Unknown.

Typical Findings of the HPI
Marked alterations in arousal (**irritability**, reckless behavior, hypervigilance, exaggerated startle response, poor concentration, and sleep disturbances) are a core feature of PTSD. Other features include intrusive symptoms, persistent avoidance to stimuli associated with traumatic event, and negative alterations in thoughts and mood.

Typical Findings on Physical and Mental Status Exam

Findings on physical exam may include

- Cardiovascular: elevated blood pressure, tachycardia
- Dermatologic: sweating
- Musculoskeletal: twitching, psychomotor agitation

Findings on mental status exam may include tense, guarded appearance, reckless behavior, intentionally sitting with back to the wall and the exit to the room in sight, sensitive startle response, avoidance behavior relevant to the context of trauma, distorted thoughts about the cause or consequences of the event, altered perceptions including reexperiencing the event or hallucinations related to the event, altered memory of the event, detached, anxious, or depressed mood, anxious, depressed, labile, or restricted affect, limited insight into the cause or consequences of the event, and impaired judgment characterized by reckless or self-harming behavior.

Typical Laboratory/Radiological Findings

There are no notable diagnostic laboratory or radiological findings.

Personality Disorders

Irritability appears in two diagnoses under the DSM-5-TR diagnostic category personality disorders: antisocial personality disorder and borderline personality disorder.

Antisocial Personality Disorder

Incidence/Prevalence

Twelve-month prevalence rates of antisocial personality disorder are between 0.2% and 3.3% [32–34].

Incidence/Prevalence of Diagnosis Presenting with Irritability

Unknown.

Typical Findings of the HPI

Irritability and aggressiveness are core features of antisocial personality disorder. Additional features include a pervasive pattern of disregard for and violation of the rights of others, deceitfulness, impulsivity, or failure to plan ahead, reckless disregard for the safety of self or others, consistent irresponsibility, and lack of remorse for harming others.

Typical Findings on Physical and Mental Status Exam

Findings on mental status exam may include behavior such as repeated lying, aggression, attempts at exploitation (stealing, sexual advances, stalking) with lack of remorse, impulsivity, and **irritable** mood and affect.

Typical Laboratory/Radiological Findings

There are no notable diagnostic laboratory or radiological findings.

Borderline Personality Disorder

Incidence/Prevalence

The median population prevalence of borderline personality disorder is estimated to be 1.6% [34] but may be as high as 5.9% [35].

Incidence/Prevalence of Borderline Personality Disorder Presenting with Irritability

Unknown.

Typical Findings of the HPI

Affective instability due to a marked reactivity of mood (e.g., intense episodic dysphoria, **irritability**, or anxiety) is a core feature of borderline personality disorder. Additional features include a pervasive pattern of instability of interpersonal relationships, self-image, and affects, marked impulsivity, frantic efforts to avoid real or imagined abandonment, pattern of unstable and intense interpersonal relationships characterized by alternating between extremes of idealization and devaluation, identity disturbance, impulsivity in at least two areas that are potentially self-damaging (e.g., spending, sex, substance abuse, reckless driving, binge eating), recurrent suicidal behavior, gestures, or threats, or self-mutilating behavior, chronic feelings of emptiness, inappropriate, intense anger or difficulty controlling anger, and transient, stress-related paranoid ideation or severe dissociative symptoms.

Typical Findings on Physical and Mental Status Exam

Findings on mental status exam may include extreme idealization or devaluation of clinicians, nonsuicidal self-injurious behavior, reckless or impulsive behavior, recurrent suicide attempts, chronic suicidal thoughts, chronic feelings of emptiness, transient paranoia, mood or affective instability including inappropriate, intense anger.

Typical Laboratory/Radiological Findings

There are no notable diagnostic laboratory or radiological findings.

Substance Use Disorders

Caffeine Withdrawal

Incidence/Prevalence

Prevalence up to 30% in small general population studies [16].

Incidence/Prevalence of Diagnosis Presenting with Irritability

Unknown.

Typical Findings of the HPI

Prolonged daily use of caffeine with abrupt cessation of or reduction in caffeine use, followed within 24 hours by **irritability**, headache, marked fatigue or drowsiness, dysphoric mood, depressed mood, difficulty concentrating, or flu-like symptoms (nausea, vomiting, or muscle pain/stiffness).

Typical Findings on Physical and Mental Status Exam

Physical exam may show evidence of tachycardia (associated with intoxication), tremor, or hypertension.

Findings on mental status exam may include dysphoric or depressed mood, irritability, and difficulty with concentration.

Typical Laboratory/Radiological Findings

There are no notable diagnostic laboratory or radiological findings; caffeine is not routinely used as part of a screening panel for drugs of abuse.

Cannabis Withdrawal

Incidence/Prevalence

Among individuals who have used cannabis regularly during some period of their lifetime, up to one-third report having experienced cannabis withdrawal [36–38].

Incidence/Prevalence of Cannabis Withdrawal Presenting with Irritability

Unknown.

Typical Findings of the HPI

Cessation of cannabis use that has been heavy and prolonged with three or more of the following symptoms developing within 1 week of discontinuation: **irritability**, anger, or aggression; nervousness or anxiety; sleep difficulty; decreased appetite or weight loss; restlessness; depressed mood; abdominal pain, shakiness/tremors, sweating, fever, chills, or headache.

Typical Findings on Physical and Mental Status Exam

Physical exam may reveal tachycardia and tremor.

Mental status exam may show irritability, anger or aggression, anxiety, depressed mood, restlessness.

Typical Laboratory/Radiological Findings

Drug screen may be positive for cannabis.

Tobacco Withdrawal

Incidence/Prevalence

Approximately 20% of US adults identified as current users in 2018. Approximately 50% of tobacco users who quit for 2 or more days will have symptoms that meet the criteria for tobacco withdrawal [39].

Incidence/Prevalence of Tobacco Withdrawal Presenting with Irritability

Unknown.

Typical Findings of the HPI

Abrupt cessation of tobacco use or reduction in tobacco use after at least a few weeks of use, which is followed within 24 h by **irritability**, frustration, anger, anxiety, difficulty concentrating, increased appetite, restlessness, depressed mood, and insomnia.

Typical Findings on Physical and Mental Status Exam

Physical exam findings may show stained teeth and fingertips.

Mental status exam may be notable for smoke smell, irritability, anxiety, and nicotine cravings.

Typical Laboratory/Radiological Findings

There are no notable diagnostic laboratory or radiological findings.

Irritability is a feature associated with many other DSM-5-TR diagnoses, in which it is not one of the core diagnostic criteria [1]**. These include:**

Schizophrenia Spectrum and Other Psychotic Disorders:

- Delusional disorder—Many individuals develop an **irritable** or dysphoric mood in reaction to their delusional beliefs.

Neurodevelopmental Disorders:

- Attention deficit hyperactivity disorder—A persistent pattern of inattention and/or hyperactivity-impulsivity that interferes with functioning or development. Associated features may include low frustration tolerance, **irritability**, or mood lability.

Disruptive, Impulse-Control, and Conduct Disorders:

- Conduct disorder: A repetitive and persistent pattern of behavior in which the basic rights of others or major age-appropriate societal norms or rules are violated. Personality features of trait negative emotionality and poor self-control, including poor frustration tolerance, **irritability**, temper outbursts, suspiciousness, insensitivity to punishment, thrill-seeking, and recklessness, frequently cooccur with conduct disorder.

Substance Use Disorders:

- Alcohol use disorder—In addition to the diagnostic criteria, severe problematic alcohol use also contributes to disinhibition and feelings of sadness and **irritability**, which contribute to suicide attempts and completed suicides.
- Alcohol withdrawal—In addition to the diagnostic criteria, which include psychomotor agitation and anxiety, among other signs and symptoms, individuals experiencing alcohol withdrawal often also present with **irritability**.

- Opiate withdrawal—In addition to the diagnostic criteria, individuals experiencing opiate withdrawal often also present with **irritability** due to the physical and psychological discomfort associated with withdrawal.
- Stimulant withdrawal—Findings on mental status exam may include disheveled clothing, poor hygiene, weight loss, restlessness, excess motor activity, rapid speech, grandiosity, paranoia, delusions of persecution, euphoric or **irritable** mood, tearfulness, inattention, poor insight, and judgment.
- Stimulant use disorder—Findings on mental status exam may include disheveled clothing, poor hygiene, weight loss, restlessness, excess motor activity, rapid speech, grandiosity, paranoia, delusions of persecution, euphoric or **irritable** mood, tearfulness, inattention, poor insight, and judgement.

Neurocognitive Disorders:

- Delirium—In addition to the diagnostic criteria, individuals with delirium may exhibit emotional disturbances, such as anxiety, fear, depression, **irritability**, anger, euphoria, and apathy. There may be rapid and unpredictable shifts from one emotional state to another. The disturbed emotional state may also be evident in calling out, screaming, cursing, muttering, moaning, or making other sounds. These behaviors are especially prevalent at night and under conditions in which stimulation and environmental cues are lacking.
- Major and mild neurocognitive disorders—Irritability often occurs in response to the cognitive decline and loss of independence associated with these disorders.
- Sleep-wake disorders—Irritability often occurs in response to the sleep deprivation associated with sleep-wake disorders.

A Medical Differential Diagnosis for Irritability

Many medical conditions cause physical signs and symptoms that can be irritating such as pain, reduced appetite, fatigue, and fever. Therefore, patients presenting with a broad array of medical conditions may have chief complaints that include irritability. The following medical conditions, listed in order of prevalence, are commonly associated with irritability.

Obstructive Sleep Apnea

See Chap. 4.

Polycystic Ovarian Syndrome (PCOS)

PCOS is the most common endocrine disorder in women of reproductive age. Clinical features include menstrual abnormalities, hyperandrogenism, polycystic ovaries, weight gain and associated metabolic and cardiovascular risks, and mood changes. **Irritability** is one of the mood-related symptoms experienced by women with PCOS.

Incidence/Prevalence
(6–10%) [40].

Incidence/Prevalence of Polycystic Ovarian Syndrome Presenting with Irritability
Unknown.

Typical Findings in the HPI
Typical findings include lifetime irregular menses, unexplained weight gain, hirsutism, and infertility.

Typical Physical Exam Findings
Typical findings include acne, obesity, and hirsutism.

Typical Laboratory/Radiological Findings (Should Typically Be Deferred to Primary Care or Endocrine Specialist)
- Elevated serum testosterone.
- Elevated morning serum 17-hydroxyprogesterone in the early follicular phase of the menstrual cycle.
- Transvaginal ultrasound showing 12 or more follicles in either ovary measuring 2–9 mm in diameter and/or increased ovarian volume (>10 mL).

Screening Tools with Sensitivity and Specificity
Clinical Tool for Diagnosis of Polycystic Ovarian Syndrome (sensitivity 85.4%, specificity 93.4%) [41].

Hyperthyroidism

Hyperthyroidism is excessive production and secretion of thyroid hormone. The physical symptoms of hyperthyroidism, such as tachycardia, tremor, and heat intolerance, mimic the physiological components of emotions such as **irritability**, anger, and anxiety. Physiological states involving hyperarousal, such as these, are known to induce their corresponding psychological symptoms. Additionally, hyperthyroidism may induce **irritability** directly through direct effects of excessive thyroid hormone and its biological sequelae on the nervous system.

Incidence/Prevalence
The incidence of hyperthyroidism is 2% in females and 0.2% in males across their lifetimes. Eighty to ninety percent of all cases of hyperthyroidism are due to Graves' disease (diffuse toxic goiter). Hyperthyroidism can also be due to toxic multinodular goiter (more common than Graves' disease in women >55 years old), toxic

adenoma, factitious (abuse of synthetic thyroid hormone), iatrogenic, or transient (in the cases of subacute thyroiditis or Hashimoto thyroiditis). Rarer causes are secondary to neoplasms that are secreting TSH, carcinoma of the thyroid, side effect of amiodarone, or hydatidiform mole [42].

Incidence/Prevalence of Hyperthyroidism Presenting with Irritability

Unknown.

Typical Findings in the HPI

Patients with hyperthyroidism may also complain of anorexia, tachycardia, tremor, anxiety, irritability, emotional lability, panic attacks, heat intolerance, increased or decreased appetite, diarrhea, weight loss, and menstrual dysfunction. In the case of Graves' ophthalmopathy, the patient may have blurring of vision, photophobia, increased lacrimation, double vision, and deep orbital pressure. Elderly patients may develop apathetic hyperthyroidism, where they will present with lethargy, weight loss, tachycardia, brittle nails, and fine skin. Insight about weight loss is present. No intentional caloric restriction.

Typical Physical Exam Findings

Physical exam may show tachycardia, tremor, hyperreflexia, or pretibial myxedema. In the case of Graves' disease, exophthalmos, lid retraction, and lid lag may be present. Periosteal new bone formation (Graves' acropachy) may lead to clubbing of fingers.

Typical Laboratory/Radiological Findings

Laboratory testing will show elevated T4 (free thyroxine), elevated T3 (free triiodothyronine), and low TSH (except in rare cases of TSH hypersecretion from a pituitary adenoma).

Radiography can be used to differentiate the cause of hyperthyroidism. An overactive thyroid gland will have increased uptake of radioactive iodine, whereas a normal thyroid (in cases of iatrogenic or factitious thyroid ingestion or subacute thyroiditis) will have normal or decreased uptake.

Screening Tools

TSH (low), T_4 (high).

Positive Predictive Values

TSH sensitivity 98%, specificity 92%.

Recommended to do multiple tests over a 3–6 month interval to confirm or rule out abnormal findings.

Hypothyroidism

Hypothyroidism is insufficient thyroid hormone due to inadequate synthesis and secretion. Hypothyroidism is a known cause of depression, of which **irritability** is a core feature. Additionally, the physical symptoms of hypothyroidism, such as fatigue, weakness, and subjective cognitive impairment can be **irritating** due to their negative impact on function.

Incidence/Prevalence

Overall, approximately 1 in 300 patients in the United States has hypothyroidism (0.003%). Patients over 60-years old are more likely to develop this disease, and up to 20% of the elderly may have subclinical hypothyroidism [38].

Incidence/Prevalence of Hypothyroidism Presenting with Irritability

Unknown.

Typical Findings in the HPI

In addition to anorexia, common presenting symptoms include fatigue, weakness, constipation, weight gain (modest, e.g., 2–5 kg, despite decreased appetite), cold intolerance, and difficulty with thinking clearly.

Typical Physical Exam Findings

Physical exam may show brittle, coarse hair, thickened tongue, possibly palpable thyroid gland, bradycardia, muscle stiffness, delayed relaxation phase of deep tendon reflexes, cerebellar ataxia, and peripheral neuropathies with paresthesia. Mental status exam may show poor memory and slowed thought processes.

Typical Laboratory/Radiological Findings

Laboratory testing will show an increased TSH in primary hypothyroidism, but it may be normal in secondary or tertiary hypothyroidism if the patient is on dopamine or corticosteroids, or after a severe illness. Free T4 will also be decreased (may be normal in subclinical cases). Additionally, hyperlipidemia, hyponatremia, and anemia may also be found.

Screening Tools

TSH (high), T_4 (low).

Positive Predictive Values

TSH sensitivity 98%, specificity 92%.

Recommended to do multiple tests over a 3–6 month interval to confirm or rule out abnormal findings.

Adrenal Insufficiency (Addison's Disease)

Adrenal insufficiency is due to the inadequate secretion of corticosteroids that occurs in primary adrenal failure (partial or complete destruction of the adrenal glands) or secondary cortisol deficiency due to critical illness and pituitary insufficiency. Acute adrenal crisis is unlikely to present as a chronic condition in a psychiatry office, as it is characterized by cardiovascular collapse and hemodynamic instability. Chronic adrenal insufficiency however will present with nonspecific symptoms, especially initially, such as **irritability.** The most common cause is autoimmune adrenalitis [43]. However, malignancy, infection (tuberculosis, cytomegalovirus, HIV, candidiasis, histoplasmosis), and genetic causes also occur.

Incidence/Prevalence

The prevalence of chronic primary adrenal insufficiency is increasing but this disease remains rare, with a prevalence of approximately 1 in 20,000 persons in the US and Western Europe (0.00005%) [44] and an annual incidence of approximately 4 per million in Western populations [45]. It is seen twice as often in females as in males. In patients with diagnosed adrenal insufficiency, 6–8% will have an adrenal crisis annually [46].

Incidence/Prevalence of Adrenal Insufficiency Presenting with Irritability

Anorexia, weakness, tiredness, fatigue: 100%.

Gastrointestinal symptoms: 92%.

Nausea: 86% [47].

Typical Findings in the HPI

Symptoms can be subtle preceding a crisis, but most patients with this disease will present with unspecified weakness and anorexia with weight loss. Additional symptoms likely to occur include other gastrointestinal symptoms such as abdominal pain, nausea, vomiting, and changes in bowel movements (diarrhea or constipation). Eighty-eight to ninety-four percent of patients have hypotension and subsequent postural dizziness. Hyperpigmentation is common and vitiligo is less common (10–20%) [47].

Typical Physical Exam Findings

Physical exam is significant for skin and mucosal membrane pigmentation changes, which is more prominent in palmar creases, buccal mucosa, pressure points, perianal mucosa, and around areolas of nipples.

Typical Laboratory/Radiological Findings

Laboratory findings will include electrolyte disturbances such as hyponatremia, hyperkalemia, hypercalcemia, azotemia (increased BUN/Cr ratio), anemia (less than half of patients), and eosinophilia (less than 1 in 5). Hypercalcemia and hypoglycemia may also be present. A low early morning serum cortisol (<3 μg/dL) is diagnostic, and if the cortisol is between 3 and 15 μg/dL, a rapid adrenocorticotropic hormone (ACTH) test can be used for confirmation.

Radiological studies are not necessary for diagnosis but may be helpful to identify underlying causes.

Screening Tools

Short 250 μg ACTH stimulation test.

Early morning salivary cortisol concentration (>16 nmol/L excludes adrenal insufficiency) [45].

Positive Predictive Values
Early morning salivary cortisol concentration 33% sensitivity, 20% specificity [48].

Cushing's Syndrome

Cushing's syndrome results from chronic exposure to excess glucocorticoid. It is divided into ACTH-dependent Cushing's syndrome and ACTH-independent Cushing's syndrome.

ACTH-dependent Cushing's syndrome is caused by pituitary hypersecretion of ACTH (65–70% of cases), ectopic secretion of ACTH by nonpituitary tumors (10–15% of cases), ectopic secretion of CRH by nonhypothalamic tumors causing pituitary hypersecretion of ACTH (<1% of cases), and iatrogenic or factitious Cushing's syndrome due to administration of exogenous ACTH (<1% of cases).

ACTH-independent Cushing's syndrome is caused by iatrogenic or factitious Cushing's syndrome (most common cause, due to prescribed prednisone), adrenocortical adenomas and carcinomas (20% of cases), primary pigmented nodular adrenocortical disease (<1% of cases), or bilateral macronodular adrenal hyperplasia (<1% of cases).

Cushing's syndrome is often difficult to diagnose because few of the signs or symptoms are diagnostic in isolation and most of the signs and symptoms are also common in individuals without the diagnosis. An important clinical clue to the presence of glucocorticoid excess is the simultaneous development and increasing severity of several of the symptoms listed below. Both the physiological hormone abnormalities as well as their clinical sequelae can cause **irritability**.

Incidence/Prevalence
0.6–0.7/100,000/year or 0.000006–0.000007% [49].

Incidence/Prevalence of Cushing's Syndrome Presenting with Irritability
Unknown.

Typical Findings in the HPI
Typical findings include menstrual irregularities, unexplained weight gain (face, posterior neck, supraclavicular area), and emotional lability.

Typical Physical Exam Findings
Physical exam is significant for posterior nuchal fat, facial plethora, proximal muscle weakness, central obesity, easy bruising, violaceous striae wider than 1 cm, and hirsutism.

Typical Laboratory/Radiological Findings

Bedtime salivary cortisol >550 ng/dL (PPV 93%) [50].

Side Effects of Medications and Supplements

Medications and supplements can also lead to **irritability** when initiated, uptitrated, or discontinued.

Classes of medications associated with **irritability** include antiepileptics, antidepressants, stimulants, benzodiazepines, immunomodulatory agents, and anabolic steroids [51].

Supplements that have been associated with **irritability** include angel's trumpet, belladonna, betel nut, caffeine, coca, cowhage, creatine, ephedra, fever bark, jimson weed, khat, manganese, rauvolfia vomitoria, Scopolia, St John's wort, and cordifolia [51].

Below is a broader differential diagnosis for irritability. This includes medical conditions with either lower prevalence of disease than those listed above or lower likelihood of irritability being included in a diagnostically ambiguous chief complaint.

Nervous System

- Chronic pain
- Vision or hearing loss
- Seizures
- Migraine
- Multiple sclerosis
- Normal-pressure hydrocephalus
- Parkinson's disease
- Limbic encephalitis
- Brain tumors
- Corticobasal degeneration
- Creutzfeldt-Jakob disease

Endocrine

- Hypoglycemia
- Primary hyperparathyroidism
- Acromegaly

Cardiopulmonology

- Hypoxia

Hepatic

- Hepatic encephalopathy

Renal

- Uremia

Infectious Disease

- HIV/AIDS
- Syphilis
- Late lyme disease

Systemic

- Wilson's disease
- Acute intermittent porphyria and porphyria variegata

Vitamin Deficiencies

- Vitamine B12 deficiency
- Pellagra

Toxic Exposures

- Arsenic poisoning (acute or chronic)
- Carbon monoxide poisoning (chronic, low-dose exposure; late-appearing symptoms)
- Lead poisoning
- Mercury poisoning

References

1. American Psychiatric Association. Diagnostic and statistical manual of mental disorders. 5th ed., text rev. Washington, DC: American Psychiatric Association; 2022.
2. Insel T, Cuthbert B, Garvey M. Research Domain Criteria (RDoC): toward a new classification framework for research on mental disorders. Am J Psychiatry. 2010;167:748–51.
3. Irritability. In: Oxford English Dictionary Online [Internet]. Oxford University Press. 2021 [cited 2021 Dec 19]. https://www.oxfordlearnersdictionaries.com/us/definition/english/irritability.
4. Vidal-Ribas P, Brotman M, Valdivieso I, Leinbluft E, Stringaris A. The status of irritability in psychiatry: a conceptual and quantitative review. J Am Acad Child Adolesc Psychiatry. 2016;55(7):556–70.
5. Stringaris A, Goodman R. Three dimensions of oppositionality in youth. J Child Psychol Psychiatry. 2009;50:216–23.
6. Bettencourt B, Talley A, Benjamin A, Valentine J. Personality and aggressive behavior under provoking and neutral conditions: a meta-analytic review. Psychol Bull. 2006;132:751–77.
7. Lengua LJ. Growth in temperament and parenting as predictors of adjustment during children's transition to adolescence. Dev Psychol. 2006;42:819–32.
8. Rothbart M. Temperament, development, and personality. Curr Dir Psychol Sci. 2007;16:207–12.

9. Tupes E, Christal R. Recurrent personality factors based on trait ratings. USAF ASD Tech Rep. 1961;60:225–51.
10. Norman W. Toward an adequate taxonomy of personality attributes: replicated factors structure in peer nomination personality ratings. J Abnorm Soc Psychol. 1963;66(6):574–83.
11. Costa P, McCrae R. Four ways five factors are basic. Personal Individ Differences. 1992;13:653–65.
12. Freud S. Mourning and melancholia. London: The Hogarth Press; 1917.
13. Adelman N, Fromm S, Razdan V. Cross-sectional and longitudinal abnormalities in brain structure in children with severe mood dysregulation or bipolar disorder. J Child Psychol Psychiatry. 2012;53:1149–56.
14. Brotman M, Rich B, Guyer A. Amygdala activation during emotion processing of neutral faces in children with severe mood dysregulation versus ADHD or bipolar disorder. Am J Psychiatry. 2010;167:61–9.
15. Stoddard J, Hsu D, Reynolds R. Aberrant amygdala intrinsic functional connectivity distinguishes youths with bipolar disorder from those with severe mood dysregulation. Psychiatry Res. 2015;231:120–5.
16. Thomas L, Brotman M, Bones B. Neural circuitry of masked emotional face processing in youth with bipolar disorder, severe mood dysregulation, and healthy volunteers. Dev Cogn Neurosci. 2014;8:110–20.
17. Tseng W, Thomas L, Harkins E, Pine D, Leibenluft E, Brotman M. Neural correlates of masked and unmasked face emotion processing in youth with severe mood dysregulation. Soc Cogn Affect Neurosci. 2016;11:78–88.
18. Seroczynski A, Bergeman C, Coccaro E. Etiology of the impulsivity/aggression relationship: genes or environment? Psychiatry Res. 1999;86(1):41–57.
19. Stringaris A, Zavos H, Leibenluft E, Maughan B, Eley T. Adolescent irritability: phenotypic associations and genetic links with depressed mood. Am J Psychiatry. 2012;169:47–54.
20. Toohey M. Irritability characteristics and parameters in an international sample. J Affect Disord. 2020;263:558–67.
21. Merikangas KR, Akiskal HS, Angst J. Lifetime and 12-month prevalence of bipolar spectrum disorder in the National Comorbidity Survey Replication. Arch Gen Psychiatry. 2007;64(5):543–52.
22. Merikangas KR, Jin R, He J-P. Prevalence and correlates of bipolar spectrum disorder in the World Mental Health Survey Initiative. Arch Gen Psychiatry. 2011;68(3):241–51.
23. Brotman M, Schmajuk M, Rich B. Prevalence, clinical correlates, and longitudinal course of severe mood dysregulation in children. Biol Psychiatry. 2006;60(9):991–7.
24. Kessler RC, Bergland P, Demler O. The epidemiology of major depressive disorder: results from the National Comorbidity Survey Replication (NCS-R). JAMA. 2003;289(23):3095–105.
25. Gehlert S, Song I, Chang C, Hartlage D. The prevalence of premenstrual dysphoric disorder in a randomly selected group of urban and rural women. Psychol Med. 2009;39(1):129–36.
26. Wittchen H, Becker E, Lieb R, Krause P. Prevalence, incidence and stability of premenstrual dysphoric disorder in the community. Psychol Med. 2002;32(1):119–32.
27. Kessler RC, Petukhova M, Sampson NA. Twelve-month and lifetime prevalence and lifetime morbid risk of anxiety and mood disorders in the US. Int J Methods Psychiatr Res. 2012;21(3):169–84.
28. Gleason M, Fox N, Drury S. The validity of evidence-derived criteria for reactive attachment disorder: indiscriminately social/disinhibited and emotionally withdrawn/inhibited types. J Am Acad Child Adolesc Psychiatry. 2011;50(3):216–31.
29. Classen C, Koopman C, Hales R, Spiegel D. Acute stress disorder as a predictor of posttraumatic stress symptoms. Am J Psychiatry. 1998;155(5):620–4.
30. Elklit A, Christiansen D. ASD and PTSD in rape victims. J Interpers Viol. 2010;25(8):1470–88.
31. Kessler RC, Berglund P, Demler O. Lifetime prevalence and age-of-onset distributions of DSM-IV disorders in the National Comorbidity Survey Replication. Arch Gen Psychiatry. 2005;62(6):593–602.

32. Goldstein R, Dawson D, Saha T. Antisocial behavioral syndromes and DSM-IV alcohol use disorders: results from the National Epidemiologic Survey on Alcohol and Related Conditions. Alcohol Clin Exp Res. 2007;31(5):814–28.
33. Lenzenweger M, Lane M, Loranger A, Kessler RC. DSM-IV personality disorders in the National Comorbidity Survey Replication. Biol Psychiatry. 2007;62(6):553–64.
34. Torgersen S, Kringlen E, Cramer V. The prevalence of personality disorders in a community sample. Arch Gen Psychiatry. 2001;58(6):590–6.
35. Grant B, Chou S, Goldstein R. Prevalence, correlates, disability, and comorbidity of DSM-IV borderline personality disorder: results from the Wave 2 National Epidemiologic Survey on Alcohol and Related Conditions. J Clin Psychiatry. 2008;69(4):533–45.
36. Agrawal A, Pergadia M, Lynskey M. Is there evidence for symptoms of cannabis withdrawal in the National Epidemiologic Survey of Alcohol and Related Conditions? Am J Addict. 2008;17(3):199–208.
37. Budney A, Hughes J. The cannabis withdrawal syndrome. Curr Opin Psychiatry. 2006;19(3):233–8.
38. Hasin D, Keyes K, Alderson D. Cannabis withdrawal in the United States: results from NESARC. J Clin Psychiatry. 2008;69(9):1354–63.
39. Hughes J. Effects of abstinence from tobacco: valid symptoms and time course. Nicotine Tob Res. 2007;9(3):315–27.
40. Bozdac G, Mumusoglu S, Zengin D, Karabulut E, Yildiz B. The prevalence and phenotypic features of polycystic ovary syndrome: a systematic review and meta-analysis. Hum Reprod. 2016;31(12):2841–55.
41. Pedersen S, Brar S, Faris P, Corenblum B. Polycystic ovary syndrome validated questionnaire for use in diagnosis. Can Fam Physician. 2007;53(6):1041–7.
42. Hallowell J, Staehling N, Flanders W, Hannon W, Gunter E, Spencer C, et al. Serum TSH, T4, and thyroid antibodies in the United States population (1988-1994): National Health and Nutrition Examination Survey (NHANES III). J Clin Endocrinol Metab. 2002;87(2):489.
43. Chakera A, Vaidya B. Addison disease in adults: diagnosis and management. Am J Med. 2010;123(5):409–13.
44. Michels A, Michels N. Addison disease: early detection and treatment principles. Am Fam Physician. 2014;89(7):563–8.
45. Charmandari E, Nicolaides N, Chrousos G. Adrenal insufficiency. Lancet. 2014;383(9935):2152–67.
46. Rushworth R, Torpy D, Falhammar H. Adrenal crisis. N Engl J Med. 2019;381(9):852–61.
47. Erichson M, Levas K, Skinningsrud B, Wolff A, Undlien D, Svartberg J, et al. Clinical, immunological, and genetic features of autoimmune primary adrenal insufficiency: observations from a Norwegian registry. J Clin Endocrinol Metab. 2009;92(12):4889.
48. Langelaan M, Kisters J, Oosterwerff M, Boer A. Salivary cortisol in the diagnosis of adrenal insufficiency: cost efficient and patient friendly. Endocr Connect. 2018;7(4):550–66.
49. Broder M, Neary M, Chang E, Cherepanov D, Ludlam W. Incidence of Cushing's syndrome and Cushing's disease in commercially-insured patients <65 years old in the United States. Pituitary. 2015;18(3):283–9.
50. Papanicolaou D, Mullen N, Kyrou L, Neiman L. Nighttime salivary cortisol: a useful test for the diagnosis of Cushing's syndrome. J Clin Endocrinol Metab. 2002;87(10):4515–21.
51. Golebiewski K, Wick J. Patient safety: aggression, irritability, and violence: drug-induce behaviors [Internet]. University of Connecticut School of Pharmacy. 2020. https://pharmacy.uconn.edu/wp-content/uploads/sites/2740/2021/04/ACCESSIBLE-CPPR-Aggression-Irritability-and-Violence-JAN2020-FINALsmaller.pdf.

Anxiety

3

Anand Jayanti, Jatin Julakanti, Robert Wieck, and Kael A. Kuster

Defining Anxiety

Historical Conceptions of Anxiety

Throughout history and across cultures, mythology has anthropomorphized our basic impulses into deities and their supporting characters. In these conceptions, historians find clues about how our ancestors understood their inner psychological worlds.

In Hindu mythology, the goddess Kali is an embodiment of divine wrath. Professor of religious studies David Kinsley characterizes Kali's role as countering the serene influence of Parvati on Shiva (their common spouse and the destroyer of worlds) [1]. It is notable that Kali, a force to neutralize anxiety and other negative emotions, is written about not as a placid force like Parvati, but as a focused, integrated, superlative elaboration of the same chaos she seeks to subdue [2]. An

A. Jayanti · J. Julakanti · R. Wieck
Psychiatry and Behavioral Medicine, University of Texas Health Science Center, Tyler, TX, USA
e-mail: anand.jayanti@uthct.edu; jatin.julakanti@uthct.edu; robert.wieck@uthct.edu

K. A. Kuster (✉)
Baylor Scott and White Health, Temple, TX, USA
e-mail: kael.kuster@bswhealth.org

E. G. Meyer et al. (eds.), *The Medical Evaluation of Psychiatric Symptoms*,
https://doi.org/10.1007/978-3-031-14372-4_3

understanding of Kali's image may be a powerful psychological tool, as it suggests that a robust conception of that which is frightening is the best defense against the object of that fear.

In *The Drama of the Gifted Child*, published in 1979, psychologist Alice Miller describes the development of an anxious child into an adult who is never certain of their worth. She traces anxiety, as well as depression, narcissistic personality disorder, and substance use back to a singular choice a child grows accustomed to making. When a child is forced to choose between procuring psychological care (attachment) or expressing their true feelings (authenticity), he chooses attachment if he is afraid his parents will reject him for those feelings, paving the way to insecurely parenting his own children, whose feelings he never learned how to confront. Miller theorized that therapy aimed at "grieving" the lost childhood is the only way to stop this cycle of deprivation [3].

In several of his writings, psychiatrist Carl Jung, active from 1900 to 1961, described anxiety with prescriptions for its resolution. While he acknowledges the contribution of family matters, such as those described by Miller, he does not focus on the past and rather directs his attention to the present resolution of these complexes [4]. He writes in his text *The Theory of Psychoanalysis:*

> *In constructing a theory which derives the neurosis from causes in the distant past, we are first and foremost following the tendency of our patient to lure us as far away as possible from the critical present... It is mainly in the present that the affective causes lie, and here alone are the possibilities of removing them.*

Here Jung highlights avoidance as a common maladaptive response to anxiety and suggests work in the present moment as remedy. His writing is a precursor to current therapies focused on present moment awareness, acceptance of symptoms and past insults, and need for *approaching* (versus *avoiding*) problems which arise in the current milieu of a patient's life.

Author C.S. Lewis, active from 1924 to 1963, explored anxiety through the perspective of a demon expounding upon torture and tribulation to a more junior demon in *The Screwtape Letters*, commenting on how to foil the plan of the "Enemy" (i.e., Biblical God). First published in 1942 amid the chaos and anxiety of war, his text explores themes of anxiety and offers a paradigm for peace amid chaos. To thwart this, the advising demon professes that "there is nothing like suspense and anxiety for barricading a human's mind against the Enemy. He wants men to be concerned with what they do; our business is to keep them thinking about what will happen to them." Thus C.S. Lewis presents a model for acceptance that promotes diffusion from anxiety, allowing for more adaptive thoughts and behaviors to proceed unfettered [5].

Eastern philosopher Jiddu Krishnamurti, active from 1909 to 1986, questioned whether the mind can ever be truly free of fear. Although he distinguishes fear of the outer world from fear of the inner world, he teaches that both come from seeking maladaptive escape. He resolves that to understand fear, all escape must come to an end. Krishnamurti teaches that the fear of death, for example, comes from thinking about not having lived a complete life and worrying that death will intersect life too soon. He offers the "cessation of thought" to eliminate the conflict, conceptualizing that it is thought itself which is responsible for the division between life and death.

When this "cessation" is accomplished, there is "no movement," between life and death, as they are both brought without conflict into the present moment [6].

Psychiatrist Irvin Yalom (active from 1963 to present) identified four ultimate concerns for the individual in his text *Existential Psychotherapy*. The first, *death*, pertains to the inescapable fate of all life. The second concern, *freedom*, comes from the injunction to navigate through a realm of cosmic indifference; it asks—*in a universe wherein anything is possible, how does one know which way to act? Isolation*, the third concern, is defined as fundamental to the nature of reality, the inevitability that we will never be truly one with others or even ourselves. An individual in balance with their isolation anxiety seeks connection with others without worrying whether she will ever totally arrive at this destination. Yalom has written about "needs-free love," which is an approach to interpersonal relationships that seeks to fill the others' needs, rather than one's own, as a way to form healthy connections in the face of interpersonal isolation. The final concern, *meaninglessness*, comes from the thrust of a meaning-seeking creature into a world seemingly without meaning [7]. In their manuscript "*Natural disasters and existential concerns: a test of Tillich's theory of existential anxiety*," Scott and Weems found that "different facets of existential concerns were shown to be related to both PTSD symptoms and suicidal ideation and so supports a multifaceted conceptualization of existential anxiety in relation to psychological distress" [8].

"Anxiety" has left a vast footprint across cultures, and throughout art, philosophy, and medicine, yet evades succinct definition. Nevertheless, the DSM-5-TR [9] provides clinicians a scaffolding upon which to organize physical and mental symptoms common to anxiety or related disorders, explored in detail in the next section. Likewise, the American Psychological Association frames anxiety as "an emotion characterized by feelings of tension, worried thoughts and physical changes like increased blood pressure" [10]. Merriam-Webster, in turn, calls it "apprehensive uneasiness or nervousness usually over an impending or anticipated ill" [11].

Pathophysiology of Anxiety

According to the National Institute of Mental Health (NIMH), anxiety disorders affect nearly 1 in 5 adults in the United States [12]. Anxiety has a distinctive fingerprint on the hippocampus, amygdala, thalamus, and hypothalamus, together called the limbic system, and is integrated by the prefrontal cortex. Individuals with anxiety disorders tend to have heightened activity in the limbic system, specifically the amygdala. In a state of anxiety, the amygdala signals the hypothalamus to release norepinephrine, in the process called "fight or flight," increasing the body's heart rate, blood pressure, respirations, and more [13]. Additional symptoms of sympathetic arousal include dry mouth, dry eyes, dilated pupils, cold hands, decreased gastrointestinal motility, urinary retention, shivering, and piloerection.

In addition to sympathetic muscle activation, there are musculoskeletal effects of anxiety. Those with anxiety disorders may exhibit behaviors like clenching their hands and grinding their teeth and may have headaches, neck pain, and excessive intercostal muscle use.

In Seligman's landmark experiment [14], dogs were tested for the circumstances that cause "learned helplessness." In one group, dogs were kept in a harness and later released. Dogs in the second and third groups were paired so that a shock was given to them at the same time. Dogs in the second group, however, were given a lever that would terminate the shock for both groups. The dogs in the third group had a lever that did not have any effect on the shock. Later, all of these groups were placed in an apparatus that delivered shocks until they jumped over a partition. The dogs in groups one and two learned this maneuver quickly. However, the dogs in group three simply laid down in response to this situation. In order to change this response, experimenters had to physically move the dogs' legs, replicating the actions of escape, in order to train them to willfully traverse the barrier themselves. Today, this experiment is often used to describe the effects of chronic anxiety on behavior; persons with chronic anxiety may "learn helplessness" and cease behaviors which might eventually improve their situation.

Nassim Taleb coined the term "anti-fragility" to describe the quality of becoming stronger with new challenges. In their sprawling manuscript "*Antifragility and tinkering in biology (and in business) flexibility provides an efficient epigenetic way to manage risk*," Dachin et al. draw parallels all the way down to the molecular level, proposing that antifragility promotes cellular survival through flexible response to variable environments [15].

A parallel conceptualization is posttraumatic growth, found across cultures, and studied often in the wake of extreme stressors, such as Hurricane Katrina or the Kobe earthquake in Japan. Evidence of posttraumatic growth includes a positive change in appreciation for life, relationships with others, openness to possibilities in life, personal change, and spiritual change [16, 17]. Appropriately contextualized stressing of a system promotes positive change and growth; whereas, maladaptive avoidance (rampant in anxiety disorders) causes loss of footing and stagnation.

Variants of Anxiety Based on Patient Population and Medical Specialty

Recapitulating the definition of anxiety from earlier in this chapter—"an emotion characterized by feelings of tension, worried thoughts and physical changes like increased blood pressure"—the task of defining anxiety against other symptoms becomes complicated. Few presentations of anxiety are truly primary, and more often implicate either biological, psychological, or social phenomena. In the following sections, we will tease anxiety apart from its mimics in various medical contexts.

Adult Primary Care The presentation of anxiety in primary care as is often considered to be from one of three sources (although it is often multiple): *primary* anxiety (anxiety in relation to concious or unconcious psychosocial constructs), anxiety *about* a potential or actual medical diagnosis, or anxiety *due to* a medical etiology. Since the etiology is rarely clear, primary care physicians are taught to begin with an exploration of the possible systemic medical etiologies. These include, but are not limited to, cardiac, endocrine, and toxicological factors that must be considered before a well-informed psychiatric investigation can begin. Specific systemic medical causes of anxiety include anoxia due to a variety of conditions (e.g., pulmonary embolism, anoxia), myocardial infarction, excessive thyroid hormone, pheochromocytoma, or pain. Additionally, delirium, specifically mild hyperactive delirium, may mimic anxiety to a degree and should be considered as a serious medical condition that may be misreported to a consulting physician as "anxiety." Examination for changes in the level of consciousness and/or attention found in delirium (to help differentiate from anxiety), and evaluating for underlying systemic medical causes to explain delirium is critical. Medical-adjacent psychiatric factors such as sleep, exercise, and diet form a watershed between general medicine and psychiatry that are crucial to explore on the way to diagnosis and medication management.

Life-threatening/Dangerous Conditions that Cause or Worsen Anxiety	
Asthma	Thyrotoxicosis
Pulmonary embolism	Pheochromocytoma
Myocardial infarction	Delirium

Pediatrics In children, anxiety should carefully be assessed against many similar presentations including fussiness, irritability, and agitation, depending on the age of the child. As is the case in adult medicine, a careful differential should be constructed for the "anxious" child to evaluate the many possible sources of unease that may not find verbal expression, particularly accidental ingestion.

Psychiatry Research initiatives to better understand mental illness as dysfunction in physiologic and biological systems have introduced the Research Domain Criteria initiative (RDoC), which uses a system of six domains of human experience [18]. Of the six, the construct of anxiety is located in the Negative Valence System and defined as "activation of a brain system in which harm may potentially occur but is distant, ambiguous, or low/uncertain in probability, characterized by a pattern of responses such as enhanced risk assessment (vigilance)."

The RDoC, interestingly, differentiates the construct of *anxiety* from the construct of *fear*, which is defined as "Activation of the brain's defensive motivational system to promote behaviors that protect the organism from perceived danger. Normal fear involves a pattern of adaptive responses to conditioned or unconditioned threat stimuli (exteroceptive or interoceptive). Fear can involve internal representations and cognitive processing and can be modulated by a variety of factors."

The sustained threat construct is defined as "an aversive emotional state caused by prolonged (i.e., weeks to months) exposure to internal and/or external condition(s), state(s), or stimuli that are adaptive to escape or avoid. The exposure may be actual or anticipated; the changes in affect, cognition, physiology, and behavior caused by sustained threat persist in the absence of the threat and can be differentiated from those changes evoked by acute threat." The RDoC system teases apart these phenomena not arbitrarily, but because of identifying unique parameters in each in the categories of genes, molecules, cells, circuits, physiology, behavior, self-report, and paradigms.

Variants of Anxiety Based on Culture

The conceptualization and nomenclature for anxiety and its related symptoms vary greatly across cultures. In their cross-sectional qualitative study, Andrew et al. write that while "somatic symptoms were by far the most frequent presenting problems… a substantial proportion of informants used the psychological construct of 'tension' or 'worry' to label their illness, but did not consider themselves as suffering from a 'mental disorder'" [19]. "*Ataque de nervios*" is a condition found in Hispanic populations, predominantly affecting females. It includes the symptoms of panic attacks with the inclusion of additional symptoms such as dissociation, crying, anger, and seizure-like or fainting behavior [20]. Consideration of cultural constructs is an important first step to disentangling symptoms and making a diagnosis. Far from impairing the clinical precision of such a diagnosis, cultural constructs offer richer context and additional information to the attentive clinician. Given the unfortunate centrality of anxiety to the human condition, these constructs are extensive in their diversity and prevalence. For each person with a chief complaint of "anxiety," the first, and most important, clinical question to answer is "what does *anxiety* mean to *you*?"

Differential for Anxiety

In many cases, generalized anxiety disorder and major depressive disorder may only be a cultural or language barrier apart, rather than truly distinct brain states. In fact, two patients may suffer from what we call major depressive disorder and be nearly noncontiguous in their symptom profiles. Whereas in diagnosing diabetes mellitus, we need only rely on the precision and accuracy of the glucometer, in diagnosing major depressive disorder, we need both physician and patient to understand what symptoms mean, communicate openly about how distressing they are, and share a sense of time.

Anxiety Disorders

Generalized Anxiety Disorder

Generalized anxiety disorder features anxiety as its defining quality, but importantly, requires a duration of 6 months, more than half of which is characterized by anxiety encompassing a great breadth of a patient's life, rather than any single aspect. According to the DSM-5-TR, this anxiety has to furthermore interfere with the patient's life in specific, often physical ways, including at least three out of the following six symptoms: (1) Restlessness or feeling keyed up or on edge. (2) Being easily fatigued. (3) Difficulty concentrating or mind going blank. (4) Irritability. (5) Muscle tension. (6) Sleep disturbance (difficulty falling or staying asleep, or restless, unsatisfying sleep) [9, p. 222].

It is important to rule out life-threatening, hormonal, metabolic, and substance-induced anxiety, while also determining if the anxiety hinges purely on social interactions (such as a public presentation) or from some “trigger,” or "out of the blue" or while in solitude. Obsessive-compulsive disorder contrasts with GAD in that OCD requires attempts to ignore or neutralize intrusive thoughts, urges, or images by performing some thought or action. Posttraumatic stress disorder requires several antecedent experiences that GAD does not, and these will be explored in a further section.

Generally, by the time we encounter GAD as physicians, it has had the opportunity to have many insidious effects on our patients' health. Chronic stress has been linked to myriad metabolic disorders, inflammatory disorders, and psychiatric comorbidities, including but not limited to other anxiety disorders and unipolar depressive disorders.

Incidence/Prevalence of Disorder

The 12-month prevalence in the United States is 2.9% in adults and 0.9% in adolescents. Lifetime morbid risk is 9.0% [9, p. 223]. It is twice as common in women. GAD is strongly associated with other anxiety disorders—odds ratio for having panic disorder or specific phobia is around 7 in persons with GAD. GAD may predict the onset of other anxiety disorders (e.g., panic disorder, social phobia, specific phobia, agoraphobia) with a hazard ratio of 4:14. Comorbid depressive disorder is less common, with HR of about 2 for prediction of depressive disorder onset in persons with GAD [21].

Typical Findings in the HPI

Symptoms include excessive anxiety and worry which is out of proportion in duration, frequency, and intensity to impact of actual event according to the DSM-5-TR, and must interfere with socio-occupational functioning. To meet full criteria for GAD, adults present with at least three and children present with at least one of the following symptoms: restlessness, fatigue, difficulty concentrating, irritability, sleep disturbances, and muscle tension.

Typical Mental Status Exam Findings

Patients have variable presentation on appearance but in severe cases can present with psychomotor agitation, diaphoresis, dyspnea, hyperventilation, GI upset, and angina. Speech is generally unaffected in generalized anxiety disorder. Mood can be anxious or fearful and their effect may be intense or frightened-appearing. Thought process is generally linear and goal-directed. Thought content can involve obsessive, preservative thoughts and feature suicidal ideation, delusions, and hallucinations in extreme cases. Cognitive symptoms may present with distractibility over the course of the interview. Insight is generally good as they understand anxiety is out of proportion to danger. Judgment is variable.

Typical Laboratory/Radiological Findings

Laboratory findings are used to rule out specific systemic medical causes and should especially be performed with weight loss, cognitive impairment, and late-onset anxiety. These tests include complete blood count, metabolic panel, TSH, EKG, urinalysis, and urine toxicology.

Rating Scales

The GAD seven-item scale can be used in clinical settings with sensitivity to diagnosis and symptom severity change. The Hospital Anxiety and Depression Scale is widely used to assess and monitor GAD with further distinction from other medical conditions. The Penn State Worry Questionnaire (PSWQ) can identify excessive worrying but is less sensitive to change than the GAD seven-item scale. At a cut-off score of 10, the GAD-7 has a sensitivity of 89% and specificity is 82% with the GAD-7 [22].

Pitfalls/Differential Diagnoses

- Anxiety disorder due to another medical condition
- Substance/medication-induced anxiety disorder
- Social anxiety disorder
- Obsessive-compulsive disorder
- Posttraumatic stress disorder
- Acute stress disorder
- Adjustment disorder
- Depressive disorder
- Bipolar disorder
- Psychotic disorder

Panic Attacks and Panic Disorder

Panic attacks and panic disorder occur with select symptoms, frequency, and the subject's concern about their recurrence. Three of the 13 symptoms explicitly involve anxiety—fear of losing control, fear of dying, and feelings of derealization/depersonalization. The other 9 symptoms are more corporeal, including trembling, sweating, nausea, chest pain, and shortness of breath. The patient must endorse at least 4 of the 13 symptoms. Panic attacks can occur in response to a sudden danger or illness or "out of the blue." To diagnose panic disorder, versus "panic attacks," patients who suffer from panic disorder have panic attacks that are followed by 1 or more months of persistent worry of further attacks, often accompanied by maladaptive changes in behavior, and are not attributed to substance use or other mental disorder. Complete differential will include medical explanations for distress including myocardial infarction. Sporadic presentation differentiates panic attacks from generalized anxiety disorder (GAD being more chronic or constant anxiety).

Panic disorder (versus panic attack) is diagnosed with recurrent panic attacks followed by at least 1 month of persistent, significant, worry about subsequent attacks and/or significant maladaptive changes in behavior.

Incidence/Prevalence of Disorder

The 12-month prevalence in the United States is 2–3% in adults and adolescents. Females are affected at about a 2:1 rate compared to males. Before age 14, the overall rate is low at less than 0.4%. Rate increases in adolescence, peaks in adulthood, then decreases in later life (i.e., 0.7% in ages over 64) [9, p. 210].

Typical Findings in the HPI

Symptoms include recurrent and unexpected panic attacks characterized by intensive fear or discomfort presenting with palpitations, sweating, trembling, shortness of breath, choking, chest pain, nausea, dizziness, chills, paresthesias, derealization, or fear of losing control/dying.

To diagnose panic *disorder* (versus panic *attacks*), patients need to be queried about 1 or more months of persistent worry of further attacks or maladaptive changes in behavior not attributed to substance use or other mental disorder.

Typical Mental Status Exam Findings

Patients have variable presentation on appearance, but in severe cases can be restless and present with psychomotor agitation, diaphoresis, shortness of breath, hyperventilation, GI upset, and chest pain. Speech may be affected by severe anxiety or a precipitating panic attack resulting in stammering or vocal tremor. Their mood can be anxious, irritable, nervous, and fearful and their affect may be intense, frightened-appearing, and increased emotional lability. Thought process is generally linear and goal-directed. Thought content can involve obsessive, preservative thoughts and feature suicidal ideation, delusions, and hallucinations in extreme cases. Cognitive symptoms may present with distractibility over the course of the interview. Insight is generally good as they understand panic is out of proportion to danger. Judgment is variable.

Typical Laboratory/Radiological Findings

Laboratory findings are used to rule out systemic medical causes and include complete blood count, metabolic panel, TSH, EKG, urinalysis, and urine toxicology.

Rating Scales

The Panic Disorder Severity Scale (PDSS) is a seven-item gold standard for screening which measures attack frequency, attack intensity, anticipatory anxiety, phobic avoidance, avoidance of internal bodily sensations, relationship impairment, and work impairment. Optimal cut-off is a score of >8, with a sensitivity of 83.3% and specificity of 64% [23].

Pitfalls/Differential Diagnoses

- Anxiety disorder due to a medical condition
- Somatic symptom disorder
- Illness anxiety disorder
- Substance/medication-induced anxiety disorder
- Other mental disorders with panic attacks as an associated feature (other anxiety and psychotic disorders)

Specific Phobia

Specific phobias are those where an object, person, creature, or situation almost always provokes immediate anxiety and therefore is actively avoided. This anxiety must be out of proportion to the actual danger posed and must cause significant distress. Common objects of phobia are spiders, insects, dogs, heights, storms, or water. Situations that commonly induce phobic avoidance are airplanes, elevators, and enclosed spaces.

Because specific phobias are relatively common, it is difficult to know what it means for a response to a stimulus to be out of proportion. The tendency of humans to have common objects of phobia suggest a likely evolutionary utility to this anxiety, as discussed in the opening paragraphs of this chapter. We must be very careful to understand how much impairment the phobia actually causes the patient and treat them proportionately. Specific phobias are very fertile spaces to explore with the patient the utility of our anxiety to protect us from danger, reframing the disorder as a defense and a tool they can learn to wield better with time.

Incidence/Prevalence of Disorder

Twelve-month prevalence in the United States is 7–9%. Prevalence rates are highest in adolescents at 16%. Lifetime prevalence is estimated at about 12.5% [24]. Specific phobias are the most common anxiety disorder. Females are affected at a 2:1 rate as males with phobias of animal, natural environment, or situations more specific to females. Blood-injection-injury phobia however is nearly equally experienced by females and males [9, p. 199].

Typical Findings in the HPI

Symptoms include the fear or anxiety about a specific object or situation which is provoked immediately, avoided actively, out of proportion with danger, persistent for greater than 6 months, and causes socio-occupational impairment. This disturbance cannot be explained by any substances, medical disorders, or other mental disorders.

Typical Mental Status Exam Findings

Patients may present with restlessness and psychomotor agitation if exposed to the specific feared object or situation. Speech may be affected by the presence of the object/situation resulting in stammering or vocal tremor. Their mood can be anxious, irritable, nervous, and fearful and their affect may be intense, frightened-appearing, and increased emotional lability. Thought process is generally linear and goal-directed. Thought content can involve irrational and ego-dystonic fear of specific situation, activity, or object. Cognitive symptoms may present with distractibility over the course of the interview. Insight is generally good as they understand specific phobia is out of proportion to actual threat. Judgment is variable and best assessed in review of patients' actions.

Typical Laboratory/Radiological Findings

There are no laboratory studies or imaging currently recommended for diagnosing specific phobias.

Functional magnetic resonance imaging has found neuroanatomical pathways associated with specific phobia through hyperactivation of amygdala and insula as well as a greater activation of stria terminalis and the right anterior cingulate cortex in response to an unpredicted threat.

Rating Scales

Specific Phobia Questionnaire [25] can be used to determine the range of fears associated with the five specific types. The Circumscribed Fear Measure [26] can be used to assess specific phobia across different phobia types. The Severity Measure for Specific Phobia similarly also assesses the intensity of symptoms across the five specific phobia types.

Pitfalls/Differential Diagnoses

- Agoraphobia
- Social anxiety disorder
- Separation anxiety disorder
- Panic disorder
- Obsessive-compulsive disorder
- Trauma and stressor-related disorders
- Eating disorders
- Schizophrenia spectrum and other psychotic disorders

Social Phobia

Social phobia is defined as anxiety about being scrutinized by others in such situations as conversations, meetings, or presentations. The patient consequently avoids such situations.

It is a common belief that people are more afraid of public speaking than of death. Whether or not this is true (the prevalence of social phobia is 7% in the US), it makes sense that anxiety about one's social standing would predominate among our stressors. It is not unlike death to be rejected by one's peers, because our reputation determines our survival in a tribe and it is only through our peers that our genes will be passed on to the next generation by way of mating. It may be helpful for our patients to understand these roots of social phobia to promote psychological diffusion from such fears. It is important to distinguish performance anxiety from a generalized anxiety type. The latter can more commonly overlap with avoidant personality disorder, which is discussed in a latter section.

Incidence/Prevalence of Disorder

Twelve-month prevalence in the United States is 7%, with children, adolescents, and adults having comparable rates. Twelve-month prevalence decreases later in life ranging from 2% to 5% in older adults [9, p. 204].

Typical Findings in the HPI

Symptoms include the fear or anxiety about one or more social situations which is provoked immediately, avoided actively, out of proportion with danger, persistent for greater than 6 months, and causes socio-occupational impairment. This disturbance cannot be explained by any substances, medical disorders, or other mental disorders.

Typical Mental Status Exam Findings

Patients have a variable presentation on appearance but may present with restlessness and psychomotor agitation if in presence of another individual or social situation. Speech may have a stammering or vocal tremor. Their mood can be anxious, irritable, nervous, fearful and their effect may be intense, frightened-appearing, and increased emotional lability. Thought process is generally linear and goal-directed. Thought content can involve irrational and ego-dystonic fear of specific social situations. Cognitive symptoms may present with distractibility over the course of the interview. Insight is generally good as they understand social anxiety is out of proportion to actual threat. Judgment is variable and best assessed in the review of patients' actions.

Typical Laboratory/Radiological Findings

There are no laboratory studies or imaging currently recommended for diagnosing social phobias.

Imaging shows hyperactivity of limbic and paralimbic fear circuitry in response to social threat stimuli. Functional magnetic resonance imaging studies have found hyperactivation of amygdala and insula when engaged with public speaking or viewing socially threatening images. There is also a dysfunction in the default mode network near the medial parietal, medial prefrontal, and occipital cortical regions.

Rating Scales

Mini-Social Phobia Inventory demonstrates (Mini-SPIN) has high sensitivity (88.7%) and specificity (90.0%) for determination of social phobia (cut-off score of 6 or greater)—positive predictive value was 52.5% and negative predictive value was 98.5%. Other longer (20 questions) scales are also sometimes used, for instance, the Social Interaction Anxiety Scale (SIAS) and the Social Phobia Scale (SPS). The Mini-Social Phobia Inventory is much shorter but still shows positive correlations with the SIAS and SPS ($r = 0.81$ and $r = 0.77$, respectively) [27].

Pitfalls/Differential Diagnoses

- Normal shyness
- Agoraphobia
- Panic disorder
- Generalized anxiety disorder
- Separation anxiety disorder
- Specific phobias
- Selective mutism
- Major depressive disorder
- Body dysmorphic disorder
- Delusional disorder
- Autism spectrum disorder

- Personality disorders
- Oppositional defiant disorder

Other Psychiatric Disorders with Prominent Anxiety

Acute Stress Disorder and Posttraumatic Stress Disorder

Patients with acute stress disorder (ASD) and posttraumatic stress disorder (PTSD) have an antecedent experience of a traumatic event. Furthermore, the trauma is followed by intrusive memories, dreams, flashbacks, or distress in response to cues, and by negative alterations in mood and avoidance of associated stimuli. These two stress-related disorders differ in their time, course, and outcome.

The anxiety of posttraumatic stress disorder is variable among patients. This is easy to imagine as the particular traumas can be so variable in nature. It is often the case that traumatic events can create a constellation of disorders, of which posttraumatic stress disorder is just one, making it hard to capture or tease apart from a depressive disorder or a substance use disorder, for example. It is 80% more likely that a patient with PTSD has another comorbid psychiatric illness than a patient without PTSD. It is also often the case that victims of trauma will not readily discuss their experiences, making the diagnosis even more difficult, perhaps leading to equivocal paths of assessment. Our precise approach in discussing a patient's trauma is of utmost importance in properly diagnosing it.

Incidence/Prevalence of Disorder

Prevalence of acute stress disorder varies according to the nature and context of the event. Assault, rape, or witnessing a mass shooting correlates with a 20–50% rate of developing acute stress disorder; whereas, non-interpersonal traumatic events generally have rates of acute stress disorder below 20% [9, p. 284]. The 12-month prevalence of posttraumatic stress disorder in the United States is 3.5% in adults. Lifetime risk by age of 75 is 8.7%. Rates are higher among veterans and first responders. Highest rates, from around 1/3 to more than 1/2 of those exposed are found in survivors of rape, military combat/captivity, ethically or politically motivated internment, and genocide [9, p. 276].

Typical Findings in the HPI

Patients have exposure to serious trauma including death, injury, or sexual violence either directly or through indirect immersion. Symptoms include recurrent, involuntary, intrusive distressing memories or dreams, dissociative reactions through flashbacks, and marked physiological and psychological reactions to internal/external cues to trauma. Patients have persistent avoidance of stimuli associated with events through efforts of avoiding distressing memories or external reminders such as people or places. Negative alterations in cognition and mood associated with events are accompanied with inability to remember important aspects, persistent negative beliefs, blaming themselves or others, feelings of detachment, and inability to experience positive emotions. Marked alterations in arousal are found in irritable, reckless, self-destructive behavior, hypervigilance, sleep disturbances, and problems with concentration. Dissociative symptoms such as depersonalization and derealization may also be found.

Typical Mental Status Exam Findings

Patients may appear to be restless and present with psychomotor agitation, increased vigilance, increased startle response, poor eye contact and difficulty engaging with physicians, and increased arousal when discussing trauma. Their mood can be anxious or fearful and their affect may be blunted with decreased range of positive emotions and persistent negative emotions. Thought processes tend to be organized. Thought content may involve obsessive ruminations, distortions of self concept, or, in extreme cases, suicidal/homicidal ideation, delusions, and hallucinations. Feature suicidal and homicidal ideation, delusions, and hallucinations in extreme cases. Cognitive symptoms may present with decreased concentration over the course of the interview.

Typical Laboratory/Radiological Findings

There are no laboratory studies or imaging currently recommended for diagnosing patients with PTSD.

Some studies have demonstrated MRI finding alterations in the anterior cingulate gyrus, as well as amygdala, hippocampus, and insular cortex in patients with PTSD [28].

Rating Scales

The Clinician-Administered PTSD scale for DSM-5-TR (CAPS-5) is a time-consuming structured interview offering the "gold standard" for diagnosis. The 20-question PTSD Checklist for DSM-5-TR (PCL-5) correlates well with the CAPS-5 with an $r = 0.94$, making the PCL-5 a viable brief option. At an optimal cut-off score of 30, sensitivity for the PCL-5 is 94.3, specificity is 93.9, PPV is 80.10, and NPV is 98.50 [29]. The Primary Care PTSD Screen for DSM-5-TR (PC-PTSD-5) is a shorter option that also performs with good sensitivity and specificity [30].

Pitfalls/Differential Diagnoses

- Adjustment disorders
- Acute stress disorder
- Anxiety disorders
- Obsessive-compulsive disorder
- Major depressive disorder
- Personality disorders
- Dissociative disorders
- Functional neurological symptom disorder
- Psychotic disorders
- Traumatic brain injury

Obsessive-Compulsive Disorder

OCD is a disorder that is characterized by recurrent, disturbing thoughts paired with attempts to suppress these thoughts with repetitive behaviors that interfere with the patient's life in significant ways. The latter compulsion need not always be acted upon.

As mentioned above, the anxiety of OCD may be creative, as it involves imagined gestures—images or actions—that need not always occur in a realistic world. Examples include violent gestures or sexual gestures or even verbal gestures that are inappropriate for the patient's context. This makes OCD a very interesting context in which to think about anxiety. It may be useful to the patient to consider exactly where this anxiety begins in their thought process.

Incidence/Prevalence of Disorder

Twelve-month prevalence in the United States is 1.2%. Females are affected at a higher rate in adulthood than men at 1.5% (female) versus 1.0% (male) [9, p. 239]. In childhood, OCD is more prominent in men. Lifetime prevalence in the United States is 2.3% [31].

Typical Findings in the HPI

Symptoms include the presence of obsessions—recurrent thoughts or urges difficult to neutralize—and compulsions—repetitive behaviors or mental acts in response to urges. These findings are time-consuming or cause socio-occupational impairment. They cannot be better explained by any substance, medical condition, or another mental disorder.

Typical Mental Status Exam Findings

Patients appear variably, but up to 30% will present with vocal or motor tics during their lifetime. The "classic" OCD behaviors are compulsions that can lead to dry hands from frequent hand washing. Speech and language tend to be less impacted in comparison to other mental conditions. Mood may be described as distressed, annoyed, or various others as a consequence of living with obsession and compulsions. Affect can also be variable in expression of emotional range. OCD typically does not cause disorganization in the thought process. Perceptual disturbances are not inherent to OCD; however, in very severe OCD, imaginative obsessions may be difficult to discern from psychotic delusions. For this reason, very severe cases of OCD may be misdiagnosed as psychotic disorders. Severe OCD may impact cognition and can lead to difficulty concentrating on anything other than urges. Because OCD is ego-dystonic, patients typically have good insight that their OCD is irrational, and are often quite bothered by their compulsive behaviors. Judgment can be variable.

Typical Laboratory/Radiological Findings

There are no laboratory studies or imaging currently recommended for diagnosing OCD. Positron emission tomography and functional magnetic resonance imaging have found abnormalities in the cortico-striatal-thalamic loop circuit, specifically in the orbitofrontal cortex, the anterior cingulate cortex, and the striatum. Further abnormalities in the dorsomedial prefrontal cortex, the inferior frontal gyrus, and cerebellum have also been noted [32].

Rating Scales

The Yale-Brown Obsessive-Compulsive Scale (Y-BOCS) is the gold standard for diagnosis which covers 54 common obsessions and compulsions that are scaled to produce a total severity score. Cut-off score of 13 was optimal with sensitivity ranging from 85% to 90% and specificity between 94% and 97% [33].

Pitfalls/Differential Diagnoses

- Anxiety disorders
- Major depressive disorder
- Other obsessive-compulsive and related disorders
- Eating disorders
- Tics and stereotyped movements
- Psychotic disorders
- Other compulsive-like behaviors
- Obsessive-compulsive personality disorder
- Somatic delusional disorder

Substance Use Disorders

Symptoms of anxiety or panic can be precipitated by the use or withdrawal from various substances. Patients can present with palpitations, dizziness, shaking, dyspnea, and diaphoresis. Mechanism of action should be considered—generally activating drugs may provoke anxiety during intoxication, and sedating drugs during withdrawal. Substances that may cause anxiety during use may include caffeine, amphetamines, cocaine, or PCP. Substances that may cause anxiety during withdrawal may include alcohol, sedatives, opioids, or anticholinergics. The specifics of each are beyond the scope of this chapter. In general, an astute clinician will ask about substance use including onset, duration, severity, and timing. Recent days of use (or since used in the case of withdrawal) are important to number and correlate with symptom onset. Specific drug clearance should be correlated to onset of symptoms—for instance, anxiety manifesting during withdrawal from a long-acting benzodiazepine such as clonazepam may onset 4–5 days after stopping the use of the substance. In general, cessation of the responsible substance is generally the primary treatment for reduction of anxiety. In the case of withdrawal, time away from substance is generally sufficient for anxiety symptoms to resolve—as long as monitoring for withdrawal seizures (with alcohol, benzodiazepines, and barbiturates), and management of patient timeline expectations occurs (as this may be considered in some circumstances of prolonged or severe substance use).

Treatment varies widely based on the causes of anxiety, and treatment guidelines should be consulted. In the United States in 2019, the 1-year prevalence of substance use disorder (including both alcohol and illicit drug use disorders) was 4.5% among ages 12–17, 14.1% for ages 18–25, and 6.7% for ages 26 and above [34]. The Alcohol Use Disorder Identification Test (AUDIT) is used to screen for hazardous use (scores 7–14) and presence of a moderate to severe use disorder (scores 15 and above). A cut-off of 8 has greater than 90% sensitivity and specificity for indicating hazardous drinking [35].

Personality Disorders

The personality disorders make for an interesting terrain to examine anxiety and its various forms. Persons with paranoid personalities harbor suspicion, without basis, that others are exploiting or harming them. They may also be reluctant to confide in people because of an unwarranted fear this information will be used against them. Paranoid personality disorder prevalence estimates range from 2.3% to 4.4%. Borderline personality disorder (BPD) is characterized by frantic efforts to avoid real or imagined abandonment. Distrust for others, sensitivity to rejection, and neuroticism are also prominent. Prevalence for BPD is estimated at 1.6–5.9% in the general population, though it may range from 10% (outpatient) to 20% (inpatient) in psychiatric settings. Next, histrionic personalities (prevalence 1.84%) are uncomfortable in situations where they are not the center of attention and therefore adopt provocative behaviors. Avoidant personality disorder has a pervasive pattern of social inhibition, feelings of inadequacy, and hypersensitivity to negative evaluation. Prevalence is 2.4%. Finally, dependent personality disorder is characterized by difficulty making decisions without excessive support from others. The patients may also have difficulty expressing disagreement with others or initiating projects on their own. These qualities stem from an exaggerated fear of being unable to care for themselves. Prevalence estimates range from 0.49% to 0.6% [9, pp. 651–677].

Anxiety clearly takes many forms in these disorders but centers on the theme of imagining ways in which the world is not set up for one's success. It may be difficult to tease apart the anxiety of personality disorders from other disorders, such as generalized anxiety or depression, or even in some cases psychosis. Some of these personality disorders can even be adaptive to a narrow social or professional context (e.g., the narcissistic CEO or the histrionic actor) making it very difficult for some individuals to understand the dysfunction in their lives and for the people surrounding them.

The McLean Screening Instrument for Borderline Personality Disorder (MSI-BPD) may be particularly useful given the frequent occurrence of BPD in medical and psychiatric offices. At a cut-off of 7, it has a sensitivity of 80% and a specificity of 85%; younger ages (25 and below) have even better sensitivity (90%) and specificity (93%) [36]. Also, please keep in mind that diagnosis of any personality disorder requires more than occasional symptomatic presentation, rather, prior to making a diagnosis, the astute clinician notes maladaptive patterns that are pervasive, inflexible, stable over time, often present in adolescence or early adulthood, found in a variety of contexts, and significantly impair social, occupational, or other functioning.

Systemic Medical Differential

Myocardial Infarction

Myocardial infarction is an event characterized by limited oxygen supply to the heart which leads to injury. This can be detected by symptomatic changes such as chest pain, the rise and fall of cardiac enzymes such as troponin, changes to the electrocardiogram, and imaging changes to myocardium.

Incidence/Prevalence of Disorder

The annual incidence rate is approximately 600 cases per 100,000 people. Coronary artery disease, a major risk factor for having MI, occurs in 6.7% of adults age 20 or over in the United States [37].

Typical Findings in the HPI

The most common presentation is chest pain or discomfort, characteristically tightness or pressure in the substernal area with radiation to the left arm or jaw. This can be accompanied by shortness of breath, sweating, weakness, and anxiety.

Typical Physical Exam Findings

Physical examination findings look at auscultation of heart and lungs, measurement of blood pressure in both arms, presence of all major pulses, heart failure, and circulation.

This can reveal evidence of systemic hypoperfusion with hypotension, tachycardia, cold, clammy skin, and delirium. Delirium can be potentiated by the subclinical vascular dementia common in vasculopathic patients. It can also show evidence of heart failure with JVD, pulmonary crackles, hypotension, tachycardia, S3 gallop, and mitral regurgitation murmur.

Typical Laboratory/Radiological Findings

Laboratory tests include ECG, cardiac enzymes including troponin, creatinine, urea, electrolytes, glucose, complete blood count, blood arterial gal, lipid studies, and CK-MB.

Rating Scales

For the diagnosis of acute MI, Cardiac troponin I has a sensitivity of 90.2%, a specificity of 95.7%, a positive predictive value of 92.5%, and a negative predictive value of 94.3% [38].

Pitfalls/Differential Diagnoses

- Pneumothorax
- Anxiety disorders
- Costochondritis
- GERD

Pulmonary Embolism

Pulmonary embolism is a vascular obstruction of the pulmonary artery or its branches by thrombus, air, or fat that travels to the lungs from somewhere else in the body.

Incidence/Prevalence of Disorder

The overall age-adjusted incidence is higher in males compared with females (130 versus 110 per 100,000, respectively). Incidence rates increase markedly with age for both male and female [39].

Typical Findings in the HPI

Most common presentation is dyspnea (73%) followed by pleuritic chest pain (66%), and cough (37%). Patients also report orthopnea (28%), calf or thigh pain (44%), wheezing (21%), and hemoptysis (13%). Patients furthermore rarely present with shock, arrhythmia, and syncope.

Typical Physical Exam Findings

The typical findings on physical examination include tachypnea (54%), tachycardia (24%), rales (18%), decreased breath sounds (17%), accentuated pulmonic component of the second heart sound (15%), jugular venous distension (14%), and fever, mimicking pneumonia (3%), usually associated with calf or thigh swelling to include erythema, edema, tenderness, and palpable, cordlike deep veins (47%) [40].

Typical Laboratory/Radiological Findings

CT angiography of the chest may show normal findings but may also display pleural effusions, wedge-shaped infarcts known as Hampton hump, and an avascularity distal to the embolism known as Westermark sign.

An ECG may show S1Q3T3 which displays an S wave in lead I and Q wave and inverted T wave in lead III. This may be accompanied by T-wave inversions in V1–V4, atrial fibrillation, right ventricular strain, and sinus tachycardia.

Arterial blood gas may show respiratory alkalosis, hypoxemia, hypocapnia, and elevated alveolar-arterial gradient.

Rating Scales

CT angiography of the chest is the imaging choice in diagnostic evaluation as it has a 90% sensitivity and 95% specificity. V/Q scan may be performed if the patient has a high pre-test probability but is unable to undergo CT angiogram. Venous duplex ultrasound of lower extremities may be done to evaluate for DVTs.

Pitfalls/Differential Diagnoses

- Pneumothorax
- Myocardial infarction
- Anxiety disorders
- Costochondritis
- GERD

Hyperthyroidism

Hyperthyroidism is the result of excessive production and secretion of thyroid hormone. While less common than hypothyroidism with lithium use, it can be seen in patients on lithium therapy, usually presenting as thyrotoxicosis early in the course of treatment. The majority of these patients will go on to develop hypothyroidism.

Incidence/Prevalence of Disorder

The prevalence of hyperthyroidism ranges from 0.2% to 1.3% in iodine-sufficient parts of the world. European studies estimate a mean prevalence rate of 0.75% for males and females combined and an incidence rate of 51 cases per 100,000 per year [41].

Typical Findings in the HPI

In addition to anorexia, patients will complain of tachycardia, tremor, anxiety, irritability, emotional lability, panic attacks, heat intolerance, increased or decreased appetite, diarrhea, weight loss, and menstrual dysfunction. In the case of Graves' ophthalmopathy, the patient may have blurring of vision, photophobia, increased lacrimation, double vision, and deep orbital pressure. Elderly patients may develop apathetic hyperthyroidism, where they will present with lethargy, weight loss, tachycardia, brittle nails, and fine skin. The patients maintain insight about weight loss and do not intentionally restrict calorie intake.

Typical Physical Exam Findings

Physical examination may show tachycardia, tremor, hyperreflexia, or pretibial myxedema. In the case of Graves' disease, exophthalmos, lid retraction, and lid lag may be present. Periosteal new bone formation (Graves' acropachy) may lead to clubbing of fingers.

Typical Laboratory/Radiological Findings

Laboratory testing will show elevated T4 (free thyroxine), elevated T3 (free triiodothyronine), and low TSH (except in rare cases of TSH hypersecretion from a pituitary adenoma).

Radiography can be used to differentiate the cause of hyperthyroidism. An overactive thyroid gland will have increased uptake of radioactive iodine, whereas a normal thyroid (in cases of iatrogenic or factitious thyroid ingestion or subacute thyroiditis) will have normal or decreased uptake.

Rating Scales

TSH alone has a sensitivity of 98% and specificity of 92% for the diagnosis of hyperthyroidism however a low positive predictive value of 12%. Use of thyroxine (T4) alone with TSH increased the PPV to 67% (study in the elderly population). It is recommended to do multiple tests over a 3- to 6-month interval to confirm or rule out abnormal findings [42].

Pitfalls/Differential Diagnoses

- Panic disorder
- Anxiety disorder

Pheochromocytoma

Incidence/Prevalence of Disorder

The incidence of pheochromocytoma is approximately 0.8 in 100,000 people in a year. Males and females have an equal incidence. As many as 0.1–1.0% of patients with hypertension may have pheochromocytoma [43].

Typical Findings in the HPI

Patients typically present with episodic symptoms of pressure, pain, pallor, palpitations, and perspiration (commonly remembered as the "5 Ps"). Their hypertension is treatment-resistant.

Typical Physical Exam Findings

Patients have an elevated diastolic blood pressure. If the pheochromocytoma is associated with another underlying condition such as NF1, they may have skin hyperpigmentation presenting in cafe-au-lait spots.

Typical Laboratory/Radiological Findings

Plasma-free metanephrine levels are increased. Twenty-four hour urine collection shows increased vanillyl mandelic acid and increased metanephrines. Imaging can show an adrenal mass on CT or MRI. MIBG scanning can further detect adrenal involvement. Histology will display chromaffin cells with enlarged dysmorphic nuclei.

Rating Scales

Best initial test is to test free metanephrine levels in plasma. This is confirmed by 24-h urine collection (sensitivity 99%, specificity 89%) [44].

Pitfalls/Differential Diagnoses

- Functional adrenal tumors
- Hyperthyroidism
- Carcinoid tumors
- Generalized anxiety disorder
- Panic disorder
- Obstructive sleep apnea

Akathisia

Akathisia is a side effect most often associated with antipsychotic treatment, although it can also be seen with other medications such as serotonergic agents (e.g., SSRIs, SNRIs, TCAs, MAOIs), calcium channel blockers, stimulants, and anti-nausea medications (promethazine). It can be described as restlessness that takes the form of fidgeting movements of the legs, rocking, pacing, and an inability to sit or stand still. Oftentimes, the patient is consequently unable to sleep. If it persists it can cause significant dysphoria and even suicidal ideation. Anxiety is often present, although this is not always the case. Treatments for akathisia range from common agents such as beta-adrenergic blockers or benzodiazepines to mindfulness techniques and even hypnosis, to help the patient get to sleep. Of course, it is also important to consider tapering the offending medication or switching to a different agent.

References

1. Kinsley D. Tantric visions of the divine feminine: the ten Mahavidyas. Berkeley: University of California Press; 1997.
2. Jagadiswarananda S. Devi Mahatmyam. Ramakrishna Math; 1953.
3. Miller A. The drama of the gifted child. New York: Basic Books; 1986.
4. Jung CG. In: Read H, et al., editors. The theory of psychoanalysis (Hull RFC, Trans.). Princeton University Press. (Original work published 1955); 1967. https://doi.org/10.1515/9781400850938.83.
5. Lewis CS. The screwtape letters. William Collins; 2012.
6. Krishnamurti Foundation Trust. Thought is fear's origin. 2020. www.youtube.com/watch?v=5ucCdfMzXwU.
7. Yalom ID. Existential psychotherapy. Basic Books; 1980.
8. Scott BG, Weems CF. Natural disasters and existential concerns: a test of Tillich's theory of existential anxiety. J Humanist Psychol. 2013;53(1):114–28.
9. American Psychiatric Association. Diagnostic and statistical manual of mental disorders. 5th ed., text rev. Washington, DC: American Psychiatric Association; 2022. https://doi.org/10.1176/appi.books.9780890425596.
10. American Psychiatric Association. Anxiety. American Psychological Association; 2022. www.apa.org/topics/anxiety
11. Anxiety. Merriam-Webster.com Dictionary. Merriam-Webster. https://www.merriam-webster.com/dictionary/anxiety. Accessed 16 Mar 2021.
12. Harvard Medical School, 2007. National Comorbidity Survey (NCS). Data Table 2: 12-month prevalence DSM-IV/WMH-CIDI disorders by sex and cohort. 2017. https://www.hcp.med.harvard.edu/ncs/index.php.
13. Martin EI, Ressler KJ, Binder E, Nemeroff CB. The neurobiology of anxiety disorders: brain imaging, genetics, and psychoneuroendocrinology. Psychiatr Clin North Am. 2009;32(3):549–75. https://doi.org/10.1016/j.psc.2009.05.004.
14. Seligman ME. Learned helplessness. Annu Rev Med. 1972;23(1):407–12. https://doi.org/10.1146/annurev.me.23.020172.002203.
15. Danchin A, Binder PM, Noria S. Antifragility and tinkering in biology (and in business) flexibility provides an efficient epigenetic way to manage risk. Genes. 2011;2(4):998–1016. https://doi.org/10.3390/genes2040998.
16. Lowe SR, Manove EE, Rhodes JE. Posttraumatic stress and posttraumatic growth among low-income mothers who survived Hurricane Katrina. J Consult Clin Psychol. 2013;81(5):877–89. https://doi.org/10.1037/a0033252d.
17. Tominaga Y, Goto T, Shelby J, Oshio A, Nishi D, Takahashi S. Secondary trauma and posttraumatic growth among mental health clinicians involved in disaster relief activities following the 2011 Tohoku earthquake and tsunami in Japan. Couns Psychol Q. 2020;33(4):427–47. https://doi.org/10.1080/09515070.2019.1639493.
18. Definitions of the RDoC domains and constructs. National Institute of Mental Health, U.S. Department of Health and Human Services. www.nimh.nih.gov/research/research-funded-by-nimh/rdoc/definitions-of-the-rdoc-domains-and-constructs.shtml.
19. Andrew G, Cohen A, Salgaonkar S, et al. The explanatory models of depression and anxiety in primary care: a qualitative study from India. BMC Res Notes. 2012;5:499. https://doi.org/10.1186/1756-0500-5-499.

20. Liebowitz MR, Salmán E, Jusino CM, Garfinkel R, Street L, Cárdenas DL, Silvestre J, Fyer AJ, Carrasco JL, Davies S. Ataque de nervios and panic disorder. Am J Psychiatry. 1994;151(6):871–5. https://doi.org/10.1176/ajp.151.6.871.
21. Beesdo K, Pine DS, Lieb R, Wittchen HU. Incidence and risk patterns of anxiety and depressive disorders and categorization of generalized anxiety disorder. Arch Gen Psychiatry. 2010;67(1):47–57. https://doi.org/10.1001/archgenpsychiatry.2009.177.
22. Löwe B, Decker O, Müller S, Brähler E, Schellberg D, Herzog W, Herzberg P. Validation and standardization of the generalized anxiety disorder screener (GAD-7) in the general population. Med Care. 2008;46(3):266–74. https://doi.org/10.1097/MLR.0b013e318160d093.
23. Shear MK, Rucci P, Williams J, Frank E, Grochocinski V, Vander Bilt J, Houck P, Wang T. Reliability and validity of the Panic Disorder Severity Scale: replication and extension. J Psychiatr Res. 2001;35(5):293–6. https://doi.org/10.1016/s0022-3956(01)00028-0.
24. Harvard Medical School, 2007. National Comorbidity Survey (NCS). 2017. https://www.hcp.med.harvard.edu/ncs/index.php.
25. Ovanessian MM, Fairbrother N, Vorstenbosch V, McCabe RE, Rowa K, Antony MM. Psychometric properties and clinical utility of the specific phobia questionnaire in an anxiety disorders sample. J Psychopathol Behav Assess. 2018;41(1):36–52. https://doi.org/10.1007/s10862-018-9687-1.
26. McCraw KS, Valentiner DP. The Circumscribed Fear Measure: development and initial validation of a trans-stimulus phobia measure. Psychol Assess. 2015;27(2):403–14. https://doi.org/10.1037/pas0000046.
27. Seeley-Wait E, Abbott MJ, Rapee RM. Psychometric properties of the mini-social phobia inventory. Prim Care Companion J Clin Psychiatry. 2009;11(5):231–6. https://doi.org/10.4088/PCC.07m00576.
28. Kunimatsu A, Yasaka K, Akai H, Kunimatsu N, Abe O. MRI findings in posttraumatic stress disorder. J Magn Reson Imaging. 2020;52(2):380–96.
29. Geier TJ, Hunt JC, Nelson LD, Brasel KJ, deRoon-Cassini TA. Detecting PTSD in a traumatically injured population: the diagnostic utility of the PTSD Checklist for DSM-5. Depress Anxiety. 2019;36(2):170–8. https://doi.org/10.1002/da.22873.
30. Prins A, Bovin MJ, Smolenski DJ, Marx BP, Kimerling R, Jenkins-Guarnieri MA, Kaloupek DG, Schnurr PP, Kaiser AP, Leyva YE, Tiet QQ. The primary care PTSD screen for DSM-5 (PC-PTSD-5): development and evaluation within a veteran primary care sample. J Gen Intern Med. 2016;31(10):1206–11. https://doi.org/10.1007/s11606-016-3703-5.
31. Ruscio AM, Stein DJ, Chiu WT, Kessler RC. The epidemiology of obsessive-compulsive disorder in the National Comorbidity Survey Replication. Mol Psychiatry. 2010;15(1):53–63. https://doi.org/10.1038/mp.2008.94.
32. Cortico-striatal-thalamic loop circuits of the salience network: a central pathway in psychiatric disease and treatment. Front Syst Neurosci. 10. https://doi.org/10.3389/fnsys.2016.00104.
33. Castro-Rodrigues P, Camacho M, Almeida S, Marinho M, Soares C, Barahona-Corrêa J, Oliveira-Maia A. Criterion validity of the Yale-Brown Obsessive-Compulsive Scale second edition for diagnosis of obsessive-compulsive disorder in adults. Front Psychiatry. 2018;9 https://doi.org/10.3389/fpsyt.2018.00431.
34. SAMHSA. 2019 National Survey on Drug Use and Health. 2019. https://www.samhsa.gov/data/sites/default/files/reports/rpt29393/2019NSDUHFFRPDFWHTML/2019NSDUHFFR090120.htm#sud11.
35. Saunders JB, Aasland OG, Babor TF, de la Fuente JR, Grant M. Development of the Alcohol Use Disorders Identification Test (AUDIT). WHO Collaborative Project on early detection of persons with harmful alcohol consumption—II. Addiction. 1993;88(6):791–804. https://doi.org/10.1111/j.1360-0443.1993.tb02093.x.
36. Zanarini M, Vujanovic A, Parachini E, Boulanger J, Frankenburg F, Hennen J. A screening measure for BPD: the McLean Screening Instrument for Borderline Personality Disorder (MSI-BPD). J Personal Disord. 2003;17(6):568–73. https://doi.org/10.1521/pedi.17.6.568.25355.
37. Virani SS, Alonso A, Aparicio HJ, Benjamin EJ, Bittencourt MS, Callaway CW, et al. Heart disease and stroke statistics—2021 update: a report from the American Heart Association. Circulation. 2021;143:e254–743.

38. Chang CC, Ip MP, Hsu RM, Vrobel T. Evaluation of a proposed panel of cardiac markers for the diagnosis of acute myocardial infarction in patients with atraumatic chest pain. Arch Pathol Lab Med. 1998;122(4):320–4.
39. Silverstein MD, Heit JA, Mohr DN, Petterson TM, O'Fallon WM, Melton LJ III. Trends in the incidence of deep vein thrombosis and pulmonary embolism: a 25-year population-based study. Arch Intern Med. 1998;158(6):585–93. https://doi.org/10.1001/archinte.158.6.585.
40. French A. Clinical characteristics of patients with acute pulmonary embolism: data from PIOPED II. J Emerg Med. 2008;34(4):491. https://doi.org/10.1016/j.jemermed.2008.02.034.
41. Taylor PN, Albrecht D, Scholz A, Gutierrez-Buey G, Lazarus JH, Dayan CM, Okosieme OE. Global epidemiology of hyperthyroidism and hypothyroidism. Nat Rev Endocrinol. 2018;14(5):301–16. https://doi.org/10.1038/nrendo.2018.18.
42. Sawin CT. Low serum thyrotropin (thyroid-stimulating hormone) in older persons without hyperthyroidism. Arch Intern Med. 1991;151(1):165. https://doi.org/10.1001/archinte.1991.00400010159025.
43. https://www.cancer.gov/types/pheochromocytoma/hp/pheochromocytoma-treatment-pdq#_25_toc.
44. Lenders JW, Pacak K, Walther MM, Linehan WM, Mannelli M, Friberg P, Keiser HR, Goldstein DS, Eisenhofer G. Biochemical diagnosis of pheochromocytoma: which test is best? JAMA. 2002;287(11):1427–34. https://doi.org/10.1001/jama.287.11.1427.

Insomnia

4

Lan-Anh T. Tran, Kyle J. Gray, Shram D. Shukla, Michael J. Goldstein, and Vincent F. Capaldi II

Introduction

History of Insomnia

Sleep disorders first appeared in medical literature as early as 400 BCE in the writings of Hippocrates and are noted in literary classics including Shakespeare's *Macbeth* (1603) and Cervantes's *The Ingenious Hidalgo Don Quixote of La Mancha* (1605). It was not until 1869 when insomnia was first described as "persistent wakefulness" when Hammond published *Sleep and Its Derangements* [1]. In 1934, W.R. Harrison described sleep onset and sleep maintenance insomnia in a series of papers.

In 1981, Thomas Roth and colleagues reported on multiple diseases associated with insomnia, which introduced the term "comorbid insomnia" to the literature on

L.-A. T. Tran (✉)
Mental Health, Naval Hospital Jacksonville, Jacksonville, FL, USA
e-mail: Lananh.t.tran3.mil@health.mil

K. J. Gray
Marine Corps Medical Home New River, United States Navy, Jacksonville, NC, USA
e-mail: Kyle.j.gray6.mil@health.mil

S. D. Shukla
3rd Marine Division, United States Navy, Okinawa, Japan
e-mail: Shram.d.shukla.mil@health.mil

M. J. Goldstein
School of Medicine, Uniformed Services University of the Health Sciences, Bethesda, MD, USA
e-mail: Michael.j.goldstein.mil@health.mil

V. F. Capaldi II
Department of Psychiatry, School of Medicine, Uniformed Services University of the Health Sciences, Bethesda, MD, USA
e-mail: Vincent.f.capaldi.mil@health.mil

E. G. Meyer et al. (eds.), *The Medical Evaluation of Psychiatric Symptoms*,
https://doi.org/10.1007/978-3-031-14372-4_4

the subject [2]. One year later, the National Institutes of Health (NIH) held the first consensus symposium conference on insomnia, which acknowledged insomnia's heterogeneous origin and the importance of systematic diagnostic inquiry to evaluate for primary medical, psychiatric, and other causes of insomnia. The terms "transient insomnia," "short-term insomnia," and "long-term insomnia" were introduced. "Transient insomnia" was considered for people who are otherwise normal sleepers but experience acute stress for several days which impacts their sleep. "Short-term insomnia" was associated with situational stress and may last up to 3 weeks. "Long-term insomnia" was considered secondary to another medical or psychiatric condition and an extensive differential diagnostic workup prior to treatment was recommended [3].

In 2005, the NIH held a second consensus conference on management of insomnia. During this conference, insomnia was further defined as "disturbed sleep in the presence of adequate opportunity to sleep" [4]. The disturbances may have one or more features including difficulty initiating sleep, difficulty maintaining sleep, or waking up too early. The criterion of nonrestorative or poor-quality sleep was dropped from the definition. Insomnia was further delineated into acute and chronic insomnia where chronic insomnia was considered when symptoms persist for 30 days or more. Insomnia was classified based on its specific symptom (i.e., sleep onset or sleep maintenance) or the duration of the disorder [4]. With the International Classification of Sleep Disorders—Third Edition (ICSD-3), the classification of primary and secondary insomnia was substituted for a more globally descriptive term of "comorbid insomnia" [5].

Today, there are still many definitions and ways to diagnose insomnia as a condition which depend upon various nosological systems and their approach to classifying insomnia. These classification systems include the International Classification of Diseases (ICD), the Diagnostic and Statistical Manual of Mental Disorders Text Revision (DSM-5-TR) by the American Psychiatric Association, the International Classification of Sleep Disorders (ICSD), and the Research Diagnostic Criteria (RDC). The lack of agreement on the definition and classification of insomnia is demonstrative of the complex, yet nonspecific nature of the chief complaint of "insomnia."

Defining Insomnia

We define insomnia as difficulty initiating sleep, difficulty in maintaining sleep, and/or early morning awakening, resulting in a sleep deficiency despite adequate opportunity for sleep and no change in the patient's baseline "need for sleep." Insomnia, therefore, is a *symptom*, reported in a patient's history, and there is no standard objective measure of insomnia through polysomnography (PSG) or other means. The routine use of PSG *alone* to evaluate insomnia is *not* recommended, but it is important to note that a patient's sleep report and objective data may not always agree, and the misperception of sleep quality or quantity may be an issue [6]. This chapter also endeavors to isolate sleep disruption as the primary symptom of focus, while definitions of insomnia as a disorder often describe secondary effects and impact on daytime functioning. Given the complexity of insomnia as a symptom, we discuss these secondary effects to some degree, but mainly to clarify the primary issue of sleep disturbance.

We consider disturbed sleep for >30 min to be a helpful rule of thumb to mark when insomnia is occurring. That is, it takes longer than 30 min to fall asleep; or the patient is awake for longer than 30 min after sleep has been initiated; or the patient awakens 30 min or more before the desired time at least three times per week for at least 3 months or more. This definition is most like the ICSD-3 definition of chronic insomnia as most patients presenting to our psychiatric offices have long-standing symptoms outside of the window of acute insomnia. Notably, we have used the word "or" in describing these sleep difficulties, but often troubles with falling and staying asleep occur in the same patient—though, as we will describe, understanding the time course of sleep disruptions is important to determining underlying pathophysiology.

Models of Insomnia

No single model of insomnia explains all forms of insomnia, as much of the etiology and pathophysiology of insomnia remain unknown. In efforts to better understand insomnia, we begin to conceptualize insomnia by both physiological and psychological models.

The predominant psychological model of insomnia is the Spielman 3-P Model of Insomnia. Under the Spielman Model, while insomnia may present acutely, *Predisposing, Precipitating, and Perpetuating* factors contribute to acute sleep loss becoming a chronic and self-perpetuating problem [7]. The 3-P model was the first to gain widespread acceptance and explains insomnia through two lenses: factors that lead to insomnia *acutely* (predisposing and precipitating factors) and those that lead to *chronic* insomnia (perpetuating factors). Predisposing factors cover the whole biopsychosocial spectrum and include increased basal metabolic rate, neurotransmitter responsiveness, worry or rumination, and sleep partner disturbances [8]. The presence of one or more of these factors creates a state in which one is vulnerable to sleep disturbance in the setting of a precipitating event, which involves an acute stressor such as medical or psychiatric illness. This acute insomnia then leads to adaptive and maladaptive behaviors, which perpetuate sleep disturbance through conditioned arousal [8, 9].

From a physiological standpoint, neurobiological changes that lead to hyperarousal and circadian dysregulation may contribute to the predisposition, precipitation, and/or perpetuation of insomnia in susceptible patients [10]. In the Two-Process Model of sleep, the interaction of two distinct drivers of sleep and wakefulness are described. The two processes are known as homeostatic sleep debt (process S) and the circadian pacemaker (process C). In brief, sleep debt builds throughout the day, creating a "sleep pressure." As it reaches the upper threshold of process C (Fig. 4.1), sleep is initiated via ventrolateral preoptic nucleus (VLPO) and median preoptic nucleus (MnPO) inhibition of the ascending reticular activating system (ARAS). As

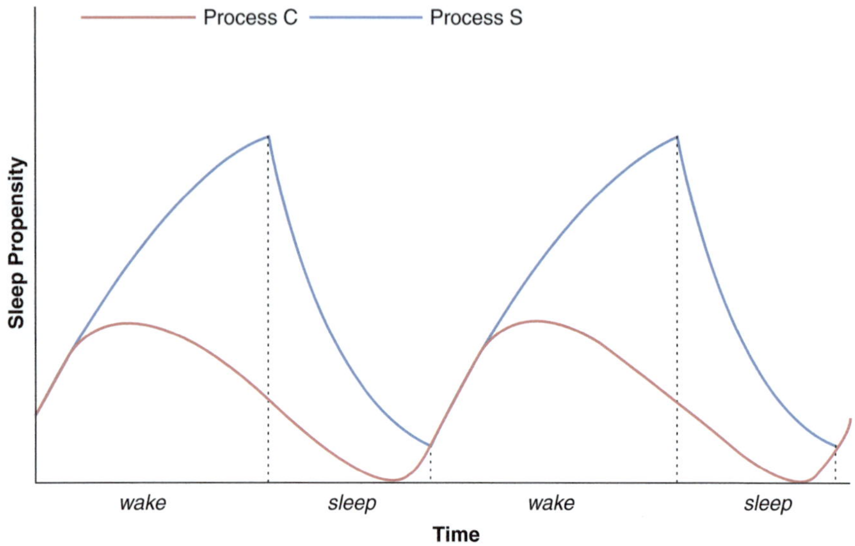

Fig. 4.1 Two-process model of sleep. Process S (blue line) is the homeostatic sleep drive. Process C (red line) is the circadian pacemaker

sleep progresses, process S approaches the lower threshold of process C, at which point the wake drive takes over and sleep is terminated [11, 12]. The neurocognitive model hypothesizes acute and chronic changes in the ARAS and VLPO perpetuate sleep disturbances, leading to the manifestation of chronic insomnia [10]. Clinically, we find it helpful to educate the patient on the two basic sleep drives and consider how either (or both) may be dysregulated in their case. For example, discussing how caffeine affects their homeostatic sleep drive applies to process S while continuous shift work affects their circadian rhythm in process C.

Initial Sleep Evaluation and Differentiating Insomnia from Other Symptoms

Given the complex nature of insomnia as a symptom, it can easily be associated with and confused with other symptoms. Understanding that sleep is integral to overall health and that insomnia appears to be associated with a general predisposition for hyperarousal, there is often a bidirectional relationship between sleep difficulties and associated symptoms. Common associated symptoms include fatigue, daytime sleepiness, attention deficits, mood disturbances, and decreased motivation. Importantly, each of these associated symptoms can have other causes, so differentiating cause and effect through careful history taking, proper screening, and complete evaluation is paramount. As this can be a daunting task, we created an algorithmic approach (see section "Insomnia Assessment Decision Tree" at the end of this chapter) as a framework. As with any medical algorithm, it does not replace sound clinical judgment.

First, we differentiate insomnia from a lack of sleep *opportunity*. Insomnia is *poor sleep despite adequate opportunity*; thus, it is important to understand a person's bedtime routine to determine whether they are allowing for sufficient sleep opportunity. There are multiple sleep diaries available at no cost on the Internet, but essential elements include time in bed; time to fall asleep; number of awakenings and duration; and ultimate wake-up time. We prefer the American Academy of Sleep Medicine (AASM) version, which yields a quick visual representation of a person's sleep for a 2-week period (http://yoursleep.aasmnet.org/pdf/sleepdiary.pdf).

In addition to sleep diaries, adequate opportunity for sleep can be measured with actigraphy, which involves having a patient wear a wristwatch-like device that typically contains accelerometers, a clock, internal memory, and a photo sensor. A patient's sleep data can be transferred to a computer for analysis which typically reveals a patient's sleep-wake cycle which can be interpreted in conjunction with sleep diary data [2]. If a clinical actigraph is not available, the use of a consumer-grade actigraph found in most smartwatches can approximate accurate information. All actigraphs underestimate sleep onset latency (SOL); however, these devices are useful in tracking treatment success over time.

Next, determine the effect of consistently disrupted sleep on the patient's feeling of restfulness. If the patient consistently sleeps less than 7 h but feels adequately rested, they may simply be a "short sleeper," that is, they fall on the "left side" of the bell curve of the population in terms of sleep need. Indeed, the National Sleep Foundation revised its sleep time duration recommendations in 2015 to reflect a widening of the range of possible "appropriate" sleep time durations [13].

Conversely, if a patient is consistently getting the median recommended 7–9 h (for adults), but is still tired, they may be "long sleepers" on the "right side" of the bell curve. In these cases, one should again attempt to determine if there is an appropriate sleep opportunity for the increased need or if insomnia is present. Finally, if a patient experiences a significant change from their baseline sleep need, such that there is a decreased need for sleep and feeling more energized, one strongly considers a diagnosis of a manic or hypomanic episode.

DSM vs. RDoC Conceptualization

Changes in sleep are ubiquitous in almost every diagnostic category in the DSM-5-TR. In addition to sleep disturbances subsumed within other psychiatric disorders, there is an additional diagnostic section referenced as "sleep-wake disorders," pertaining to sleep disorders that are distinct from other psychiatric conditions. Of the sleep disorders referenced in this DSM-5-TR section, insomnia disorder is the most common. Insomnia disorder is characterized by dissatisfaction with sleep quantity or quality. It is associated with difficulty initiating sleep, maintaining sleep which is characterized by frequent awakenings or problems returning to sleep after awakenings, and early morning awakening with an inability to return to sleep. These symptoms cause clinically significant distress or functional impairment. The sleep difficulties occur at least three nights per week and are present for at least 3 months despite adequate opportunity for sleep. These symptoms are not better explained by and do not occur exclusively during the course of another sleep-wake disorder, substance use, or coexisting medical or psychiatric condition [14].

In comparison, the National Institute of Mental Health (NIMH) established the Research Domain Criteria (RDoC) to address the limitations of the current categorical nosology within the DSM. Sleep-wakefulness is primarily classified as a construct within the "arousal and regulatory systems" domain. The RDoC describes sleep-wakefulness as "endogenous, recurring, behavioral states that reflect coordinated changes in the dynamic functional organization of the brain and that optimize physiology, behavior, and health." Sleep is reversible and has a complex architecture with predictable cycling of non-rapid eye movement (NREM) and rapid eye movement (REM) states. The intensity and duration are affected by homeostatic regulation and experiences during wakefulness, which are evident at the cellular, circuit, and system levels. Sleep has restorative and transformative effects that optimize neurobehavioral functions during wakefulness [15]. However, even within the RDoC system, sleep is inconsistently conceptualized [16].

Cultural Considerations for "Insomnia"

Most people experience insomnia as a temporary condition exacerbated by an acute stressor which becomes chronic for about 10% of the population. Insomnia has a biological basis as discussed in the above sections with the Two-Process Model of Sleep, but insomnia is also shaped by the prevailing cultural, historical, and societal influences. In the Western world, different perspectives of insomnia have existed during the preindustrial period, industrial period, postindustrial period, and the modern world.

In the preindustrial period, people lived ritualized lives to take advantage of the available natural light and higher daytime temperatures which translated into a regimented day and night routine. Routine produced familiar environmental and cultural cues that led to conditioned responses of sleep. In addition, during this period, sleep was celebrated as a time for restoration of the body and spirit after a long day of work. During the industrial period, society romanticized insomnia and coined the term "involuntary sleeplessness." Involuntary sleeplessness was valued and associated with imagination, intellectual creativity, and a period of enlightenment that few individuals experienced while the rest of the world slept. Conversely, in the postindustrial period, views of insomnia shifted to a negative connotation. It was identified as a product of nervous stimulation. An article in *The Lancet* by Morison identified a pathological archetype of the "neurotic insomniac" [17].

Today, society continues to be more connected through technological advances leading to a 24-h working civilization. Taking us further away from the preindustrial period's routine lifestyle, environmental cues for restful sleep are being removed. In addition, current society views sleep in a negative context, using phrases such as "wake-up call" for Americans who were "lulled to sleep by misguided conviction" during the bombing of the Twin Towers [18]. Our technologically connected world and negative undertones regarding sleep perpetuate an unnatural degree of wakefulness and help explain the increase in prevalence of insomnia. Paying attention to the historical and cultural contexts may help clue physicians into how sleep and sleeplessness are experienced by patients.

Differential Diagnosis for Insomnia

When evaluating patients with insomnia, it is important to consider medical, psychiatric, substance use, or medication causes. The following sections review these conditions in each of these categories, organizing them by if they typically present with disruptions in the early, middle, or late phases of sleep. Table 4.1 comprises each of these diagnostic considerations and provides a quick reference for the busy clinician.

Table 4.1 Diagnostic considerations for Early, Middle, and Late Insomnia

Insomnia subtype	Early	Middle	Late
Psychiatric	Generalized anxiety disorder Schizophrenia and other psychotic disorders Bipolar disorder TBI Delirium Major neurocognitive disorder	Posttraumatic stress disorder Acute stress disorder Delirium	Major depressive disorder Delirium
Substance use	Alcohol withdrawal Caffeine intoxication Cannabis intoxication Cannabis withdrawal Stimulant intoxication Stimulant withdrawal	Alcohol[a] intoxication	See reminder below[a]
Medications	SSRI, SNRI, MAOI, TCA, DNRI Stimulants Decongestants and antihistamines Opioid analgesics Alpha adrenergic agonists and antagonists Antihypertensive agents Beta adrenergic antagonists Calcium channel blockers Diuretics Lipid-lowering agents Pulmonary medications (e.g., beta adrenergic agonists, theophylline) Corticosteroids Thyroid hormone Cholinesterase inhibitors		
Systemic	Restless leg syndrome Delayed sleep-wake phase disorder Chronic obstructive pulmonary disease	Obstructive sleep apnea Benign prostatic hyperplasia/ lower urinary tract symptoms Overactive bladder Gastroesophageal reflux disease Chronic pain	Advanced sleep-wake phase disorder

[a] Reminder: The Early, Middle, and Late categories are meant as a general rule and these disorders often cause insomnia in multiple phases of sleep. The substance use syndromes and medications listed in early insomnia can alter middle and late phases of sleep as well and should be considered for any insomnia presentation

SSRI selective serotonin reuptake inhibitor; *SNRI* serotonin and norepinephrine reuptake inhibitor; *MAOI* monoamine oxidase inhibitors; *DNRI* norepinephrine and dopamine reuptake inhibitor

Psychiatric Differential Diagnosis for Subtypes of Insomnia

The psychiatric differential for each type of insomnia could include a remarkable number of diagnoses from the DSM. Here, we limit our discussion to the most common and clinically relevant ones. It is worth emphasizing that there may be significant overlap across insomnia types, and furthermore comorbidities among both psychiatric and other systemic medical illnesses can complicate the picture. Despite this muddying of boundaries, we find it clinically useful to lump diagnoses into the category where the problems *predominantly* exist or first developed. These categories include early insomnia (sleep-onset insomnia), middle insomnia (mid-sleep awakenings with difficulty returning to sleep), and late insomnia (early morning awakenings).

The DSM-5-TR diagnosis of insomnia disorder specifically invites the physician to consider if the patient is suffering from early, middle, or late insomnia. The diagnosis should be applied when the insomnia is not better explained and does not occur exclusively during another sleep-wake disorder, is not attributable to the physiological effects of a psychoactive substance, and coexisting mental disorders and medical conditions do not adequately explain the predominant complaint of insomnia [14]. However, if other diagnoses are thoroughly explored and do not apply, this diagnosis can help bring clinical attention to the problem.

Early Insomnia Psychiatric Differential

Generalized Anxiety Disorder (GAD)

Epidemiology

One to four percent annual incidence reported [19]. In the United States, the 12-month prevalence of GAD is 2.9% in adults [20]. There is a reported lifetime prevalence of 4–7% [21]. There is a 3% estimated lifetime prevalence in children and 10.8% in adolescents [19].

Incidence of Generalized Anxiety Disorder Presenting as Insomnia

Sleep disturbances have been reported in up to 75% of patients with GAD. The symptom is heterogeneous in nature and includes difficulty initiating sleep (36.3%), difficulty maintaining sleep (33%), or restless sleep. The severity of GAD was found to be the strongest independent factor related to insomnia [22].

Typical Findings of the HPI

Excessive anxiety and worry occurring more days than not for at least 6 months with difficulty controlling worries. Associated symptoms include restlessness, easily fatigued, difficulty concentrating, irritability, muscle tension, and sleep disturbances (difficulty falling or staying asleep, or restless, unsatisfying sleep). Other possible symptoms include gastrointestinal discomfort, headaches, dizziness, and lightheadedness. This presentation is also associated with significant distress and impairment in psychosocial function.

Typical Findings on Physical Exam

Physical exam:

- Cardiac: tachycardia, chest pain [21]
- Musculoskeletal: muscle tension, trembling [23]
- Dermatologic: diaphoresis [23]

Typical Laboratory/Radiological Findings

None. Ensure that symptoms are not attributable to the physiological effects of a substance or another medical condition.

Substance-Induced Sleep Disorder

Substance intoxication or withdrawal can significantly impact different stages of sleep. According to the DSM-5-TR, sleep is affected at the onset of intoxication and onset of withdrawal for the substances below (Table 4.2). For the purposes of this section, we will focus on substance intoxication and withdrawal that primarily affect SOL.

Alcohol Withdrawal

Epidemiology

Approximately 50% of middle-class, highly functional individuals with alcohol use disorder (AUD) have experienced a full alcohol withdrawal syndrome. Individuals with AUD who are hospitalized or homeless experience rates of alcohol withdrawal that may exceed 80% [24].

Table 4.2 Substances that impact sleep at the onset of intoxication and at the onset of withdrawal, collated from DSM-5-TR [24]

Substances	Onset of intoxication	Onset of withdrawal
Alcohol	X	X
Caffeine	X	X
Cannabis	X	X
Hallucinogens		
Phencyclidine		
Other hallucinogens		
Inhalants		
Opioids	X	X
Sedatives, hypnotics, or anxiolytics	X	X
Stimulants (amphetamine-type substances, cocaine, and other unspecified stimulants)	X	X
Tobacco		X
Other (or unknown)	X	X

Incidence of Alcohol Withdrawal Presenting as Insomnia

Symptoms occur in four clinical stages with insomnia presenting as a minor withdrawal symptom (stage 1) which is typically seen in the first 6–12 h after discontinuing alcohol [25]. Insomnia was reported by 36–91% of patients who admitted alcohol dependence and may persist up to 2 years after alcohol withdrawal [26]. Sleep alterations with alcohol withdrawal include increased SOL, decreased total sleep time, increased REM, decreased sleep efficiency, decreased REM latency, increased wake after sleep onset, and decreased slow wave sleep [27].

Typical Findings of the HPI

Cessation or reduction in alcohol use that has been heavy and prolonged with associated symptoms to include autonomic hyperactivity (sweating and tachycardia); hand tremor; insomnia; nausea or vomiting; transient visual, tactile, or auditory hallucinations or illusions; psychomotor agitation, anxiety, or generalized tonic-clonic seizures. These symptoms cause significant distress or impairment in social, occupational, or other important areas of functioning and are not attributable to another medical or psychiatric condition.

Typical Findings on Physical Exam

Physical exam:

- General: hypertension, tachycardia, hyperthermia [25]
- Neurologic: dilated pupils, tremors [25]
- Dermatologic: diaphoresis [25]

Typical Laboratory/Radiological Findings [28]

- Blood alcohol level: elevated
- Complete blood count: anemia, megaloblastic anemia, thrombocytopenia
- Comprehensive metabolic panel: metabolic acidosis, hypocalcemia, hypoglycemia
- Magnesium: hypomagnesemia
- Creatine kinase and cardiac troponin: elevation from demand ischemia secondary to hypertension from alcohol withdrawal
- Liver-associated enzymes: transaminitis
- Amylase and lipase: elevation
- Urinalysis: ketonuria
- Urine or serum drug screen: coingestion of other drugs
- Prothrombin time: increased demonstrating coagulopathy

Caffeine Intoxication

Epidemiology

Approximately 7% of the United States population may experience five or more symptoms along with functional impairment consistent with a diagnosis of caffeine intoxication [29].

Incidence of Caffeine Intoxication Presenting as Insomnia

There is an unknown incidence of caffeine intoxication presenting as insomnia. Sleep alterations include decreased REM, increased REM latency, decreased slow wave sleep, decreased total sleep time, and increased SOL [27, 29].

Typical Findings of the HPI

Recent consumption of caffeine in excess (>250 mg) with five or more associated symptoms including restlessness, nervousness, excitement, insomnia, flushed face, diuresis, GI disturbances, muscle twitching, rambling flow of thought/speech, tachycardia or arrhythmia, periods of inexhaustibility, and psychomotor agitation. Symptoms cause impairment in social, occupation, or other important areas of function and are not attributable to another medical or psychiatric condition.

Typical Findings on Physical Exam

Physical exam:

- General: restlessness, psychomotor agitation
- Cardiac: tachycardia, arrhythmia
- Musculoskeletal: muscle twitching

Typical Laboratory/Radiological Findings

None.

Cannabis Intoxication

Epidemiology

There is a 21–43% reported lifetime prevalence of cannabis use in the United States [30].

Incidence of Cannabis Intoxication Presenting as Insomnia

There is an unknown incidence of cannabis intoxication presenting as insomnia. Sleep alterations with heavy THC intoxication include increased SOL, decreased REM, and decreased slow wave sleep [27].

Typical Findings of the HPI

Recent use of cannabis is associated with problematic behavioral or psychological changes (e.g., impaired motor coordination, euphoria, anxiety, sensation of slowed time, impaired judgment, social withdrawal) that developed during, or shortly after, cannabis use. Two or more of the following signs or symptoms develop within 2 h of use: conjunctival injection, increased appetite, dry mouth, and tachycardia. Symptoms are not attributable to another medical or psychiatric condition.

Typical Findings on Physical Exam

Physical exam:
- Head, Ears, Eyes, Nose Throat: conjunctival injection
- Cardiac: tachycardia in nonchronic users. Chronic users may have decreased heart rate, lower blood pressure, and postural hypotension [31]
- Psychiatric: anxiety, euphoria, perceptual disturbances

Typical Laboratory/Radiological Findings

Positive urine or serum drug screen for cannabis.

Cannabis Withdrawal

Epidemiology

In frequent cannabis users, the prevalence of cannabis withdrawal syndrome (CWS) was 12.1% [32].

Incidence of Cannabis Withdrawal Presenting as Insomnia

Sleep difficulty was reported in 68.2% of individuals who experience CWS [32]. Sleep alterations include increased SOL, decreased slow wave sleep, increased REM, decreased REM latency, decreased total sleep time, and decreased sleep efficiency [27].

Typical Findings of the HPI

Cessation of cannabis use that has been heavy and prolonged with three or more of the following symptoms developing within 1 week after discontinuation: irritability, anger, or aggression; nervousness or anxiety; sleep difficulty; decreased appetite or weight loss; restlessness; depressed mood; and at least one of the following physical symptoms of discomfort: abdominal pain, shakiness/tremors, sweating, fever, chills, or headache. Symptoms cause impairment in social, occupation, or other important areas of function and are not attributable to another medical or psychiatric condition.

Typical Findings on Physical Exam

Physical exam:
- Psychiatric: anxiety, psychomotor agitation
- Neurologic: tremors
- Dermatologic: diaphoresis

Typical Laboratory/Radiological Findings

Possible positive urine or serum drug screen for cannabis.

Stimulant Intoxication

Epidemiology

There is an unknown incidence and prevalence of stimulant intoxication.

Incidence of Stimulant Intoxication Presenting as Insomnia

There is an unknown incidence of stimulant intoxication presenting as insomnia. Sleep alterations with cocaine intoxication include increased SOL, decreased total sleep time, decreased REM, and increased REM latency [27].

Typical Findings of the HPI

Recent use of amphetamine-type substance, cocaine, or other stimulants that is associated with significant problematic behavioral or psychological changes (e.g., euphoria or affective blunting; changes in sociability; hypervigilance; interpersonal sensitivity; anxiety, tension, or anger; stereotyped behaviors; impaired judgment) that developed during, or shortly after, use of a stimulant. Two or more of the following symptoms develop after use: tachycardia or bradycardia; pupillary dilation; elevated or lowered blood pressure; perspiration or chills; nausea or vomiting; weight loss; psychomotor agitation or retardation; muscular weakness, respiration depression, chest pain, or cardiac arrhythmia; and confusion, seizures, dyskinesias, dystonia, or coma. Symptoms cause impairment in social, occupation, or other important areas of function and are not attributable to another medical or psychiatric condition.

Typical Findings on Physical Exam

Physical exam [33]:

- General: agitation, hyperthermia
- Cardiac: tachycardia, hypertension
- Dermatologic: diaphoresis
- Neurologic: mydriasis, choreoathetoid movements
- Psychiatric: psychosis, delusion, paranoia

Typical Laboratory/Radiological Findings

Positive urine or serum drug screen for stimulants. QRS widening and dysrhythmias on ECG.

Stimulant Withdrawal

Epidemiology

There is an unknown incidence and prevalence of stimulant withdrawal.

Incidence of Stimulant Withdrawal Presenting as Insomnia

There is an unknown incidence of stimulant withdrawal presenting as insomnia. Sleep alterations with subacute cocaine withdrawal include increased SOL, decreased sleep efficiency, decreased total sleep time, decreased REM, and increased slow wave sleep [27].

Typical Findings of the HPI

Cessation or reduction of dose in prolonged use of amphetamine-type substance, cocaine, or other stimulants which is associated with dysphoria and two or more of the following physiological changes, developing within a few hours to several days: fatigue; vivid, unpleasant dreams; insomnia or hypersomnia; increased appetite, and psychomotor retardation or agitation. Symptoms cause impairment in social, occupation, or other important areas of function and are not attributable to another medical or psychiatric condition.

Typical Findings on Physical Exam

Physical exam:

- General: fatigue
- Cardiac: bradycardia
- Psychiatric: dysphoria, anhedonia, psychomotor agitation/retardation

Typical Laboratory/Radiological Findings

Positive urine or serum drug screen for stimulants.

Medication-Induced Sleep Disorder

In addition to substances, the following medications may cause early insomnia [34–36].

- Antidepressants: SSRI, SNRI, MAOI, TCA, DNRI
- Stimulants
- Decongestants and antihistamines
- Opioid analgesics
- Alpha adrenergic receptor agonists and antagonists
- Antihypertensive agents
- Beta adrenergic receptor antagonists
- Calcium channel blockers
- Diuretics
- Lipid-lowering agents
- Pulmonary medications: beta adrenergic agonists, theophylline
- Corticosteroids
- Thyroid hormone
- Cholinesterase inhibitors

Schizophrenia Spectrum and Other Psychotic Disorders

Epidemiology

The global lifetime prevalence for schizophrenia spectrum illness is 0.3–0.7% [37, 38].

Incidence of Schizophrenia Presenting as Insomnia

Insomnia is commonly disrupted in schizophrenia and other psychotic disorders. Most common complaints include an increase in both SOL and time awake after sleep onset, as well as decreased total sleep time and sleep efficiency. Sleep often worsens during relapses of psychosis [39]. Sleep is often also disrupted by daytime sleeping and nighttime activity which demonstrates a sleep-wake cycle reversal [24].

Typical Findings of the HPI

Hallmark features include delusions, hallucinations, disorganized thinking and/or speech, grossly disorganized or abnormal motor behavior, and negative symptoms. Symptoms cause impairment in social, occupational, or other important areas of function and are not attributable to another medical or psychiatric condition.

Typical Findings on Physical Exam

Physical exam:

- Psychiatric: constricted to flat affect, disorganized thought process, delusions, hallucinations, appearance of responding to internal stimuli

Typical Laboratory/Radiological Findings

None. Ensure that symptoms are not attributable to the physiological effects of a substance or another medical condition.

Bipolar Disorder

Epidemiology

The 12-month prevalence estimate in the continental United States was 0.6% for bipolar I disorder as defined in 2007 using DSM-IV criteria [40]. Estimated prevalence for bipolar disorder across 11 countries is 2.4% with 0.6% for bipolar I disorder, 0.4% for bipolar II disorder, and 1.4% for subthreshold bipolar disorder [41, 42].

Incidence of Bipolar Disorder Presenting as Insomnia

In the manic phase, 66–99% of patients experience a reduced need for sleep [43] and increased SOL [44].

Typical Findings of the HPI

A distinct period of abnormally and persistently elevated, expansive, or irritable mood and abnormally and persistently increased activity or energy, lasting at least 1 week and present most of the day, nearly every day (or any duration if hospitalization is necessary). At least three or more of the following symptoms are present to a significant degree and represent a noticeable change from usual behavior: inflated self-esteem or grandiosity; decreased need for sleep (e.g., patient feels rested after only 3 h of sleep); more talkative than usual or pressure to keep talking; flight of ideas or subjective experience that thoughts are racing; distractibility; increase in goal-directed activity or psychomotor agitation; and excessive involvement in activities that have a high potential for painful consequences. Symptoms cause impairment in social, occupation, or other important areas of function and are not attributable to another medical or psychiatric condition. The manic episode may be preceded by or followed by a hypomanic or major depressive episode.

Typical Findings on Physical Exam

Physical exam:

- Psychiatric: restlessness, agitation, rapid speech, grandiosity, distractibility, tangentiality

Typical Laboratory/Radiological Findings

None. Ensure that symptoms are not attributable to the physiological effects of a substance or another medical condition.

Traumatic Brain Injury (TBI)

Epidemiology

In the United States, it is estimated that 1.7 million TBIs occur annually, with males accounting for 59% of cases. Approximately 2% of the United States population lives with TBI-associated disability [24].

Incidence of Traumatic Brain Injury Presenting as Insomnia

About one-third of patients who are in the acute and subacute phases of a TBI report sleep-wake complaints within the first 10 days after injury. The acute phase of TBI increases the risk of delirium for up to 30 days which may further complicate sleep disturbances. Up to 50% of patients report sleep disturbances 6 weeks after the injury. About 40% of patients continue to report sleep disturbances 1 year after their initial injury. Notably, insomnia was more prevalent in mild TBI cases compared to moderate or severe TBI [45].

Typical Findings of the HPI

History of head trauma with at least one of the following: loss of consciousness, posttraumatic amnesia, disorientation and confusion, and/or neurological signs (positive neuroimaging, new onset seizures or marked worsening of existing seizure disorder, visual field deficits, anosmia, and/or hemiparesis). Cognitive presentation may be variable depending on the type of injury. There may be deficits in attention, executive function, learning, memory, information processing, and/or social cognition [24].

Typical Findings on Physical Exam

Physical exam [24]:

- General: fatigue.
- Head, Ears, Eyes, Nose, Throat: abnormalities in retina, smooth pursuit eye movements, repetitive saccadic eye movements, loss of vestibulo-ocular reflex, abnormal near point of convergence, and decreased accommodation [46]. Visible signs of injury to scalp, underlying skull fracture, Battle's sign, decreased range of motion of head and jaw. Tenderness of C-spine.
- Gastrointestinal: nausea, vomiting.
- Psychiatric: personality changes (e.g., disinhibition, apathy, suspiciousness, aggression), inattention, impaired memory, impaired executive function, delirium, disorientation, anterograde, and/or retrograde amnesia [47].
- Neurological: disrupted coordination, gait, balance and vestibular function, oculomotor function [48]. Impairment in cranial nerves, muscle tone, and strength [49].

Typical Laboratory/Radiological Findings

Abnormal head and C-spine imaging (CT, MRI) may be present.

Middle Insomnia Psychiatric Differential

Posttraumatic Stress Disorder (PTSD)

Epidemiology

According to the DSM-IV criteria, PTSD in the United States has a lifetime prevalence of about 8%. In a survey conducted in the United States in 2012–2013 based on the DSM-IV criteria, lifetime prevalence of PTSD in the US was 6.1% in adults [19, 20, 49, 50]. Special populations such as the United States military service members involved in Operation Iraqi Freedom/Operation Enduring Freedom are estimated to have a prevalence of 7.1–12.9% [51].

Incidence of Posttraumatic Stress Disorder Presenting as Insomnia

In a study of Operation Iraqi Freedom, Operation Enduring Freedom, and Operation New Dawn veterans with PTSD, 56% of the PTSD group reported severe insomnia while 44% reported moderate insomnia [52]. PTSD can manifest with a variety of sleep disruptions, including SOL, a feature of early insomnia. However, according to a meta-analysis of studies of polysomnogram data in patients with PTSD, SOL did not have a significant mean effect size while the overall mean effect sizes were largest in showing increased stage 1 sleep, less slow wave sleep and greater REM density (REMD) [53], which are all better indicators of middle insomnia. The latter of these measures, REMD, has also been directly associated with level or arousal, while additional studies have shown that patients with PTSD have elevated central measures of hyperarousal during sleep [54–56]. Thus, it appears patients with PTSD are hyper-aroused during sleep and have increased REM density, and we can hypothesize that REM density may be related to recurrent nightmares. We can further postulate that for individuals with PTSD who complain of sleep onset difficulties, it is more likely secondary to these middle insomnia features, and an associated fear of sleep.

Typical Findings of the HPI

Patients report exposure to actual or threatened traumatic event either through direct experience, witnessing an event, learning about an event that occurred to a close family member or friend, or experiencing repeated or extreme exposure to aversive details of a traumatic event. Other symptoms present include intrusive symptoms (involuntary thoughts, distressing dreams, dissociative reactions, intense psychological distress to internal or external reminders, and marked physiological reactions to internal or external reminders), persistent avoidance of stimuli associated with a traumatic event, negative alterations in thoughts and mood (inability to recall important aspects of event, persistent negative beliefs, persistent distorted thoughts about cause or consequences, persistent negative emotional state, diminished interest in significant activities, detachment, and inability to feel positive emotions), and marked alterations in arousal (irritability, hypervigilance, exaggerated startle response, poor concentration, and sleep disturbances). Symptoms persist for more than 1 month and are not attributable to other medical or psychiatric conditions.

Typical Findings on Physical Exam

Physical Exam [50]:

- Cardiac: elevated blood pressure, tachycardia
- Dermatologic: profuse sweating
- Musculoskeletal: twitching, psychomotor agitation

Typical Laboratory/Radiological Findings

None.

Alcohol Intoxication

Epidemiology

Most alcohol consumers are likely to have been intoxicated at some point in their lives [24]. It is estimated that two-thirds of US adults consume alcohol with up to 10% of adults abusing alcohol [57].

Incidence of Alcohol Intoxication Presenting as Insomnia

The nonspecific diagnosis of substance/medication-induced sleep disorder from the DSM-5-TR obviously covers a vast array of possible sleep difficulties. The most common of these, however, given the prevalence of alcohol use and AUD (as high as 14% with DSM-5-TR criteria), is middle insomnia associated with problems with alcohol [58]. Patients commonly use alcohol to promote sleep—and while alcohol use in healthy nonalcoholics decreases sleep latency and increases the quality and quantity of NREM sleep during the first half of the night, it disrupts sleep during the second half of the night. Additionally, patients with AUD will have a multitude of sleep-related difficulties including disrupted sleep architecture markers of prolonged sleep latency, decreased REM %, and decreased total sleep time [59, 60]. Again, we see that the more prolonged the problem, the more severe the insomnia often becomes and the more overlap among insomnia subtypes, as demonstrated by the early insomnia marker of prolonged sleep latency in patients with AUD. Even with sustained remission, sleep disruption associated with AUD may persist for 6–12 months following cessation of alcohol use.

Typical Findings of the HPI

Recent ingestion of alcohol with clinically significant problematic behavioral or psychological changes that developed during, or shortly after, alcohol ingestion. Associated signs and symptoms include slurred speech, incoordination, unsteady gait, nystagmus, impairment in attention or memory, and stupor or coma. Signs and symptoms of intoxication are more likely to be intense when the blood alcohol level is rising. Symptoms must not be attributable to another medical condition.

Typical Findings on Physical Exam

Physical exam:

- General: vital signs, level of consciousness, signs of trauma
- Head, Ears, Eyes, Nose Throat: dry mucous membranes
- Dermatologic: signs of liver damage—caput medusa, capillary prominence, gynecomastia, jaundice, nail changes, palmar erythema, scleral icterus, spider telangiectasias
- Cardiac: ventricular tachyarrhythmias (severe intoxication), atrial fibrillation (severe intoxication)
- Gastrointestinal: abdominal pain, ascites (chronic)
- Musculoskeletal: muscular atrophy (chronic)
- Neurologic: nystagmus, incoordination, unsteady gait
- Psychiatric: slurred speech, impairment in attention and/or memory, delirium, stupor or coma

Typical Laboratory/Radiological Findings

- Elevated alcohol level in breath, blood, or urine sample
- Elevated serum osmolality, osmolar gap >20 mOsm/L
- Elevated LAEs
- Abnormal electrolytes
- Elevated blood and/or urine ketones

Late Insomnia Psychiatric Differential

Major Depressive Disorder (MDD)

Epidemiology

According to the Mental Health Surveillance Study conducted by the Substance Abuse and Mental Health Services Administration, the 12-month prevalence of MDD in the United States is estimated to be 6% [61]. The WHO World Mental Health Survey estimates the lifetime prevalence in the United States to be 17% [62]. A Danish study found the cumulative incidence over a period of 12 years (2000–2012) to be 5.6% in males and 10.2% in females [63].

Incidence of Major Depressive Disorder Presenting as Insomnia

Sleep disturbances (trouble falling asleep, staying asleep, or waking up early) have been reported in up to 88% of patients with MDD, with late insomnia being more classically associated with depression [64]. Studies find depressed patients have decreased REM sleep latency and prolonged REM sleep periods early in the night [65].

Typical Findings of the HPI

Sleep disturbances in MDD often manifest as early morning awakenings with the chance for concurrent disturbances of sleep onset and waking up after sleep onset (as compared to solely having difficulty with early insomnia or middle insomnia) [66]. Recent studies have found that MDD can cause earlier dim light melatonin onset (DLMO) resulting in an advanced phase of sleep [67]. Treatment with antidepressants can potentially result in a phase delay and correction of relatively advanced cycles [68–70]. In general for any diagnosis of MDD, DSM-5-TR guidelines for clinical presentation involve a functional impact due to a 2-week period with at least five of the following (with one symptom being either depressed mood or loss of interest): depressed mood, loss of interest or pleasure, unintended weight loss or gain, insomnia or hypersomnia, psychomotor retardation or agitation, fatigue or loss of energy, feelings of worthlessness or inappropriate guilt, diminished ability to concentrate, or recurrent thoughts of death or suicide. The presence of late insomnia in depression can therefore be a stronger marker for supporting the diagnosis of depression in older populations (as compared to younger populations).

Typical Findings on Physical Exam

Physical exam:

- General: weight changes (loss or gain), psychomotor slowing or agitation (i.e., slowed/delayed activity or restlessness) [71]
- Psychiatric: mood changes, cognitive distortions [72]

Typical Laboratory/Radiological Findings

None. Ensure that symptoms are not attributable to the physiological effects of a substance or another medical condition.

Systemic Medical Condition Differential

A vast array of medical conditions can also contribute to sleep disturbances and when considering these, our preferred process is again to first identify where in the sleep cycle the disruption predominantly occurs. From there, we can rule out (or rule in) different processes. We aim to focus on the most common systemic medical causes of sleep disruption that we consider to be of a more insidious nature, that is, conditions in which the psychiatrist is more likely to discover and diagnose upon working up a chief complaint of insomnia. A discussion of the sleep impacts on medical comorbidities is beyond the scope of this topic, with certain noted exceptions such as heart failure. This differential, which again is outlined in Table 4.1, is not an exhaustive list, but common conditions with practical screening tools that are readily available and can be easily utilized by the psychiatrist.

Early Insomnia Systemic Medical Condition Differential

Restless Leg Syndrome (RLS)/Willis-Ekbom Disease

RLS is a neurological disorder characterized by the urge to move the legs that worsen at rest and is alleviated with movement. RLS is typically divided into primary (idiopathic) or secondary to another medical condition. Common medical conditions that may cause RLS include chronic kidney disease, pregnancy, iron deficiency, spinal cord disease, multiple sclerosis, Parkinson's disease, and neuropathy.

Epidemiology

There is a reported annual incidence of 0.8–2.2% in the general population [73]. The estimated prevalence of RLS in the United States is 4–29% [74]. Data for incidence and prevalence of RLS presenting as insomnia was not available.

Typical Findings of the HPI

Patients will report an urge to move the legs which is accompanied by or in response to uncomfortable and unpleasant sensations (e.g., crawling, tingling, burning, itching) in the leg. These episodes begin or worsen during periods of rest or inactivity, partially or fully relieved by movement, and the urge is worse in the evening or at night. This occurs at least three times per week for at least 3 months. The symptoms are significantly distressing and are not better explained by another psychiatric condition, medical condition, or substance. These symptoms can delay sleep onset and awaken patients leading to sleep fragmentation [24]. Severe forms of RLS may significantly impair function and are associated with depression and anxiety which occur in about 2–3% of the population [75–78]. Other possible symptoms that have psychiatric overlap include irritability and hyperactivity [79].

Typical Findings on Physical Exam

If primary RLS, physical exam is typically normal [80, 81]. If RLS is due to a secondary cause, physical exam will be consistent with the underlying disorder (e.g., peripheral neuropathy) [80].

Typical Laboratory/Radiological Findings

For secondary RLS, evaluate for iron deficiency with complete blood count, serum ferritin, serum iron, total iron binding capacity, and percent transferrin saturation. Consider also screening for kidney disease, diabetes, vitamin B12 deficiency, folic acid deficiency, and thyroid dysfunction.

Available Rating Scales

The most reliable rating scale is the RLS-Diagnostic Index (RLS-DI) which is a 10-item questionnaire that consists of the essential diagnostic criteria established by the International RLS Study Group in addition to supportive features. Scores range from 22 (no RLS) to 20 (definite RLS) with a cut-off of ≥11 points is used to identify RLS. At the designated cut-off score of >11, the sensitivity is 93% with a specificity of 98.9% and a PPV of 98.8% [82]. Other diagnostic tests that can assist in diagnosing RLS include performing a levodopa challenge (L-Dopa test). This requires a single dose of levodopa 100 mg orally, followed by 2 h of self-reported monitoring. The levodopa challenge is considered positive if RLS symptoms reduce by ≥50% [80, 83]. It was found to have a sensitivity of 88% for improvement in leg symptoms and 80% sensitivity for improvement in urge to move the legs with a specificity of 100% for both test items [84].

Delayed Sleep-Wake Phase Disorder (DSWPD)

Epidemiology

While prevalence of DSWPD tends to vary, most studies find the range to be anywhere between 0.2% and 8% with younger ages tending to fall higher within the range [85, 86]. Data for incidence and prevalence of DSWPD presenting as insomnia was not available.

Typical Findings of the HPI

Hallmark findings of DSWPD involve trouble initiating sleep, morning sleepiness, and late morning awakenings [87, 88]. Patients may report sleeping without difficulty when asked about their sleep in the absence of sleep pressures (as in work or other similar responsibilities requiring waking up at an earlier time not in accordance with their sleep cycle) [88]. Presentation must include all of the following: chronic complaint of difficulty waking up at desired wake-time with an inability to fall asleep at the desired time, presence of symptoms for a minimum of 3 months, improved sleep quality and duration when allowed to sleep in accordance with their internal biological clock [89]. The condition must not be better explained by other medical or psychiatric conditions.

Typical Findings on Physical Exam
None.

Typical Laboratory/Radiological Findings
None.

Available Rating Scales
Tools commonly used in evaluating sleep disorders range from subjective sleep diaries to actigraphy and PSG. The AASM practice guidelines recommend with a "moderate degree of clinical certainty" that the process starts with the use of sleep logs and actigraphy [90]. Actigraphy has an overall sensitivity of 96% but an overall specificity of 33% in detecting sleep and wakefulness [91]. The low specificity is reflective of difficulty of detecting sleep-wake patterns between individuals, but the accuracy and sensitivity reflect the strong capability for screening patients in the context of clinical suspicion and, in combination with sleep diaries, can provide more robust clinical pictures for diagnosing patients [92, 93]. Current guidelines highlight that there are no other currently available evaluation tools recommended for routine use that fit the category of "high degree of clinical certainty" in the initial evaluation phase [90]. PPV for actigraphy is not readily available.

Another option to consider can be a PSG, but current guidelines do not recommend its routine use unless there is suspicion of another primary sleep disorder [90]. Additionally, the Morningness-Eveningness Questionnaire can be utilized to provide confirmatory evidence for a sleep phase disorder, but the data does not indicate it is reliable enough to be utilized as the only way to establish a diagnosis [94].

Chronic Obstructive Pulmonary Disease (COPD)

Epidemiology
COPD is the third leading cause of morbidity and mortality [95] with an estimated prevalence of 4–10% worldwide [96]. In the United States, the estimated prevalence of COPD is 6.3% [97]. Data for incidence and prevalence of COPD presenting as insomnia was not available.

Typical Findings of the HPI
Patients will typically present with complaints of progressive symptoms of dyspnea, cough, wheezing, breathlessness, and sputum production that may be variable from day to day. Symptoms may worsen with exertion and have a significant impact on daily life to include physical limitations, work impairment, social impairment, depression, anxiety, impairment in sexual activity, and sleep disturbances [95]. Approximately 75% of COPD patients report nocturnal disturbances with COPD symptoms disrupting SOL and sleep architecture. Given overlap with obstructive sleep apnea, increased nighttime awakenings have also been observed in patients with COPD [98].

Typical Findings on Physical Exam

There is insufficient evidence to support a specific physical exam for COPD as physical signs of airflow limitations may not manifest until lung function is substantially compromised. Listed below are typical physical exam signs of COPD:

- General: muscle wasting, cachexia
- Dermatologic: central cyanosis [99]
- Cardiac: barrel chest
- Pulmonary: use of accessory respiratory muscles, pursed-lip breathing, reduced chest expansion, reduced breath sounds, expiratory time ≥4 s, wheezing, hyperresonance [100]

Typical Laboratory/Radiological Findings

- Complete blood count may demonstrate anemia or polycythemia
- Chest X-Ray may show diaphragmatic flattening, increased lung length, increased rib space, bronchial wall thickening, increased lung markings, prominent vessels, hyperlucency [95]

Available Rating Scales

The COPD Assessment Test (CAT) is an 8-item questionnaire that may be used to assess the impacts of COPD on a person's quality of life and how it changes over time. In a multicenter study, total CAT scores were higher in the COPD patients and the "soundly sleeping" item was the most significant item associated with CAT. Sensitivity and specificity to estimate COPD diagnosed with spirometry were 66.67% and 75.15%, respectively. The positive predictive value and negative predictive value were 10.53% and 98.09%, respectively [101]. In a cross-sectional study, CAT scores were also significant predictors of insomnia [102]. The gold standard for diagnosing COPD is spirometry.

Middle Insomnia Systemic Medical Condition Differential

Obstructive Sleep Apnea (OSA)

The first of the more "occult" conditions to consider for middle insomnia is OSA. OSA is the most common sleep-related breathing disorder and is characterized by obstructive or hypopneic events that occur during sleep due to repetitive collapse of the upper airway. OSA requires PSG for diagnosis but there are certain clinical features that must also be present and should lead the physician to consider testing.

Epidemiology

Prevalence estimates vary according to which OSA metrics are collected and the distribution of risk factors in the population. The estimated prevalence in North America is 20–30% in males and 10–15% in females when OSA is more broadly defined (apnea-hypopnea index (AHI) > 5) measured by PSG [103, 104]. Prevalence in the United States appears to be increasing in association with rising rates of obesity. Data for incidence and prevalence of OSA presenting as insomnia was not available.

Typical Findings of the HPI

The most common symptoms reported by patients with OSA are excessive daytime sleepiness (EDS), partner-reported loud snoring and related breathing abnormalities, and morning headaches. Daytime sleepiness is a core feature of insomnia; it is reliably quantified in the Epworth Sleepiness Scale which ranges from 0 to 24 with a suggested cut-off of >10 for EDS (https://epworthsleepinessscale.com/about-the-ess/). This tool can also be helpful in distinguishing fatigue from EDS but is generally not seen as a good screening tool for OSA, likely because other factors should also be present and the differential for EDS includes a number of separate diseases [105].

Taken together, snoring and related sounds (gasping, choking, snorting) have a high sensitivity in detecting OSA (80–90%) but a low specificity (50%); noted gasping or choking appears far more predictive of OSA than mere snoring with likelihood ratios (LR) of 3.3 vs. 1.1, respectively [106]. A 2013 systematic review of signs, symptoms, and composite tools for diagnosing OSA found observed gasping or choking to be the most reliable indicator of OSA, while all other indicators fell below the threshold of LR > 2.0 when more strict criteria of AHI > 10 or 15 per hour were applied. Thus, the relatively common symptom of morning headaches (affecting 10–30% or patients with OSA), also proved a relatively unreliable indicator of more severe OSA [107].

It is also notable that OSA has a bidirectional relationship with many other diseases including chronic kidney diseases [108] and type 2 diabetes mellitus [109] which also impact a patient's quality of sleep. Assessing for a thorough past medical history and ensuring other disease processes are well controlled is vital to a comprehensive sleep assessment.

Typical Findings on Physical Exam

Evidence is mixed as to how useful physical exam findings are in predicting OSA. As noted, one 2013 systematic review did not find any physical exam findings or composite tools to be reliable predictors of more narrowly defined OSA. In contrast, several previous models have found hypertension to be a reliable predictor when used with EDS [110]. For this reason, the AASM clinical practice guidelines consider hypertension to be an important parameter. They recommend testing for OSA in patients who have EDS and any two of the following three characteristics: (1) hypertension; (2) habitual loud snoring; (3) witnessed apnea or gasping or choking (the latter two of which have already been discussed above) [111]. Other exam findings that have been studied include pharyngeal anatomy, obesity, and neck circumference. The 2013 review included studies of both Mallampati class and pharyngeal narrowing, finding LRs of 1.6 and 1.4, respectively. Around the same time in 2013, the namesake for another proposed sign of OSA, Friedman, published a meta-analysis on the diagnostic value of the Friedman tongue position and Mallampati classification [112]. He concluded that these exams are significantly associated with obstructive sleep apnea severity; however, the confidence intervals for the respective correlation coefficients overlap and the study did not provide likelihood ratios or positive predictive values for the findings [112]. Similarly, BMI and neck circumference appear correlated but not reliably predictive of OSA [111].

Typical Laboratory/Radiological Findings

Apart from PSG and home sleep apnea tests (HSAT) designed to definitively diagnose OSA, there are no laboratory or radiological findings that are predictive of OSA. Once diagnostic testing for OSA is determined appropriate, we recommend allowing sleep specialists to determine the appropriateness and availability of HSAT versus the "gold standard" of PSG.

Available Rating Scales

Experts advise caution in routine use of screening tools given their low validity in settings outside of the sleep clinic and high-risk populations. Keeping these caveats in mind, their reported sensitivities can make them helpful in ruling out OSA. The STOP-BANG questionnaire performs best. Its name connotes an acronym for predictors of OSA including snoring (loud); tired (during the day); observed (choking/gasping); increased blood pressure (history of hypertension); BMI (>35 kg/m^2); age (>50); neck size (male >17 in.; female >16 in.); and gender (males are at higher risk). Each positive response is one point. For a score of 3 or higher, the questionnaire has sensitivities of 90.5% for the diagnosis of OSA using an AHI threshold of 5–14, 94.6% for a moderate/severe OSA (AHI 15–29), and 100% for severe OSA (AHI > 30) [113, 114]. The respective specificity for a score of 3 or higher for all OSA is 28.1%, 19.9% for moderate/severe OSA, and 17.4% for severe OSA. As the STOP-BANG score increases, specificity may reach up to 87.7%. PPV for a score of 3 or higher was 84.8% for all OSA, 52.2% for moderate/severe OSA, and 29.6% for severe OSA [114]. Other rating scales such as the Sleep Apnea Clinical Score (SACS), the Berlin questionnaire, the Lausanne NoSAS (Neck circumference, Obesity, Snoring, Age, Sex) score, and the Multivariable Apnea Prediction Instrument (MVAP) all combine a similar collection of variables discussed above.

Urologic Disorders

A range of urologic disorders can lead to middle sleep problems due to incontinence or nocturia. It appears the reverse may also be true, in that sleep-related problems can have downstream effects on urologic symptoms [115]. This process could be mediated by obesity, metabolic dysregulation, and increased inflammation associated with disordered sleep, all of which can also lead to or aggravate urologic illness [116–119]. OSA, a condition also associated with obesity, metabolic disturbances, and sleep disruptions, has an identified mechanism for producing nocturia. In OSA, a release of atrial natriuretic peptide (ANP) due to negative intrathoracic pressure and stretching of the myocardium leads to subsequent aldosterone inhibition and increased sodium and water excretion resulting in nocturia [120]. This may be yet another reason why OSA causes middle insomnia and should be identified and treated. On the other hand, another group concluded that patients may use "faulty *post hoc* reasoning" in misattributing their nighttime awakenings caused by OSA and other sleep disorders (e.g., RLS) as a need to urinate when in fact the awakening had a separate cause and the patient voluntarily decided to urinate while awake [121].

Thus, the diagnostic process can be complicated by the dynamic relationship between sleep and urologic disorders. Nevertheless, the psychiatrist can simplify the process by first assessing for the presence of nocturia or urinary incontinence affecting sleep, and then attempting to determine if the problem may be related to an anatomical (obstructive or storage-related symptoms) process or a functional process. For anatomical processes, we will consider the common problem of benign prostatic hyperplasia that may affect the bladder outlet; for functional abnormalities, we will consider the common problem of overactive bladder. These considerations are obviously not exhaustive and if clinical suspicion remains high for an alternative urological process, or if symptoms are severe (such as incontinence or urinary retention), consultation with a urologist is recommended.

Benign Prostatic Hyperplasia (BPH) and Lower Urinary Tract Symptoms (LUTS)

BPH is a histologic diagnosis describing hyperplasia of cells within the transition zone of the prostate. While BPH is not purely a diagnosis of exclusion in that it can be confirmed via histologic examination of a biopsy, for practical clinical purposes it can be considered as such. The only reason to diagnose this condition via biopsy is if there was reasonable suspicion of malignancy. Unfortunately, no other clinical tools are used to aid in the diagnosis other than excluding alternative causes of LUTS.

Epidemiology

According to autopsy studies, histologically proven BPH occurs in 60% of men at age 60 and 80% of men at age 80 [122]. Clinicians commonly refer to benign enlargement of the prostate (BPE) as BPH without a histologic diagnosis. When symptomatic, the condition is referred to as BPH/LUTS indicating lower urinary tract symptoms attributed to BPH. Prevalence of BPH/LUTS increases with age, affecting approximately a quarter of men in their 50s and half of men in their 80s according to one population-based survey in Minnesota [123]. Data for incidence and prevalence of BPH/LUTS presenting as insomnia was not available.

Typical Findings of the HPI

The LUTS of BPH can include urinary frequency, urgency, nocturia, and incontinence as well as voiding symptoms such as slow urinary stream, straining to void, and urinary intermittency or hesitancy. LUTS can be attributed to a wide variety of urologic concerns, and none of these symptoms from the history are specific to BPH; BPH is simply the most common cause.

Typical Findings on Physical Exam

As with findings on history, physical exam findings are not very specific to BPH. However, in addition to an abdominal and neurological exam, it is important to perform a digital rectal exam (DRE) in patients complaining of LUTS. We do not recommend the treating psychiatrist perform any sensitive exams on patients; the exam can be deferred to another physician. The DRE is generally not a helpful predictor of prostate size and prostate size does not necessarily correlate with symptoms. However, DRE can help in cases of very large prostates or prompt further exploration if the prostate is tender (prostatitis), asymmetrical, or nodular (malignancy). DRE can also be used to evaluate sphincter tone or whether perineal sensation is decreased on exam (neurological) [124, 125]. Normal size of the prostate is about the size of a walnut.

Typical Laboratory/Radiological Findings

Laboratory and imaging studies are generally used to exclude other diagnoses and to guide treatment. For evaluation of LUTS in men, experts recommend a urinalysis which can identify signs of other causes of LUTS such as infection (pyuria, bacteriuria), diabetes (glucosuria, ketonuria), or malignancy (hematuria) [126]. While BPH and other more benign conditions can cause hematuria, any level of blood in the urine, particularly in the older patient, warrants further evaluation with additional imaging or cystoscopy and urology referral if an easily identifiable cause such as menstruation cannot be found [127]. A prostate-specific antigen (PSA) is not specifically recommended in all men with LUTS but should be considered as part of shared decision-making for screening for prostate cancer or for certain BPH treatment options.[1] Urologists also recommend as a "clinical principle" (a term used due to insufficient data from studies) that patients with bothersome LUTS also undergo a post-void residual volume measurement via the use of a bedside bladder scanner (ultrasound) or straight catheterization [129]. Volumes greater than 250 mL or increasing over time may warrant surgical intervention.

Available Rating Scales

The current gold standard for evaluating severity of BPH/LUTS is the International Prostate Symptom Score (IPSS) [130]. The IPSS consists of seven questions assessing for voiding and storage symptoms. As the IPSS voiding to storage subscore ratio (IPSS-V/S) decreases, sensitivity can reach as high as 85.7% with a specificity of 45.7% and a PPV of 61%. As the IPSS-V/S increases, specificity increases to 89% with 65.9% sensitivity with a PPV of 85.4% [130].

---

[1] **Note about prostate cancer**: Prostate cancer is a rare cause of LUTS, but still the second most diagnosed cancer in men, with an overall incidence of 131 cases per 100,000 men annually in the United States [128]. Since the advent of PSA screening, most cases are discovered while still asymptomatic and localized. However, because PSA is not specific to prostate cancer, screening with PSA can lead to a variety of harms such as overdiagnosis of a condition that might not have become clinically relevant, poor biopsy outcomes, and lingering anxiety. Thus, physicians have adopted a shared decision-making model with patients in regard to screening, noting important risk factors to include such as age, race (Black men are at the highest risk), and family history. If the patient meets any of these risk factors and is interested in screening, it should be offered.

Overactive Bladder (OAB)

Like the term LUTS, OAB describes a clinical syndrome rather than a diagnosis of a specific pathological etiology. Specifically, the International Continence Society defines OAB as "urinary urgency, usually accompanied by frequency and nocturia, with or without urgency urinary incontinence, in the absence of urinary tract infection or other obvious pathology," and urgency urinary incontinence as "involuntary loss of urine associated with urgency" [131].

Epidemiology

Incidence appears to be between 10% and 15% for both men and women, although there is significant overlap with BPH/LUTS for men [132, 133]. Data for incidence and prevalence of OAB presenting as insomnia was not available.

Typical Findings of the HPI

History should focus on symptoms of urinary urgency (which are associated with worse quality of sleep and poorer quality of life), urinary frequency, precipitating factors, voiding habits, and bathroom accessibility. It should also address risk factors such obesity—obese women are three times more likely to experience incontinence, impaired functional status, comorbid MDD diabetes mellitus, recurrent urinary tract infections, and bladder symptoms in childhood [134, 135].

Typical Findings on Physical Exam

There are no physical exam signs that would predict OAB, but a few things should be ruled out according to urologists: a pelvic mass and neurologic dysfunction—particularly at S2, S3, and S4 [136].

Typical Laboratory/Radiological Findings

As with BPH/LUTS, diagnostic tests should include a urinalysis to assess for bacteriuria and hematuria, and possibly a post-void residual volume measurement if symptoms are consistent with an obstructive process or if surgical interventions are being considered.

Available Rating Scales

Several screening questionnaires exist to evaluate urinary incontinence and lower urinary tract symptoms; of these, the Michigan Incontinence Symptom Index (M-ISI) is favorable because it was validated in a well-designed study using a population that better reflects a typical screening population. The sensitivity for total incontinence is 84% with a positive predictive value of 75% [137]. The tool can be found at the Michigan Urology website: https://medicine.umich.edu/dept/urology/research/quality-life-tools/michigan-incontinence-symptom-index.

Gastroesophageal Reflux (GERD)

GERD is a common condition in the Western world and a common cause of sleep disturbance that typically resolves with treatment [138]. Because some degree of postprandial reflux is physiologic [139], GERD has been broadly defined as the condition that develops when reflux of stomach contents causes "troublesome symptoms or complications" [138] and is classified as either erosive or nonerosive based on the appearance of the esophageal mucosa. Erosive esophagitis is characterized by the presence of visual breaks in the distal esophageal mucosa, with or without symptoms. Nonerosive reflux disease is characterized by the presence of symptoms without visible changes in the esophageal mucosa [138]. Esophagogastroduodenoscopy (EGD) can classify patients into either erosive or nonerosive disease; however, EGD is not recommended in the diagnosis of GERD in patients without alarm symptoms or without risk factors for Barrett esophagus [140].

Epidemiology

Epidemiologic studies have put the prevalence between 10% and 20% [141]. That is likely an underestimate because those studies prioritize heartburn and regurgitation symptoms which are not always present, or not always the most bothersome symptoms associated with GERD [142]. Erosive esophagitis is found in only 30% of treatment-naive patients and in less than 10% of patients on a proton-pump inhibitor (PPI), and Barrett's esophagus is found in only 5–15% of patients with chronic GERD [143]. Data for incidence and prevalence of GERD presenting as insomnia was not available.

Typical Findings on HPI

The American College of Gastroenterology and Canadian Association of Gastroenterology guidelines recommend diagnosing GERD using symptomatology when "red flags" and risk factors for Barrett's esophagus are absent [144, 145]. See Table 4.3 to identify these "red flags."

Heartburn and regurgitation are the primary symptoms associated with GERD; however, there is often variability between patients in presentation. Extraintestinal manifestations such as chronic nighttime cough, asthma, and sleep disturbance may be the most prominent or only presenting symptoms [138, 146]. Patients with GERD will typically present with complaints of a bad taste in the mouth in the morning or a sensation of esophageal discomfort at nighttime. Because of this variability, nonspecialists have significantly lower sensitivity than gastroenterologists in diagnosing GERD [141].

Table 4.3 "Red flag" symptoms for gastro-esophageal reflux (GERD) and risk factors for Barrett's esophagus

GERD Red Flags	
Alarm features for malignancy	Risk factors for Barrett's esophagus
New onset dyspepsia in patient ≥60 years	Duration of GERD for 5–10 years or more[a]
Evidence of gastrointestinal bleeding	Age ≥50 years
Iron deficiency anemia	Male
Anorexia	Caucasian
Unexplained weight loss	Hiatal hernia
Dysphagia	Central obesity
Odynophagia	Nocturnal reflux
Persistent vomiting	Tobacco use (past or present)
Gastrointestinal cancer in first-degree relative	Barrett esophagus and/or adenocarcinoma in first-degree relative

Response to a trial of PPI has poor sensitivity and specificity. In a meta-analysis of 15 studies comparing PPI trials with objective measures of GERD, the combined sensitivity and specificity were 78% and 54%, respectively [147]. The PPV for these studies ranged from 68% to 100%; however, the prevalence in these studies ranged from 53% to 83% [147], which is significantly higher than the general population. As such, the PPV of a PPI trial will be lower in practice. The positive and negative likelihood ratios (+LR/−LR) give us a more consistent idea of how useful a test is based on how much they raise or lower the posttest probability for a given diagnosis or finding. For PPI trials, the +LR ranges from 1.63 to 1.87, with a pooled +LR of 1.70. The pooled −LR for PPI response is 0.41 [147]. These test characteristics indicate that a PPI trial will only change the posttest probability by around 5–10%, which makes it not very useful as a test for either ruling in or out GERD.

Typical Findings on Physical Exam

None—physical exams are typically unremarkable. There may be atypical signs of GERD present to include dental erosion, wheezing, recurrent otitis media, or laryngitis [148, 149].

Typical Laboratory/Radiological Findings

None. See above re: EGD.

Available Rating Scales

The Reflux Diagnostic Questionnaire (RDQ) and GERD Questionnaire (GerdQ) are two tools that have been validated in the evaluation and management of GERD [141, 146]. Both questionnaires have a sensitivity higher than EGD and are similar to gastroenterologists. The +LR for the GerdQ (https://www.ncbi.nlm.nih.gov/pmc/articles/PMC3851875/) is 2.24 [146], which corresponds to an increase in posttest probability of approximately 20%. This is higher than primary care physicians alone and comparable to gastroenterologists [141], making it a useful tool for nonspecialists to use in the initial evaluation and management of GERD without specialist referral. GerdQ has a sensitivity of 66.7%, specificity of 91.7%, and a PPV of 97.1% [150].

Chronic Pain

Chronic pain is defined as pain that is present on most days for at least 3 months by the International Association for the Study of Pain. The IASP is working to differentiate chronic pain into six subgroups to categorize pain that is secondary to underlying disease. This includes chronic cancer-related pain, chronic neuropathic pain, chronic secondary visceral pain, chronic posttraumatic and postsurgical pain, chronic secondary headache and orofacial pain, and chronic secondary musculoskeletal pain [151].

Epidemiology

It is estimated that 10–25% of the adult population experience chronic pain [152–154]. In the United States, 53% of adults ≥65 years old report pain symptoms that have lasted for more than 1 month [155]. The high-impact chronic pain (HICP) population consists of patients who are more severely impacted in terms of disability and pain duration within the chronic pain population. It is estimated that HICP affects 4.8% of the adult population in the United States [156]. Data for incidence and prevalence of chronic pain presenting as insomnia was not available.

Typical Findings of the HPI

Characterize pain (e.g., nociceptive, neuropathic, other) to identify underlying etiology if possible. Regardless of the medical cause for their pain, a large portion of the chronic pain population will report sleep disturbances including difficulty falling asleep and maintaining sleep [157]. Sleep disturbances are heterogeneous and difficult to measure; however, chronic pain patients experience greater sleep fragmentation demonstrated by significantly more awakenings and movement-related disruption on PSG. This patient population also had a high prevalence (up to 55%) of comorbid psychiatric disorders, specifically depression, and comorbid sleep disorders (insomnia, RLS, and OSA) [158].

Typical Findings on Physical Exam

The physical exam should focus on a complete musculoskeletal and neurological exam. This includes assessing for inflammation, weakness, neuropathy, functional limitations, and other physical signs of pain (facial grimace, tachycardia, tachypnea, or restlessness). Obtain a pain assessment scale [159].

Typical Laboratory/Radiological Findings

Imaging if appropriate in history and physical to make specific diagnosis or if "red flag" symptoms are present.

Available Rating Scales

There is a complex relationship between sleep and chronic pain and pain should be optimally controlled. The Brief Pain inventory (BPI) is one of the most widely used measurement tools for assessing clinical pain both in clinical practice and research. The BPI can be used to discriminate neuropathic and nociceptive pain, in addition, to assess for impact on a patient's daily life including sleep, mood, functioning at work and home, and enjoyment of life. Compared to the clinical assessment, the BPI has a sensitivity of 79.4%, a specificity of 46.9%, positive predictive value of 65.8%, and negative predictive value of 63.9%. It is considered a reliable and valid evaluation for both neuropathic and nociceptive pain [160].

Late Insomnia Systemic Medical Condition Differential

Advanced Sleep-Wake Phase Disorder (ASWPD)

Epidemiology

In examining the incidence and prevalence of ASWPD, a more recent New Zealand survey-based study found a prevalence to be anywhere between 0.25% and 7% [161]. Another study focusing on a sleep study population determined the prevalence of ASWPD to be 1 in 2500 [162]. Otherwise, data on the incidence and the prevalence of ASWPD tends to vary. Data for incidence and prevalence of ASWPD presenting as insomnia was not available.

Typical Findings of the HPI

Hallmark findings of ASWPD involve evening sleepiness reports and early morning awakenings [88]. Presentation must include all of the following: chronic complaint of difficulty staying awake until desired bedtime with an inability to remain asleep until the desired time, presence of symptoms for a minimum of 3 months, improved sleep quality and duration when allowed to sleep in accordance with their internal biological clock [89]. The condition must not be better explained by other medical or psychiatric conditions.

Typical Findings on Physical Exam

None.

Typical Laboratory/Radiological Findings

None. As mentioned above in DSWPD, the evaluation of DLMO as a biomarker shows promise with recent studies showing a sensitivity of 90% and specificity of 84% in typing sleep phase disruptions [163]. The clinical utility remains difficult to recommend (as in DSWPD) given that the formal diagnosis does not currently require the objective classification of a phase disruption and the inherent barriers of this test, to include requiring special environmental conditions and a time series of at least several hours for a sample collection [164].

Available Rating Scales

Screening tools for working up ASWPD are the same as for DSWPD. The focus remains on the combination of a 2-week sleep diary with actigraphy with the PSG reserved for ruling out a suspicion for other primary sleep disorders. Actigraphy has an accuracy of 86% in detecting sleep versus wake, an overall sensitivity of 96% but an overall specificity of 33% in detecting sleep and wakefulness [91]. The low specificity is reflective of difficulty with detecting sleep-wake patterns between individuals, but despite that, the accuracy and sensitivity reflect the strong capability for screening patients in the context of clinical suspicion and, in combination with sleep diaries, can provide more robust clinical pictures for diagnosing patients [92, 93]. PPV is not readily available for actigraphy. As such, current guidelines highlight that there are no other currently available evaluation tools recommended for routine use that fit the category of "high degree of clinical certainty" according to experts in the initial evaluation phase [90].

Of note, the aging process results in numerous changes to sleep architecture that can also result in an advancement of the sleep/wake cycle [165]. A key point in determining the presence of an underlying sleep disorder is the report of clinically significant distress with the expected phase advancement with aging [166]. If such distress is present, assessment and treatment for an advanced sleep-wake phase disorder should follow. The goal of treatment would be to find a more socially appropriate or desirable timing of the sleep cycle with the addition of potentially melatonin or photic treatment [166].

Insomnia Assessment Decision Tree

Sleep is a complex and largely mysterious process. There are numerous psychiatric, substance-induced, and systemic medical conditions that can affect its integrity. The task of efficiently and effectively diagnosing patients who complain of sleep problems can be a daunting one. There is no single correct approach; however, we provide a comprehensive and helpful framework for narrowing the diagnostic process. In summary, first, we need to define the problem (**Decision Tree 1**; Fig. 4.2), then focus on the predominant sleep phase (early, middle, or late) disruption. From there, psychiatric, medication, substance use, and systemic medical causes can be considered (**Decision Tree 2**; Fig. 4.3). If necessary, utilizing the rating scales we described in this chapter may further narrow down systemic medical disorders presenting as insomnia. We find most sleep

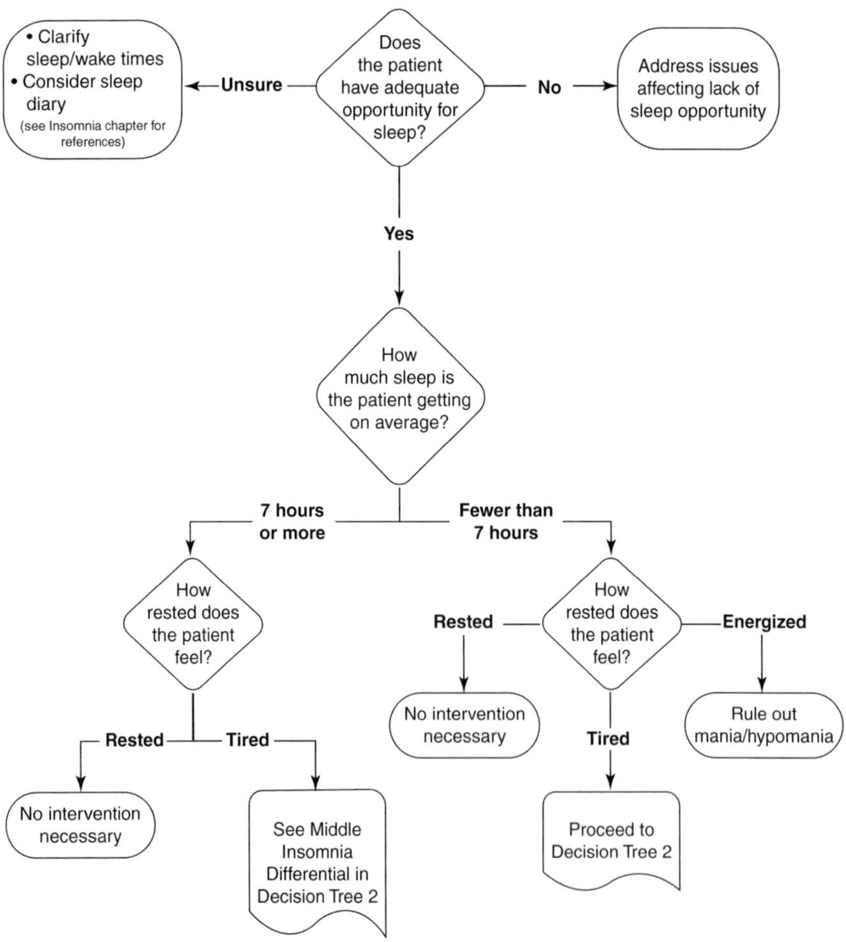

Fig. 4.2 Decision tree 1

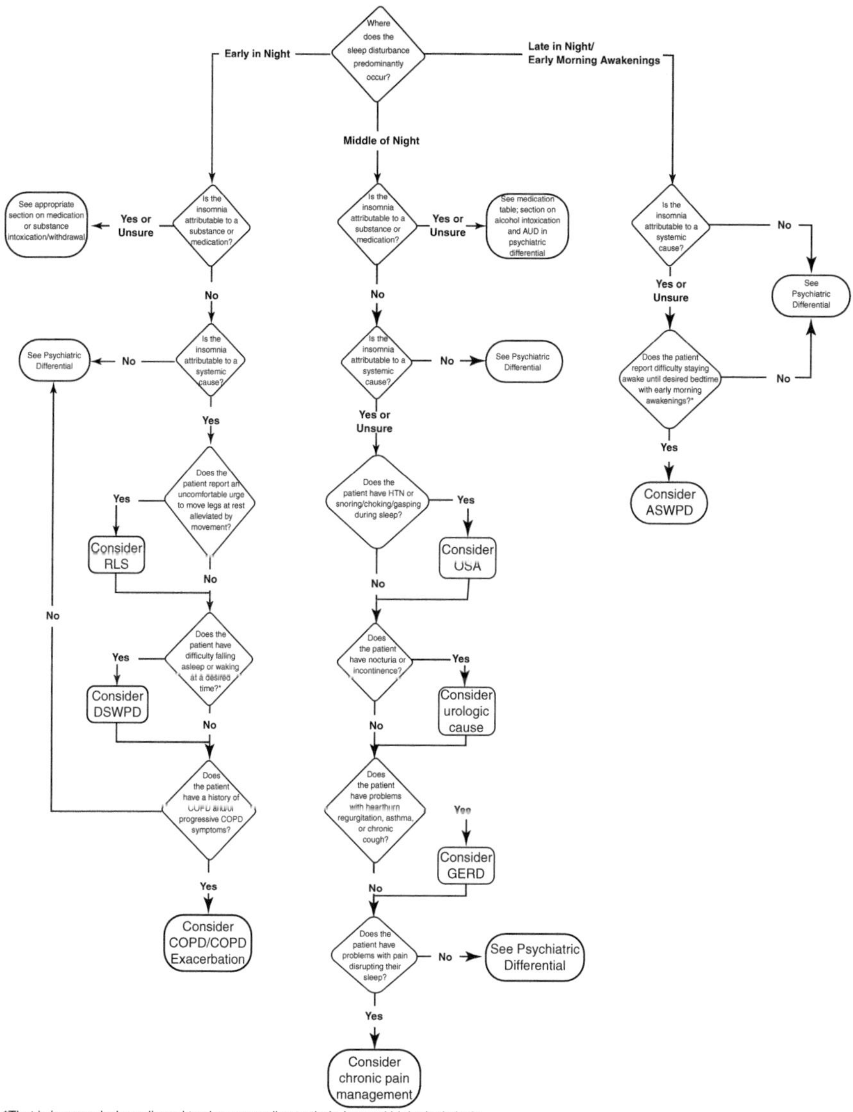

*That is improved when allowed to sleep according to their internal biological clock

Fig. 4.3 Decision tree 2

conditions predominantly affect early sleep, then middle sleep, with few affecting the late phase of sleep. We remind readers that these distinctions are meant as general guidelines as sleep complaints may be derived from—and affect—multiple phases of sleep. You may have to explore multiple diagnoses in each of the phase categories before the primary underlying cause is identified. For patients that continue to elude this diagnostic process, consultation with a sleep specialist is strongly encouraged.

Instructions: Start with **Decision Tree 1** to help differentiate insomnia from other symptoms. If you get to Question 4, determine if sleep disruption occurs predominantly in the early, middle, or late phases of sleep. Find that respective heading under **Decision Tree 2**.

References

1. Hammond WA. Sleep and its derangements. London: Forgotten Books; 2015.
2. Kryger MH. Atlas of clinical sleep medicine: expert consult - online and print. Saunders; 2014.
3. National Institutes of Health Consensus Development Conference Statement. Drugs and Insomnia: the use of medications to promote sleep [Internet]. 1983. https://consensus.nih.gov/1983/1983insomniadrugs039html.htm.
4. National Institutes of Health. National Institutes of Health State of the Science Conference statement on manifestations and management of chronic insomnia in adults, June 13–15, 2005. Sleep. 2005;28:1049–57.
5. Edinger JD, Kryger MH, Roth T. Insomnia. In: Kryger MH, editor. Atlas of clinical sleep medicine. 2nd ed. Philadelphia: Saunders; 2014. p. 148–58.
6. Kryger MH, Roth T, Dement WC. Principles and practice of sleep medicine. Philadelphia, PA: Elsevier; 2017.
7. Spielman AJ, Caruso LS, Glovinsky PB. A behavioral perspective on insomnia treatment. Psychiatr Clin North Am. 1987;10(4):541–53.
8. Perlis M, Shaw PJ, Cano G, Espie CA. Models of insomnia. In: Kryger MH, Roth T, Dement WC, editors. Principles and practice of sleep medicine. Elsevier; 2011. p. 850–65.
9. Perlis ML, Gehrman P. Types of insomnia. In: Kushida CA, editor. Encyclopedia of sleep. Academic Press: London; 2013. p. 199–202.
10. Riemann D, Spiegelhalder K, Feige B, Voderholzer U, Berger M, Perlis M, et al. The hyperarousal model of insomnia: a review of the concept and its evidence. Sleep Med Rev. 2010;14(1):19–31.
11. Bjorness TE, Greene RW. Adenosine and sleep. Curr Neuropharmacol. 2009;7(3):238–45.
12. Levenson JC, Kay DB, Buysse DJ. The pathophysiology of insomnia. Chest. 2015;147(4):1179–92.
13. Hirshkowitz M, Whiton K, Albert SM, Alessi C, Bruni O, DonCarlos L, et al. National Sleep Foundation's sleep time duration recommendations: methodology and results summary. Sleep Health. 2015;1(1):40–3.
14. "Sleep-Wake Disorders" in American Psychiatric Association. Diagnostic and statistical manual of mental disorders. 5th ed., text rev. Washington, DC: American Psychiatric Association; 2022. pp 407–76.
15. Sleep-Wakefulness [Internet]. Nih.gov. [cited 2021 Nov 23]. https://www.nimh.nih.gov/research/research-funded-by-nimh/rdoc/constructs/sleep-wakefulness.
16. Kelly MR, Killgore WDS, Haynes PL. Understanding recent insights in sleep and posttraumatic stress disorder from a research domain criteria (RDoC) framework. Curr Sleep Med Rep. 2016;2(4):223–32.
17. Whitehead K, Beaumont M. Insomnia: a cultural history. Lancet. 2018;391(10138):2408–9.
18. Summers-Bremner E. Insomnia: a cultural history. London: Reaktion Books; 2008.
19. Katzman MA, Bleau P, Blier P, Chokka P, Kjernisted K, Van Ameringen M, et al. Canadian clinical practice guidelines for the management of anxiety, posttraumatic stress and obsessive-compulsive disorders. BMC Psychiatry. 2014;14(Suppl 1):S1.
20. Kessler RC, Petukhova M, Sampson NA, Zaslavsky AM, Wittchen H-U. Twelve-month and lifetime prevalence and lifetime morbid risk of anxiety and mood disorders in the United States. Int J Methods Psychiatr Res. 2012;21(3):169–84. https://doi.org/10.1002/mpr.1359.
21. DeMartini J, Patel G, Fancher TL. Generalized anxiety disorder. Ann Intern Med. 2019;170(7):ITC49–64.

22. Ferre Navarrete F, Pérez Páramo M, Fermin Ordoño J, López Gómez V. Prevalence of insomnia and associated factors in outpatients with generalized anxiety disorder treated in psychiatric clinics. Behav Sleep Med. 2017;15(6):491–501.
23. Hoge EA, Ivkovic A, Fricchione GL. Generalized anxiety disorder: diagnosis and treatment. BMJ. 2012;345(v27 2):e7500.
24. "Substance/Medication-Induced Sleep Disorder" in American Psychiatric Association. Diagnostic and statistical manual of mental disorders. 5th ed., text rev. Washington, DC: American Psychiatric Association; 2022. pp 468–74.
25. Sachdeva A, Choudhary M, Chandra M. Alcohol withdrawal syndrome: benzodiazepines and beyond. J Clin Diagn Res. 2015;9(9):VE01–7.
26. Perney P, Lehert P. Insomnia in alcohol-dependent patients: prevalence, risk factors and acamprosate effect: an individual patient data meta-analysis. Alcohol Alcohol. 2018;53(5):611–8.
27. Garcia AN, Salloum IM. Polysomnographic sleep disturbances in nicotine, caffeine, alcohol, cocaine, opioid, and cannabis use: a focused review: polysomnographic changes in substance use. Am J Addict. 2015;24(7):590–8.
28. Withdrawal Syndromes Workup [Internet]. Medscape.com. 2021. [cited 2021 Nov 23]. https://emedicine.medscape.com/article/819502-workup.
29. Hughes JR, Oliveto AH, Liguori A, Carpenter J, Howard T. Endorsement of DSM-IV dependence criteria among caffeine users. Drug Alcohol Depend. 1998;52(2):99–107.
30. Copeland J, Pokorski I. Progress toward pharmacotherapies for cannabis-use disorder: an evidence-based review. Subst Abus Rehabil. 2016;7:41–53.
31. Rella JG. Recreational cannabis use: pleasures and pitfalls. Cleve Clin J Med. 2015;82(11):765 72.
32. Livne O, Shmulewitz D, Lev-Ran S, Hasin DS. DSM-5 cannabis withdrawal syndrome: demographic and clinical correlates in U.S. adults. Drug Alcohol Depend. 2019;195:170–7.
33. Schwartz BG, Rezkalla S, Kloner RA. Cardiovascular effects of cocaine. Circulation. 2010;122(24):2558–69.
34. Van Gastel A. Drug-induced insomnia and excessive sleepiness. Sleep Med Clin. 2018;13(2):147–59.
35. UpToDate [Internet]. Uptodate.com. [cited 2021 Nov 23]. https://www.uptodate.com/contents/risk-factors-comorbidities-and-consequences-of-insomnia-in-adults?search=insomnia&source=search_result&selectedTitle=5~150&usage_type=default&display_rank=5.
36. Schutte-Rodin S, Broch L, Buysse D, Dorsey C, Sateia M. Clinical guideline for the evaluation and management of chronic insomnia in adults. J Clin Sleep Med. 2008;4(5):487–504.
37. Edmunds AL. Psychotic and bipolar disorders: schizophrenia. FP Essent. 2017;455:11–7.
38. Kahn RS, Sommer IE, Murray RM, Meyer-Lindenberg A, Weinberger DR, Cannon TD, et al. Schizophrenia. Nat Rev Dis Primers. 2015; https://doi.org/10.1038/nrdp.2015.67.
39. Oliveira P, Coroa M, Madeira N. Treatment options for insomnia in schizophrenia: a systematic review. Pharmacopsychiatry. 2019;52(4):165–9.
40. Merikangas KR, Akiskal HS, Angst J, Greenberg PE, Hirschfeld RMA, Petukhova M, et al. Lifetime and 12-month prevalence of bipolar spectrum disorder in the national comorbidity survey replication. Arch Gen Psychiatry. 2007;64(5):543.
41. Grande I, Berk M, Birmaher B, Vieta E. Bipolar disorder. Lancet. 2016;387(10027):1561–72.
42. Yatham LN, Kennedy SH, Parikh SV, Schaffer A, Bond DJ, Frey BN, et al. Canadian Network for Mood and Anxiety Treatments (CANMAT) and International Society for Bipolar Disorders (ISBD) 2018 guidelines for the management of patients with bipolar disorder. Bipolar Disord. 2018;20(2):97–170.
43. Serretti A, Olgiati P. Profiles of "manic" symptoms in bipolar I, bipolar II and major depressive disorders. J Affect Disord. 2005;84(2–3):159–66.
44. Harvey AG, Talbot LS, Gershon A. Sleep disturbance in bipolar disorder across the lifespan. Clin Psychol (New York). 2009;16(2):256–77.
45. UpToDate [Internet]. Uptodate.com. [cited 2021 Nov 23]. https://www.uptodate.com/contents/sleep-wake-disorders-in-patients-with-traumatic-brain-injury?search=insomnia&topicRef=97867&source=see_link.

46. Haider MN, Leddy JJ, Du W, Macfarlane AJ, Viera KB, Willer BS. Practical management: brief physical examination for sport-related concussion in the outpatient setting. Clin J Sport Med. 2018;30(5):513–7.
47. Overview | Head injury: assessment and early management | Guidance | NICE. [cited 2021 Nov 23]. https://www.nice.org.uk/guidance/cg176.
48. McCrory P, Meeuwisse W, Dvorak J, Aubry M, Bailes J, Broglio S, et al. Consensus statement on concussion in sport—the 5th International Conference on Concussion in Sport Held in Berlin, October 2016. Br J Sports Med. 2017; https://doi.org/10.1136/bjsports-2017-097699.
49. VA/DoD clinical practice guidelines [Internet]. Healthquality.va.gov. [cited 2021 Nov 23]. https://www.healthquality.va.gov/guidelines/rehab/mtbi/.
50. Warner CH, Warner CM, Appenzeller GN, Hoge CW. Identifying and managing posttraumatic stress disorder. Am Fam Physician. 2013;88(12):827–34.
51. Hines LA, Sundin J, Rona RJ, Wessely S, Fear NT. Posttraumatic stress disorder post Iraq and Afghanistan: prevalence among military subgroups. Can J Psychiatr. 2014;59(9):468–79.
52. Wallace DM, Shafazand S, Ramos AR, Carvalho DZ, Gardener H, Lorenzo D, et al. Insomnia characteristics and clinical correlates in Operation Enduring Freedom/Operation Iraqi Freedom veterans with post-traumatic stress disorder and mild traumatic brain injury: an exploratory study. Sleep Med. 2011;12(9):850–9.
53. Kobayashi I, Boarts JM, Delahanty DL. Polysomnographically measured sleep abnormalities in PTSD: a meta-analytic review. Psychophysiology. 2007;44(4):660–9.
54. Barbato G, Barker C, Bender C, Giesen HA, Wehr TA. Extended sleep in humans in 14 hour nights (LD 10:14): relationship between REM density and spontaneous awakening. Electroencephalogr Clin Neurophysiol. 1994;90(4):291–7.
55. Mellman TA, Kumar A, Kulick-Bell R, Kumar M, Nolan B. Nocturnal/daytime urine noradrenergic measures and sleep in combat-related PTSD. Biol Psychiatry. 1995;38(3):174–9.
56. Woodward SH, Murburg MM, Bliwise DL. PTSD-related hyperarousal assessed during sleep. Physiol Behav. 2000;70(1–2):197–203.
57. Kanny D, Brewer RD, Mesnick JB, Paulozzi LJ, Naimi TS, Lu H. Vital signs: alcohol poisoning deaths - United States, 2010–2012. MMWR Morb Mortal Wkly Rep. 2015;63(53):1238–42.
58. Grant BF, Goldstein RB, Saha TD, Chou SP, Jung J, Zhang H, et al. Epidemiology of DSM-5 alcohol use disorder: results from the National Epidemiologic Survey on alcohol and related conditions III. JAMA Psychiat. 2015;72(8):757–66.
59. Thakkar MM, Sharma R, Sahota P. Alcohol disrupts sleep homeostasis. Alcohol. 2015;49(4):299–310.
60. Conroy DA, Arnedt JT. Sleep and substance use disorders: an update. Curr Psychiatry Rep. 2014;16(10):487.
61. Karg RS, Bose J, Batts KR, et al. Past year mental disorders among adults in the United States: results from the 2008–2012 Mental Health Surveillance Study. CBHSQ Data Review, vol. 232. Rockville, MD: Substance Abuse and Mental Health Services Administration (US); 2014. p. 10.
62. Kessler RC, Ormel J, Petukhova M, McLaughlin KA, Green JG, Russo LJ, et al. Development of lifetime comorbidity in the World Health Organization world mental health surveys. Arch Gen Psychiatry. 2011;68(1):90–100.
63. Pedersen CB, Mors O, Bertelsen A, Waltoft BL, Agerbo E, McGrath JJ, et al. A comprehensive nationwide study of the incidence rate and lifetime risk for treated mental disorders. JAMA Psychiat. 2014;71(5):573–81.
64. Murphy MJ, Peterson MJ. Sleep disturbances in depression. Sleep Med Clin. 2015;10(1):17–23.
65. Peterson MJ, Benca RM. Sleep in mood disorders. Psychiatr Clin North Am. 2006;29(4):1009–32. abstract ix
66. Bjorøy I, Jørgensen VA, Pallesen S, Bjorvatn B. The prevalence of insomnia subtypes in relation to demographic characteristics, anxiety, depression, alcohol consumption and use of hypnotics. Front Psychol. 2020;11:527.

67. Coleman MY, McGlashan EM, Vidafar P, Phillips AJK, Cain SW. Advanced melatonin onset relative to sleep in women with unmedicated major depressive disorder. Chronobiol Int. 2019;36(10):1373–83.
68. Emens J, Lewy A, Kinzie JM, Arntz D, Rough J. Circadian misalignment in major depressive disorder. Psychiatry Res. 2009;168(3):259–61.
69. McGlashan EM, Nandam LS, Vidafar P, Mansfield DR, Rajaratnam SMW, Cain SW. The SSRI citalopram increases the sensitivity of the human circadian system to light in an acute dose. Psychopharmacology. 2018;235(11):3201–9.
70. Robillard R, Carpenter JS, Rogers NL, Fares S, Grierson AB, Hermens DF, et al. Circadian rhythms and psychiatric profiles in young adults with unipolar depressive disorders. Transl Psychiatry. 2018;8(1):213.
71. American Psychiatric Association. Depressive disorders. In: American Psychiatric Association, editor. Diagnostic and statistical manual of mental disorders. 5th ed. Arlington, VA: American Psychiatric Association; 2013. p. 155–88.
72. Beck AT. The evolution of the cognitive model of depression and its neurobiological correlates. Am J Psychiatry. 2008;165(8):969–77.
73. Garcia-Borreguero D, Cano-Pumarega I. New concepts in the management of restless legs syndrome. BMJ. 2017;356:j104.
74. Innes KE, Selfe TK, Agarwal P. Prevalence of restless legs syndrome in North American and Western European populations: a systematic review. Sleep Med. 2011;12(7):623–34.
75. Cho S-J, Hong JP, Hahm B-J, Jeon HJ, Chang SM, Cho MJ, et al. Restless legs syndrome in a community sample of Korean adults: prevalence, impact on quality of life, and association with DSM-IV psychiatric disorders. Sleep. 2009;32(8):1069–76.
76. Hening W, Walters AS, Allen RP, Montplaisir J, Myers A, Ferini-Strambi L. Impact, diagnosis and treatment of restless legs syndrome (RLS) in a primary care population: the REST (RLS epidemiology, symptoms, and treatment) primary care study. Sleep Med. 2004;5(3):237–46.
77. Trenkwalder C, Högl B, Winkelmann J. Recent advances in the diagnosis, genetics and treatment of restless legs syndrome. J Neurol. 2009;256(4):539–53.
78. Winkelmann J, Prager M, Lieb R, Pfister H, Spiegel B, Wittchen H-U, et al. "Anxietas tibiarum". Depression and anxiety disorders in patients with restless legs syndrome: depression and anxiety disorders in patients with restless legs syndrome. J Neurol. 2005;252(1):67–71
79. Durmer JS, Quraishi GH. Restless legs syndrome, periodic leg movements, and periodic limb movement disorder in children. Pediatr Clin N Am. 2011;58(3):591–620.
80. Trenkwalder C, Paulus W. Restless legs syndrome: pathophysiology, clinical presentation and management. Nat Rev Neurol. 2010;6(6):337–46.
81. Garcia-Borreguero D, Stillman P, Benes H, Buschmann H, Chaudhuri KR, Gonzalez Rodríguez VM, et al. Algorithms for the diagnosis and treatment of restless legs syndrome in primary care. BMC Neurol. 2011;11(1):28.
82. Benes H, Kohnen R. Validation of an algorithm for the diagnosis of restless legs syndrome: the Restless Legs Syndrome-Diagnostic Index (RLS-DI). Sleep Med. 2009;10(5):515–23.
83. Trotti LM, Rye DB. Restless legs syndrome. Handb Clin Neurol. 2011;100:661–73.
84. Stiasny-Kolster K, Kohnen R, Möller JC, Trenkwalder C, Oertel WH. Validation of the "L-DOPA test" for diagnosis of restless legs syndrome. Mov Disord. 2006;21(9):1333–9.
85. Sivertsen B, Pallesen S, Stormark KM, Bøe T, Lundervold AJ, Hysing M. Delayed sleep phase syndrome in adolescents: prevalence and correlates in a large population based study. BMC Public Health. 2013;13(1):1163.
86. Yazaki M, Shirakawa S, Okawa M, Takahashi K. Demography of sleep disturbances associated with circadian rhythm disorders in Japan. Psychiatry Clin Neurosci. 1999;53(2):267–8.
87. Magee M, Marbas EM, Wright KP Jr, Rajaratnam SMW, Broussard JL. Diagnosis, cause, and treatment approaches for delayed sleep-wake phase disorder. Sleep Med Clin. 2016;11(3):389–401.
88. Pavlova M. Circadian rhythm sleep-wake disorders. Continuum (Minneap Minn). 2017;23(4):1051–63.

89. American Academy of Sleep Medicine. International classification of sleep disorders. 3rd ed. Darien, IL: American Academy of Sleep Medicine; 2014.
90. Morgenthaler TI, Lee-Chiong T, Alessi C, Friedman L, Aurora RN, Boehlecke B, et al. Practice parameters for the clinical evaluation and treatment of circadian rhythm sleep disorders. An American Academy of Sleep Medicine report. Sleep. 2007;30(11):1445–59.
91. Marino M, Li Y, Rueschman MN, Winkelman JW, Ellenbogen JM, Solet JM, et al. Measuring sleep: accuracy, sensitivity, and specificity of wrist actigraphy compared to polysomnography. Sleep. 2013;36(11):1747–55.
92. Morgenthaler T, Alessi C, Friedman L, Owens J, Kapur V, Boehlecke B, et al. Practice parameters for the use of actigraphy in the assessment of sleep and sleep disorders: an update for 2007. Sleep. 2007;30(4):519–29.
93. Smith MT, McCrae CS, Cheung J, Martin JL, Harrod CG, Heald JL, et al. Use of actigraphy for the evaluation of sleep disorders and circadian rhythm sleep-wake disorders: an American Academy of Sleep Medicine systematic review, meta-analysis, and GRADE assessment. J Clin Sleep Med. 2018;14(07):1209–30.
94. Sack RL, Auckley D, Auger RR, Carskadon MA, Wright KP Jr, Vitiello MV, et al. Circadian rhythm sleep disorders: Part II, Advanced sleep phase disorder, delayed sleep phase disorder, free-running disorder, and irregular sleep-wake rhythm. An American Academy of Sleep Medicine review. Sleep. 2007;30(11):1484–501.
95. Global Initiative for Chronic Obstructive Lung Disease. Global strategy for the diagnosis, management, and prevention of COPD. GOLD 2020. 2020. Fontana, WI.
96. Halbert RJ, Isonaka S, George D, Iqbal A. Interpreting COPD prevalence estimates: what is the true burden of disease? Chest. 2003;123(5):1684–92.
97. Centers for Disease Control and Prevention (CDC). Chronic obstructive pulmonary disease among adults—United States, 2011. MMWR Morb Mortal Wkly Rep. 2012;61(46):938–43.
98. Vukoja M, Kopitovic I, Milicic D, Maksimovic O, Pavlovic-Popovic Z, Ilic M. Sleep quality and daytime sleepiness in patients with COPD and asthma. Clin Respir J. 2018;12(2):398–403.
99. Stephens MB, Yew KS. Diagnosis of chronic obstructive pulmonary disease. Am Fam Physician. 2008;78(1):87–92.
100. de Mattos WLLD, Signori LGH, Borges FK, Bergamin JA, Machado V. Tital: Accuracy of clinical examination findings in the diagnosis of COPD. J Bras Pneumol. 2009;35(5):404–8.
101. Demirci H, Eniste K, Basaran EO, Ocakoglu G, Yilmaz Z, Tuna S. A multicenter family practitioners' research on chronic obstructive pulmonary disease screening using the COPD assessment test. Prim Health Care Res Dev. 2017;18(6):603–7.
102. Ban WH, Joo H, Lim JU, Kang HH, Moon HS, Lee SH. The relationship between sleep disturbance and health status in patients with COPD. Int J Chron Obstruct Pulmon Dis. 2018;13:2049–55.
103. Young T, Palta M, Dempsey J, Peppard PE, Nieto FJ, Hla KM. Burden of sleep apnea: rationale, design, and major findings of the Wisconsin Sleep Cohort study. WMJ. 2009;108(5):246–9.
104. Peppard PE, Young T, Barnet JH, Palta M, Hagen EW, Hla KM. Increased prevalence of sleep-disordered breathing in adults. Am J Epidemiol. 2013;177(9):1006–14.
105. Johns M. About the ESS [Internet]. Epworth Sleepiness Scale. [cited 2021 Dec 19]. https://epworthsleepinessscale.com/about-the-ess/.
106. Myers KA, Mrkobrada M, Simel DL. Does this patient have obstructive sleep apnea?: the rational clinical examination systematic review. JAMA. 2013;310(7):731–41.
107. Russell MB, Kristiansen HA, Kværner KJ. Headache in sleep apnea syndrome: epidemiology and pathophysiology. Cephalalgia. 2014;34(10):752–5.
108. Lin C-H, Perger E, Lyons OD. Obstructive sleep apnea and chronic kidney disease. Curr Opin Pulm Med. 2018;24(6):549–54. https://doi.org/10.1097/MCP.0000000000000525.
109. Reutrakul S, Mokhlesi B. Obstructive sleep apnea and diabetes: a state of the art review. Chest. 2017;152(5):1070–86.
110. Flemons WW, Whitelaw WA, Brant R, Remmers JE. Likelihood ratios for a sleep apnea clinical prediction rule. Am J Respir Crit Care Med. 1994;150(5 Pt 1):1279–85.

111. Kapur VK, Auckley DH, Chowdhuri S, Kuhlmann DC, Mehra R, Ramar K, et al. Clinical practice guideline for diagnostic testing for adult obstructive sleep apnea: an American Academy of Sleep Medicine clinical practice guideline. J Clin Sleep Med. 2017;13(03):479–504.
112. Friedman M, Hamilton C, Samuelson CG, Lundgren ME, Pott T. Diagnostic value of the Friedman tongue position and Mallampati classification for obstructive sleep apnea: a meta-analysis. Otolaryngol Head Neck Surg. 2013;148(4):540–7.
113. Chiu H-Y, Chen P-Y, Chuang L-P, Chen N-H, Tu Y-K, Hsieh Y-J, et al. Diagnostic accuracy of the Berlin questionnaire, STOP-BANG, STOP, and Epworth sleepiness scale in detecting obstructive sleep apnea: a bivariate meta-analysis. Sleep Med Rev. 2017;36:57–70.
114. Chung F, Yegneswaran B, Liao P, Chung SA, Vairavanathan S, Islam S, et al. STOP questionnaire: a tool to screen patients for obstructive sleep apnea. Anesthesiology. 2008;108(5):812–21.
115. Araujo AB, Yaggi HK, Yang M, McVary KT, Fang SC, Bliwise DL. Sleep related problems and urological symptoms: testing the hypothesis of bidirectionality in a longitudinal, population based study. J Urol. 2014;191(1):100–6.
116. Patel SR, Hu FB. Short sleep duration and weight gain: a systematic review. Obesity (Silver Spring). 2008;16(3):643–53.
117. Spiegel K, Leproult R, Van Cauter E. Impact of sleep debt on metabolic and endocrine function. Lancet. 1999;354(9188):1435–9.
118. Yaggi HK, Araujo AB, McKinlay JB. Sleep duration as a risk factor for the development of type 2 diabetes. Diabetes Care. 2006;29(3):657–61.
119. Simpson N, Dinges DF. Sleep and inflammation. Nutr Rev. 2007;65(12 Pt 2):S244–52.
120. Fitzgerald MP, Mulligan M, Parthasarathy S. Nocturic frequency is related to severity of obstructive sleep apnea, improves with continuous positive airways treatment. Am J Obstet Gynecol. 2006;194(5):1399–403.
121. Pressman MR, Figueroa WG, Kendrick-Mohamed J, Greenspon LW, Peterson DD. Nocturia. A rarely recognized symptom of sleep apnea and other occult sleep disorders. Arch Intern Med. 1996;156(5):545–50.
122. Wei JT, Calhoun E, Jacobsen SJ. Urologic diseases in America project: benign prostatic hyperplasia. J Urol. 2005;173(4):1256–61.
123. Chute CG, Panser LA, Girman CJ, Oesterling JE, Guess HA, Jacobsen SJ, et al. The prevalence of prostatism: a population-based survey of urinary symptoms. J Urol. 1993;150(1):85–9.
124. Roehrborn CG. Accurate determination of prostate size via digital rectal examination and transrectal ultrasound. Urology. 1998;51(4):19–22.
125. Pinsky PF, Kramer BS, Crawford ED, Grubb RL, Urban DA, Andriole GL, et al. Prostate volume and prostate-specific antigen levels in men enrolled in a large screening trial. Urology. 2006;68(2):352–6.
126. McVary KT, Roehrborn CG, Avins AL, Barry MJ, Bruskewitz RC, Donnell RF, et al. Update on AUA guideline on the management of benign prostatic hyperplasia. J Urol. 2011;185(5):1793–803.
127. Khadra MH, Pickard RS, Charlton M, Powell PH, Neal DE. A prospective analysis of 1,930 patients with hematuria to evaluate current diagnostic practice. J Urol. 2000;163(2):524–7.
128. Butler SS, Muralidhar V, Zhao SG, Sanford NN, Franco I, Fullerton ZH, et al. Prostate cancer incidence across stage, NCCN risk groups, and age before and after USPSTF Grade D recommendations against prostate-specific antigen screening in 2012. Cancer. 2020;126(4):717–24.
129. Foster HE, Barry MJ, Dahm P, Gandhi MC, Kaplan SA, Kohler TS, et al. Surgical management of lower urinary tract symptoms attributed to benign prostatic hyperplasia: AUA guideline. J Urol. 2018,200(3):612–9.
130. Liao C-H, Chung S-D, Kuo H-C. Diagnostic value of International Prostate Symptom Score voiding-to-storage subscore ratio in male lower urinary tract symptoms: diagnostic value of IPSS subscores. Int J Clin Pract. 2011;65(5):552–8. https://doi.org/10.1111/j.1742-1241.2011.02638.x.
131. Haylen BT, de Ridder D, Freeman RM, Swift SE, Berghmans B, Lee J, et al. An International Urogynecological Association (IUGA)/International Continence Society (ICS) joint report

on the terminology for female pelvic floor dysfunction: terminology for female pelvic floor dysfunction. Neurourol Urodyn. 2010;29(1):4–20.
132. Hartmann KE, McPheeters ML, Biller DH, Ward RM, McKoy JN, Jerome RN, et al. Treatment of overactive bladder in women. Evid Rep Technol Assess (Full Rep). 2009;(187):1–120, v.
133. Dmochowski RR, Gomelsky A. Overactive bladder in males. Ther Adv Urol. 2009;1(4):209–21.
134. Shamliyan T, Wyman J, Bliss DZ, Kane RL, Wilt TJ. Prevention of urinary and fecal incontinence in adults. Evid Rep Technol Assess (Full Rep). 2007;(161):1–379.
135. Fitzgerald MP, Thom DH, Wassel-Fyr C, Subak L, Brubaker L, Van Den Eeden SK, et al. Childhood urinary symptoms predict adult overactive bladder symptoms. J Urol. 2006;175(3 Pt 1):989–93.
136. Nygaard I. Clinical practice. Idiopathic urgency urinary incontinence. N Engl J Med. 2010;363(12):1156–62.
137. Suskind AM, Dunn RL, Morgan DM, DeLancey JOL, McGuire EJ, Wei JT. The Michigan Incontinence Symptom Index (M-ISI): a clinical measure for type, severity, and bother related to urinary incontinence: Incontinence Symptom Index. Neurourol Urodyn. 2014;33(7):1128–34.
138. Vakil N, van Zanten SV, Kahrilas P, Dent J, Jones R, Global Consensus Group. The Montreal definition and classification of gastroesophageal reflux disease: a global evidence-based consensus. Am J Gastroenterol. 2006;101(8):1900–20. quiz 1943
139. Richter JE. Typical and atypical presentations of gastroesophageal reflux disease. The role of esophageal testing in diagnosis and management. Gastroenterol Clin N Am. 1996;25(1):75–102.
140. Giannini EG, Zentilin P, Dulbecco P, Vigneri S, Scarlata P, Savarino V. Management strategy for patients with gastroesophageal reflux disease: a comparison between empirical treatment with esomeprazole and endoscopy-oriented treatment. Am J Gastroenterol. 2008;103(2):267–75.
141. Dent J, Vakil N, Jones R, Bytzer P, Schoning U, Halling K, et al. Accuracy of the diagnosis of GORD by questionnaire, physicians and a trial of proton pump inhibitor treatment: the Diamond Study. Gut. 2010;59(6):714–21.
142. Zagari RM, Fuccio L, Wallander M-A, Johansson S, Fiocca R, Casanova S, et al. Gastro-oesophageal reflux symptoms, oesophagitis and Barrett's oesophagus in the general population: the Loiano-Monghidoro study. Gut. 2008;57(10):1354–9.
143. Gyawali CP, Kahrilas PJ, Savarino E, Zerbib F, Mion F, Smout AJPM, et al. Modern diagnosis of GERD: the Lyon consensus. Gut. 2018;67(7):1351–62.
144. Moayyedi P, Lacy BE, Andrews CN, Enns RA, Howden CW, Vakil N. ACG and CAG clinical guideline: management of dyspepsia. Am J Gastroenterol. 2017;112(7):988–1013.
145. ASGE Standards of Practice Committee, Muthusamy VR, Lightdale JR, Acosta RD, Chandrasekhara V, Chathadi KV, et al. The role of endoscopy in the management of GERD. Gastrointest Endosc. 2015;81(6):1305–10.
146. Jones R, Junghard O, Dent J, Vakil N, Halling K, Wernersson B, et al. Development of the GerdQ, a tool for the diagnosis and management of gastro-oesophageal reflux disease in primary care. Aliment Pharmacol Ther. 2009;30(10):1030–8.
147. Numans ME, Lau J, de Wit NJ, Bonis PA. Short-term treatment with proton-pump inhibitors as a test for gastroesophageal reflux disease: a meta-analysis of diagnostic test characteristics. Ann Intern Med. 2004;140(7):518.
148. Kellerman R, Kintanar T. Gastroesophageal reflux disease. Prim Care. 2017;44(4):561–73.
149. Harnik IG. Gastroesophageal reflux disease. Ann Intern Med. 2015;163(1):ITC1–16.
150. Xu X, Chen Q, Liang S, Lv H, Qiu Z. Comparison of gastroesophageal reflux disease questionnaire and multichannel intraluminal impedance pH monitoring in identifying patients with chronic cough responsive to antireflux therapy. Chest. 2014;145(6):1264–70. https://doi.org/10.1378/chest.13-1634.
151. Treede R-D, Rief W, Barke A, Aziz Q, Bennett MI, Benoliel R, et al. Chronic pain as a symptom or a disease: the IASP classification of chronic pain for the International Classification of Diseases (ICD-11). Pain. 2019;160(1):19–27.

152. Currow DC, Agar M, Plummer JL, Blyth FM, Abernethy AP. Chronic pain in South Australia - population levels that interfere extremely with activities of daily living. Aust N Z J Public Health. 2010;34(3):232–9.
153. Goldberg DS, McGee SJ. Pain as a global public health priority. BMC Public Health. 2011;11(1):770.
154. Henderson JV, Harrison CM, Britt HC, Bayram CF, Miller GC. Prevalence, causes, severity, impact, and management of chronic pain in Australian general practice patients. Pain Med. 2013;14(9):1346–61.
155. Patel KV, Guralnik JM, Dansie EJ, Turk DC. Prevalence and impact of pain among older adults in the United States: findings from the 2011 National Health and Aging Trends Study. Pain. 2013;154(12):2649–57.
156. Pitcher MH, Von Korff M, Bushnell MC, Porter L. Prevalence and profile of high-impact chronic pain in the United States. J Pain. 2019;20(2):146–60.
157. International Association for the Study of Pain. Chronic pain management: measurement-based step care solutions. Pain Clin Updates. 2012;10:1–8.
158. Mathias JL, Cant ML, Burke ALJ. Sleep disturbances and sleep disorders in adults living with chronic pain: a meta-analysis. Sleep Med. 2018;52:198–210.
159. Reid MC, Eccleston C, Pillemer K. Management of chronic pain in older adults. BMJ. 2015;350(feb13 2):h532.
160. Erdemoglu AK, Koc R. Brief Pain Inventory score identifying and discriminating neuropathic and nociceptive pain. Acta Neurol Scand. 2013;128(5):351–8.
161. Paine S-J, Fink J, Gander PH, Warman GR. Identifying advanced and delayed sleep phase disorders in the general population: a national survey of New Zealand adults. Chronobiol Int. 2014;31(5):627–36.
162. Curtis BJ, Ashbrook LH, Young T, Finn LA, Fu Y-H, Ptáček LJ, et al. Extreme morning chronotypes are often familial and not exceedingly rare: the estimated prevalence of advanced sleep phase, familial advanced sleep phase, and advanced sleep-wake phase disorder in a sleep clinic population. Sleep. 2019; https://doi.org/10.1093/sleep/zsz148.
163. Rahman SA, Kayumov L, Tchmoutina EA, Shapiro CM. Clinical efficacy of dim light melatonin onset testing in diagnosing delayed sleep phase syndrome. Sleep Med. 2009;10(5):549–55.
164. Dijk D-J, Duffy JF. Novel approaches for assessing circadian rhythmicity in humans: a review. J Biol Rhythm. 2020;35(5):421–38.
165. Martin J, Shochat T, Ancoli-Israel S. Assessment and treatment of sleep disturbances in older adults. Clin Psychol Rev. 2000;20(6):783–805.
166. Neubauer DN. Sleep problems in the elderly. Am Fam Physician. 1999;59(9):2551–8, 2559–60.

Dizziness

5

Rohul Amin, Adam L. Bumgardner, and Matthew T. Hunter

Defining Dizziness

The definition of "dizzy," according to Merriam-Webster, is "having a feeling of being whirled about and in danger of falling down" [1]. *Synonyms* for this specific term include, "aswoon, giddy, lightheaded, reeling, swimmy, vertiginous, whirling, and woozy." *Related* words include, "faint, befuddled, confused, dazed, and groggy" [1]. This is *not* an all-encompassing list and may have cultural aspects of presentations as discussed later in this chapter [p. 833].

Patients may use the term "dizziness" to refer to various subjective experiences related to sensations of disturbed relation to one's surroundings in space. It can be described as feelings of rotation or whirling, but also non-rotary swaying, weakness, or faintness [2]. Based on the ambiguous and subjective nature of the term dizziness, creating a differential for dizziness or operationalizing it as a useful diagnostic anchor is often not useful. Due to this lack of specificity, we recommend treating this term as a "complaint" rather than an actual "symptom." This must be done without discounting the experience of the patient. Further exploring this complaint often yields evidence of more specific and clinically meaningful symptoms of vertigo, syncope/presyncope, and disequilibrium/lightheadedness [3].

To this end, the patient should be asked "*what do you feel when you experience these symptoms or what do you mean when you say that you are dizzy?*" The

R. Amin (✉) · M. T. Hunter
National Capital Consortium Psychiatry Residency Program, Department of Consultation and Education, Walter Reed National Military Medical Center, Bethesda, MD, USA
e-mail: rohul.amin.mil@health.mil; matthew.t.hunter6.mil@health.mil

A. L. Bumgardner
National Capital Consortium Combined Internal Medicine/Psychiatry Residency Program, Department of Consultation and Education, Walter Reed National Military Medical Center, Bethesda, MD, USA
e-mail: adam.l.bumgardner.mil@health.mil

E. G. Meyer et al. (eds.), *The Medical Evaluation of Psychiatric Symptoms*,
https://doi.org/10.1007/978-3-031-14372-4_5

clinician should be empathic and allow the patient to describe their personal and subjective experience without interruptions to establish a shared mental model of understanding. More close-ended questions such as "*does the room spin?*" *Or* "*does the floor move?*" may help refine the complaint into one of the more specific categories. This is quite different from asking the patient if their vision became narrow, or if they are unable to recall events surrounding the event—questions that would indicate presyncopal and syncopal etiologies, respectively.

Separating Vertigo from Other Symptoms

As previously discussed in the introduction, vertigo is a possible symptom of a patient complaining of "dizziness." Other possible etiologies of dizziness are syncope and disequilibrium. Refer to Table 5.1 for an overview.

Syncope

Syncope is defined as a transient loss of consciousness secondary to inadequate cerebral perfusion with oxygenated blood. When the patient experiences a presyncope, there are feelings of passing out without actual loss of consciousness. Most etiologies that cause syncope can cause presyncope [3, 4]. There are many causes of syncope as identified in Table 5.1. Unlike syncope, vertigo does not result in loss of consciousness, and the patient experiences the spinning sensation.

Disequilibrium

Disequilibrium is referred to unsteadiness or a sense of disconnect from the environment. Its pathophysiology is often related to a disconnect or miscommunication between the central nervous system (somatosensory cortex and the cerebellum), and the peripheral nervous system such as the visual system, sensory fibers, and proprioception. It is typically associated with aging and can be attributed to the aging vestibular system that shows a decrease in neural and sensory cells. Other implicated mechanisms include attrition of cerebellar Purkinje cells over time, neuronal and fiber loss in the extrapyramidal system, and a general decline in postural control and reaction time. Risk factors include visual impairments, muscle weakness, medications, and cognitive impairment among others. Patients may describe this as a "feeling like being on a boat" but deny spinning of the environment symptoms which differentiates it from vertigo [5]. The differential is very large as listed in Table 5.1.

Each of the aforementioned three symptoms of vertigo, syncope/presyncope, and disequilibrium/lightheadedness provide the much-needed organization to help operationalize the clinical encounter to yield a working diagnosis [6]. This allows for the determination of appropriate triage, ascertainment of clinical acuity, and accuracy of diagnosis. The three categories enable the clinician to more focally consider a more limited set of systemic medical and psychiatric differential diagnostic considerations. Table 5.1 and Fig. 5.1 provide the differential for these three symptoms. Each of these symptoms may also point to the underlying pathophysiology. For example, vertigo symptoms either occur due to a dysfunction in the vestibular apparatus (peripheral anatomy) or central nervous system lesions such as in multiple

Table 5.1 Common medical and psychiatric conditions that may present with the complaint of "dizziness." Differentiation of this nonspecific term into either vertigo, syncope, or disequilibrium allows for a narrower medical and psychiatric differential diagnosis

Dizziness			
	Vertigo	Syncope	Disequilibrium
Description	False sense of motion or a spinning sensation	*Syncope*: loss of consciousness *Presyncope*: feelings of impending passing out *without* actual loss of consciousness	A feeling of disconnect from the environment or a sense of imbalance or unsteadiness
Medical conditions	*Peripheral*: • BPPV • Vestibular neuritis/labyrinthitis • Ménière's disease • Acoustic neuroma *Central*: • Vestibular migraine • Cerebellar hemorrhage or ischemia • Vertebrobasilar insufficiency • Chiari I malformation • Head or neck trauma • Multiple sclerosis • Neoplasm • Postural-perceptual dizziness	• Arrhythmia • Aortic stenosis • Pulmonary embolism • Cerebral stroke/bleed • Hypovolemia • Hemorrhage • Vasovagal • Hypoglycemia • Medications • Substance	• TIA or stroke • Peripheral neuropathy • Demyelinating disease • Motor neuron disease • Vitamin B12 deficiency • Parkinsonism • Myelopathy • Normal pressure hydrocephalus • Infection • Medications • Substances
Psychiatric conditions in DSM-5-TR	• Substance/medication-induced anxiety disorder • Anxiety disorder due to another medical condition • Major or mild neurocognitive disorder due to: traumatic brain injury; substance-induced; vascular; due to another medical condition, and neurocognitive disorder not elsewhere classified • Cultural concepts of distress	• Specific phobia • Functional neurological symptom disorder • Major or mild neurocognitive disorder with Lewy bodies • Cultural concepts of distress	• Depersonalization/derealization disorder • Trauma spectrum disorders • Anxiety disorders • Depressive disorders • Somatic symptom disorder • Conversion disorder • Cultural concepts of distress • Major or mild neurocognitive disorder due to: vascular neurocognitive disorder, neurocognitive disorder due to another medical condition (any of the disorders listed in medical conditions), and neurocognitive disorder not elsewhere classified

BPPV benign paroxysmal peripheral vertigo

sclerosis [7, 8]. Similarly, the sudden loss of consciousness associated with syncope points to an underlying loss of blood flow to the brain which can be due to "pump" or "plumbing" issues, i.e., cardiac or vascular, respectively. A large number of

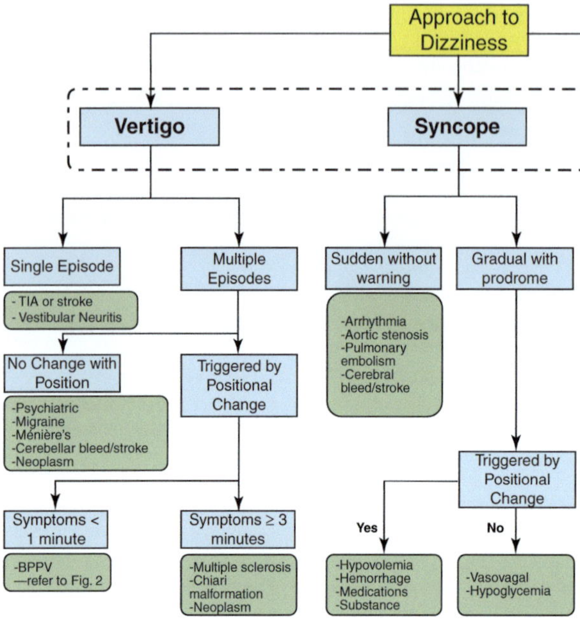

Fig. 5.1 Approach to dizziness involves clarification of the complaint into symptoms of syncope/presyncope; lightheadedness; and vertigo. Vertiginous symptoms are the most common presentation and can be approached using the algorithm based on the number of episodes, positional trigger, and duration of symptoms. Sudden syncopal episodes portend malignant etiology and immediate referral is needed. *TIA* transient ischemic attack, *BPPV* benign paroxysmal positional vertigo

etiologies such as mass, inflammatory, infectious, and metabolic etiologies can cause disruptions across these systems to result in disequilibrium.

Finally, as discussed later, the term "dizziness" may have other important clinical meanings when reviewed through a cultural lens. It is often a replacement term for various conditions such as depressive disorders, anxiety disorders, and trauma spectrum disorders.

As shown in Table 5.1, the differential for the three diagnostic categories is still broad; however, the majority of cases of dizziness end up with final diagnoses related to vertigo or psychiatric illness. One study showed that among 21,000 patients in Korea referred to a specialty dizziness clinic with dizziness complaints, 46.9% of patients were categorized into vertiginous etiologies with final diagnoses including benign paroxysmal positional vertigo (BPPV) 24.1%, vestibular migraine (10.2%), Ménière's disease (7.2%), and vestibular neuritis (5.4%). In 20.4% of the patients, the symptoms were attributed to psychiatric illnesses [9]. We only focus on vertigo, including psychiatric and cultural etiologies of this complaint in this chapter, which covers the majority of causes of "dizziness" symptoms, but the reader is encouraged to refer to additional sources on approaches to syncope/presyncope and disequilibrium/lightheadedness symptoms [10, 11].

Vertigo

Vertigo is a false sense of motion or a spinning sensation. Pathology directly affects the vestibular apparatus or how the brain processes vestibular afferent information [7]. Both benign and more concerning etiologies, such as central nervous system (CNS) malignancies, ischemia, or hemorrhage, can result in vertigo [3]. When a patient complains of "dizziness," the clinician's challenge is to appraise the underlying quality of the symptoms. The feelings of "the world" or "the room" spinning during the episode qualify the presentation as vertiginous. In the following sections, we discuss the pathophysiology of vertigo. Following that, we review important systemic medical etiologies associated with vertigo. Next, we discuss psychiatric conditions that are associated with complaints of dizziness. Finally, we further highlight the challenge of dizziness complaints in the cultural context with specific cultural phenomena that have been described in the Diagnostic and Statistical Manual, 5th edition, text revision (DSM-5-TR) [p. 833]. Interestingly, other institutions have constructed a framework for dizziness including the National Institute of Mental Health's (NIMH) Research Domain Criteria Initiative (RDoC), which categorizes multimodal perceptions such as a sense of self in space under the cognitive systems domain [12].

Pathophysiology

The vestibular apparatus is responsible for the sense of balance. This system detects head orientation and linear acceleration. The varying orientations of the hair cells that result from the different types of head movement lead to depolarization and hyperpolarization patterns that maintain equilibrium via afferent input to the vestibular nerve [7]. It also relies on input from the visual system and proprioceptive system of the head and neck. Mismatch of information from any of these systems, including integration of input in the CNS, can result in various vertigo and other dizziness symptoms. An in-depth discussion on the pathophysiology of balance and equilibrium can be found elsewhere [8].

Medical Specialty Approaches to Assessing Vertigo

Regardless of specialty, the goal of assessing a "vertiginous" complaint is to determine the correct diagnosis to establish acuity. Figure 5.1 provides an algorithm to help with identifying a specific diagnosis for symptoms of vertigo.

Medicine In medicine, including primary care, psychiatry, and the emergency department setting, the greatest emphasis is placed on identifying whether the presentation is due to a malignant etiology such as stroke, malignancy, or cardiac arrhythmia or a more benign condition such as benign paroxysmal positional vertigo (BPPV). The clinician may be less focused on the exact diagnosis, but rather ruling out conditions that require immediate interventions. Acute central dizziness variants would require acute evaluation for cerebellar stroke. Following ruling out acute concerns, primary care also typically focuses on common presentations such as BPPV.

Neurology Common conditions such as BPPV, and deadly etiologies such as strokes are often ruled out by primary care or emergency medicine physicians. Neurologists are therefore more concerned with exact neurological diagnosis of vertigo such as migraine or multiple sclerosis, or to determine the symptoms to be non-neurological.

Otolaryngology and Audiology Patients with hearing loss or tinnitus with vertigo symptoms are referred to otolaryngologists for diagnostic assessment if BPPV is ruled out by primary care. The otolaryngologists often focus on vestibular (peripheral) causes of vertigo or to determine the presentation as non-otological. This may result in a benign diagnosis such as vestibular neuritis or a more malignant process such as an acoustic schwannoma [8].

Differentiating Systemic Conditions that Present with Vertigo

When evaluating patients, it is important to consider medical, psychiatric, substance use, or medication causes. The most important first step is clarifying the ambiguous concern of *dizziness* and determining whether it is specifically *vertiginous* in nature. Most problems presenting with vertigo are episodic, and two symptoms associated with vertigo are *impulsion* and *oscillopsia*, which can help guide the physician from the vague complaint of dizziness to a more precise complaint of vertigo. *Impulsion* is defined as "a sensation that the body is being hurled or pulled in space," while *oscillopsia* is "a visual illusion of moving back and forth" [13, p. 191]. Figure 5.1 outlines an algorithm to help the physician differentiate various etiologies that present with vertiginous symptoms. Conditions that cause vertigo are usually divided into *central* and *peripheral* causes. A *peripheral* etiology (88%) is most common and results from vestibular disease. The remaining 12% have vertigo related to a *central nervous system* problem [14]. In psychiatric practice, the presence of true vertigo should cause the psychiatrist to pursue evaluation for systemic medical causes in addition to traumatic brain injury, substance or medication use, or a withdrawal syndrome (Table 5.1).

Peripheral Causes of Vertigo

Benign Paroxysmal Positional Vertigo (BPPV)

Among all the causes of nystagmus, benign paroxysmal positional vertigo (BPPV) is the most common etiology and accounts for one-quarter of all patients complaining of dizziness [9]. *It is relatively easy to diagnose based on history and examination as is described at greater length below. Given its prevalence, all clinicians should be familiar with three special maneuvers to diagnose BPPV.*

Incidence/Prevalence

BPPV is the most common cause of vertigo and has a lifetime prevalence of 2.4% [15, 16].

Typical Findings in the HPI

As the name implies, the patient complains of brief (usually less than 1 min) episodes of vertigo that are triggered by position changes such as turning over, moving the head, sitting up, or bending over.

Typical Physical Exam Findings

The goal of the exam is to confirm either spontaneous or positional nystagmus with an otherwise non-focal neurological exam. The positional nystagmus can be triggered by the Dix-Hallpike maneuver or the supine role [17].

The Dix-Hallpike maneuver is used to evaluate for any free-floating calcium carbonate crystals in the vestibular system, which disrupt the sensing mechanisms, causing vertiginous symptoms associated with BPPV [18, 19]. The sensitivity and the specificity for the Dix-Hallpike maneuver are 79% and 75%, respectively. This makes it a useful test for *ruling out* BPPV. If positive, the probability of BPPV is only 50%, but when this test is negative, the probability of the patient having BPPV is dropped to 8% [20]. To perform the Dix-Hallpike, have the patient sit with their head turned 45°, quickly and safely lower them in a supine position until their head is about 20° below the examination table. Observe ocular movements for nystagmus; the test is positive if there are a few seconds of latency, followed by transient (about 15–60 s) of upbeat, torsional nystagmus [21]. A video illustrating the Dix-Hallpike maneuver can be reviewed here: https://youtu.be/8RYB2QlO1N4

If the Dix-Hallpike maneuver is negative, the canalith (a crystalline particle derived from otoliths in the utricle of the inner ear) may be lodged within the lateral canals. To assess for this, utilize the supine roll test [21, 22]. This test begins with the patient sitting and then is brought to a supine position but the head is turned 90° and brought to a positive 20° above the table. Evaluate for nystagmus for 30 s; if negative for nystagmus, then rotate to midline for another 30 s, and then proceed to rotate their head in the opposite 90° direction [23]. A video illustrating the supine roll test can be reviewed here: https://youtu.be/ns8XZ4rKiJc

The Head Impulse, Nystagmus, and Test of Skew or HINTS exam is a brief, three-part, effective evaluation for determining if the vertiginous pathology is a central or peripheral etiology. To perform, have the patient sit across from the physician and rapidly have them rotate their head 20° in both rotational directions while trying to focus their gaze on the physician. If their gaze moves in the direction of rotation and is quickly followed by a saccade back to the physician, this is consistent with a *peripheral* cause. If their gaze is fixed then the test is *normal or concerning for a central etiology* [21].

One major component of the HINTS exam is *nystagmus*, which is defined as "rhythmic oscillation of the eyes" [13, p. 15]. If nystagmus is unidirectional when not looking straight ahead or can be suppressed by fixating on a point, then this is more consistent with a *peripheral* cause. Alternatively, if nystagmus changes direction, or is not suppressed by gaze fixation, this is more supportive of a *central* etiology [21].

The last component of the HINTS exam is a test of *skew*. Have the patient focus on a fixed point and cover and uncover one eye and repeat on the other side. If there is any rapid movement of the eye, it may be concerning for a central cause [21]. A video illustrating the HINTS exam can be reviewed here: https://youtu.be/VwmrjYuvqtQ

Typical Laboratory/Radiological Findings

There are no laboratory tests specific for vertigo. Magnetic resonance imaging (MRI) may be used to rule out vestibular lesions such as acoustic neuroma.

Screening Tools

An excellent screening questionnaire from Kim et al. can quickly help assess the presence or absence of BPPV and overall performs better than the Dix-Hallpike maneuver. It is based on three questions (see Fig. 5.2). A negative response to question #1 drops the probability of BPPV from 24% to just 4%. If the first question is positive, then the subsequent 2 questions may be used. Each additional positive question further improves the positive likelihood of BPPV. When all three questions are positive, there is a 73% probability of having BPPV [24]. Clinicians can utilize Fig. 5.2 to quickly conduct an assessment for BPPV.

Fig. 5.2 Three Question BPPV Questionnaire

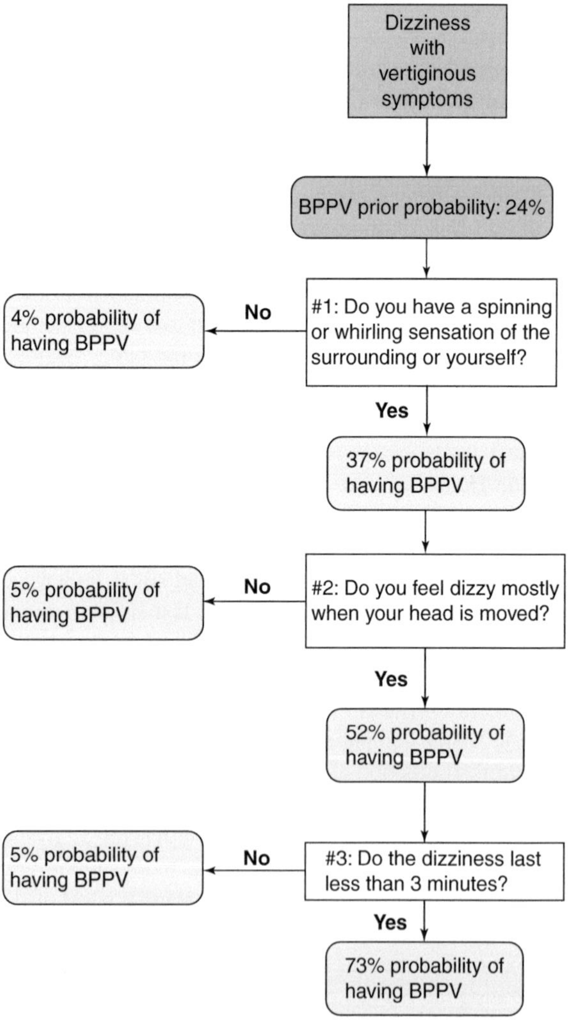

Pitfalls/Differential Diagnosis

There is a broad differential of diagnoses to consider in addition to BPPV, but most are much rarer than BPPV. Peripheral conditions include otological disorders such as Ménière's disease, vestibular neuritis, posttraumatic vertigo, and inner ear lesions or masses. Central neurological conditions that may mimic BPPV include vestibular migraines, stroke, demyelinating diseases such as multiple sclerosis, vertebrobasilar insufficiency, or central positional vertigo. Stroke syndromes are nonrecurrent and may have other associated focal neurological findings on exam. Any central infection, as well as substance use or withdrawal may also mimic BPPV. The clue to diagnostic success is in the term "paroxysmal" in "BPPV," where the symptoms are sudden, short-lived, and triggered by changes in the position of the head [25]. As outlined in Fig. 5.1, most of these conditions can be separated based on history and physical exam.

Vestibular Neuritis

Incidence/Prevalence

The annual incidence is 3.5 per 100,000 persons-year [26].

Typical Findings in the HPI

Patients typically present with sudden onset of severe vertigo with nausea, vomiting, and gait imbalance for hours to days that gradually improve over several weeks [27]. It can be preceded by a viral syndrome with a post-viral etiology being the leading theory for etiology [26]. Note that this differs from Ménière's disease since it is *not* associated with *hearing loss*, but can be uncommonly associated with a sense of aural "fullness" or tinnitus [27].

Typical Physical Exam Findings

With all peripheral etiologies of vertigo, the HINTS exam will display saccade back to a fixed point with head rotation or head impulse, unilateral nystagmus, or the resolution of nystagmus with gaze fixation, and fixed gaze with the test of skew [21]. While assessing gait and station, postural imbalance can be seen with the patient falling towards the affected ear [26]. Notably, focal limb weakness, sensory deficits, speech impairment, and memory loss are *not consistent* with vestibular neuritis [27].

Typical Laboratory/Radiological Findings

There are no specific laboratory test results. Magnetic resonance imaging (MRI) with contrast may be warranted if an acoustic neuroma or central etiology cannot be ruled out.

Screening Tools

There are no specific screening tools for vestibular neuritis.

Pitfalls/Differential Diagnosis

Differential diagnosis includes all peripheral etiologies for vertigo, including BPPV, Ménière's disease, or acoustic neuroma. CNS causes should be considered, including transient ischemic attack, cerebellar or brainstem stroke, vestibular migraine, or demyelinating disease [26]. If symptoms are episodic in nature, associated with hearing loss, change in the level of consciousness or cognition, or have peripheral motor or sensory deficits, the etiology of vertigo is *unlikely* to be vestibular neuritis.

Ménière's Disease

Incidence/Prevalence

Ménière's disease has a lifetime prevalence of 0.2%, with women affected more than men [22].

Typical Findings in the HPI

The classic triad in Ménière's disease is *episodic vertigo* without triggers that last minutes to hours, *unilateral tinnitus* and aural fullness or pain, with reversible *sensorineural hearing loss*. About 25% of patients present with *all three* symptoms [15, 28]. Frequency of vertigo episodes is variable and symptoms may occur every few weeks to every few years. Ménière's disease is associated with progressive hearing loss, and as hearing declines, vertigo severity usually lessens [29].

Typical Physical Exam Findings

Head rotation/head impulse testing will be notable for saccades back to a fixed point, unilateral nystagmus with resolution of spontaneous nystagmus with gaze fixation, and fixed gaze with test of skew [21]. Hearing loss is usually unable to be assessed at the bedside if not advanced [13, p. 204].

Typical Laboratory/Radiological Findings

There are no specific laboratory tests. MRI with contrast may be needed to differentiate if there is a peripheral mass or central etiology that is contributing to the patient's vertigo. If an MRI is obtained, endolymphatic hydrops, an increase in the volume of labyrinth endolymph, can be seen [30]. Formal audiology consultation with audiometry may need to be obtained to fully assess and monitor hearing deficits.

Screening Tools

There are no specific screening tools for Ménière's disease.

Pitfalls/Differential Diagnosis

As discussed with vestibular neuritis, peripheral causes of vertigo should be at the forefront of the differential. These include BPPV or acoustic neuroma. Other etiologies that affect the inner ear such as temporal bone fractures, infection, and otosclerosis can have a similar presentation as well [30]. The classic triad of symptoms is important but only present in a quarter of patients with Ménière's disease.

Acoustic Neuroma/Vestibular Schwannoma

Incidence/Prevalence

Incidence is 1–20 per million persons-year with the mean age at diagnosis being 50–55 years old [31]. Vertigo eventually develops in 8% of patients with acoustic neuroma [32].

Typical Findings in the HPI

Initial presentation is primarily insidious unilateral hearing loss, but poor balance, vertigo, or tinnitus can be the presenting symptom. Most cases of vestibular schwannomas are sporadic but some are genetically related with two disorders being notable, including neurofibromatosis type 2 (NF2) and schwannomatosis. NF2 is known to cause bilateral vestibular schwannomas but also additional schwannomas located in cranial and spinal nerves as well as ocular involvement including cataracts. About 25% of vestibular schwannomas are incidentally found when imaging is obtained for unrelated symptoms [32].

Typical Physical Exam Findings

Unilateral sensorineural hearing loss is common; facial palsy or sensory loss, abnormal corneal reflex, imbalance, and/or ataxia can also be seen [32].

Typical Laboratory/Radiological Findings

Cerebrospinal fluid (CSF) protein is elevated in most patients with the range typically being 50–200 mg/dL [13, p. 205]. The tumor is typically found in the internal auditory canal and/or cerebellopontine angle [32]. Gadolinium-enhanced MRI is the imaging modality of choice with a sensitivity and specificity of 96% and 88.2%, respectively [33].

Screening Tools

There is no screening test for acoustic neuromas.

Pitfalls/Differential Diagnosis

If cranial nerve V or VII impairment, or ataxia is present on examination, then other etiologies should be evaluated including other types of schwannoma, meningioma, or metastatic cancer. The progressive, continuous quality of vertigo, if present, differentiates it from other peripheral causes [32].

Central Causes of Vertigo

Vestibular Migraine

Incidence/Prevalence

Lifetime prevalence is 1% and affects women more than men with women 3.3 times more likely to suffer from vestibular migraine [34]. Vertigo is a hallmark symptom.

Typical Findings in the HPI

Vestibular migraine usually presents as vertigo with headache, nausea, emesis, photophobia, and/or phonophobia. Notably, headaches may be absent or mild. Episode length is variable from seconds to days. To formally make the diagnosis, there need to be five or more attacks with episodic or fluctuating vestibular symptoms, a history of migraines, and other associated migraine symptoms with at least half of the attacks [15, 28]. Some notable features can include triggers of vertigo with moving visual scenery or susceptibility to motion sickness, but vestibular migraine is usually *not* associated with positional changes [35].

Typical Physical Exam Findings

Examination is usually unremarkable when the patient is asymptomatic. During an episode, the patient can have persistent bilateral horizontal positional nystagmus, as well as spontaneous nystagmus worsened by fixation of gaze. Other rare findings on examination may include imbalance or hearing loss [35].

Typical Laboratory/Radiological Findings

There are no typical laboratory or radiographic findings.

Screening Tools

Celebisoy et al. published the eight-question Vestibular Migraine Diagnosis Questionnaire, which is a useful screening tool [34]. For specifics regarding this questionnaire, please see our references. With certain answer choices, the sensitivity was 82.8% with a specificity of 83.9% [34]. With a prevalence of 1%, this questionnaire has a positive likelihood ratio of 5.19 and a negative likelihood ratio of 0.20. When the questionnaire result is negative, the chance of this condition is close to 0%. If positive, the posterior probability is only 5% and clinically not helpful. Therefore, this test is most helpful in ruling out vestibular migraine.

Pitfalls/Differential Diagnosis

Ménière's disease has a significant overlap with vestibular migraine, which can make diagnosis challenging. Both conditions may present with transient vertigo symptoms with aural fullness; however, only Ménière's disease presents with hearing loss. Other considerations for differential diagnosis include BPPV, vertebrobasilar transient ischemic attack (TIA), vascular compression of the eighth cranial nerve, and acoustic schwannoma [35].

Transient Ischemic Attack

Incidence/Prevalence

The annual incidence rate of transient ischemic attacks (TIAs) in the United States is 1.1 per 1000 person-years [36]. While there are an estimated 400,000 individuals in the United States diagnosed with TIAs each year, the true number of cases is estimated to be around five million. This difference is due to under-reporting due to many patients not seeking medical attention [37]. Incidence or prevalence of vertigo with

TIAs is unknown. A nonspecific dizziness symptom is present in 3.2% of patients with stroke or TIA. Isolated dizziness, i.e., without other focal findings, is much rarer and only present in 0.7% of patients with TIA or stroke. Patients presenting with vertigo symptoms do not have higher odds of having TIAs or stroke when compared to the nonspecific complaint of dizziness. Patients with imbalance (disequilibrium) symptoms are four times more likely to have TIAs or stroke when compared to patients without disequilibrium symptoms [38]. Disequilibrium symptoms result from motor impairment of the lower extremities or cerebellar lesions. The Rapid Arterial oCclusion Evaluation (RACE) scale, which assesses leg weakness or paralysis resulting in disequilibrium, is part of some prehospital stroke assessments [39].

Typical Findings in the HPI

TIAs can present with a wide range of symptoms, including but not limited to isolated vertigo, diplopia, aphasia, dysarthria, limb weakness or sensory loss, nausea, vomiting, or ataxia [15, 40]. To be deemed a transient ischemic attack, neurologic symptoms need to occur secondary to retinal and/or focal brain ischemia and resolve fully, which usually occurs within 1 h. Additionally, patients, need to have no evidence of acute infarction [41].

Typical Physical Exam Findings

Examination findings are highly variable and are determined by specific vascular involvement. Cranial nerve palsies, sensorimotor deficits, alteration in level of consciousness, aphasia, and ataxia can be seen on physical exam [40, 41].

Typical Laboratory/Radiological Findings

There are no specific laboratory or radiographic findings with TIA. The main goal of brain imaging is to exclude acute ischemic or hemorrhagic stroke. Head Computer Tomography (CT) is helpful to rule out bleeding or subacute strokes. MRI is the most sensitive modality for excluding acute and subacute strokes. The diffusion-weighted imaging (DWI) of MR is 90% sensitive and 97% specific for acute ischemic strokes [42].

Screening Tools

There are many screening tests for TIA and stroke symptoms, with one of the most common being the Cincinnati Prehospital Stroke Severity Scale (CPSSS), which examines facial droop, arm drift, and speech. Using a cut-off of 2 on a scale of 1–4, CPSSS is 70.0% sensitive and 86.8% specific for predicting large vessel occlusion [43].

Pitfalls/Differential Diagnosis

Evaluation of serum glucose is paramount since hypoglycemia can mimic TIA symptoms [41]. If symptoms continue to evolve, then there should be a strong consideration of stroke. Additional differential diagnoses that should be considered are seizures, migraines, multiple sclerosis, neoplasm, central nervous system infection, or peripheral causes of vertigo [44].

Chiari Malformation Type I

Incidence/Prevalence

Chiari Malformation Type I (CM-I) occurs among 1 in a 1000 live births with a male to female ratio of 1.3:1. Vertigo is an unusual presentation of CM-I [45]. In one study of patients with various otological complaints (including vertigo) in an otolaryngology clinic, 0.9% of the patients were found to have Chiari malformation [46].

Typical Findings in the HPI

The most common symptom is pain in the occipital region that is exacerbated by the Valsalva maneuver. Patients with CM-I may also experience unspecified dizziness, vertigo, syncope, and disequilibrium. Patients may also complain of dysphagia and tinnitus. Additionally, patients may develop progressive muscular weakness in the extremities, as well as bowel and bladder dysfunction [47]. Patients can also be asymptomatic with incidental findings of CM-I on MRI [45].

Typical Physical Exam Findings

If there is autonomic dysfunction, bradycardia may be seen. Patients may display ataxia, dysmetria, impaired balance, limb sensorimotor dysfunction, and impaired swallowing [47]. Positional nystagmus is common. Vertigo may be induced by neck flexion, extension, or rotation similar to findings in cervical vertigo resulting in a delayed onset of positional nystagmus on the Dix-Hallpike maneuver [48].

Typical Laboratory/Radiological Findings

There are no standard laboratory findings for Chiari Malformation Type I. MRI shows greater than 5 mm tonsillar descent and herniation (6 mm in children) through the foramen magnum. These cut-offs are 92% sensitive and 100% specific [49].

Screening Tools

There are no routine screening tools for Chiari Malformation Type I.

Pitfalls/Differential Diagnosis

Differential diagnosis includes other Chiari malformations (Types II–IV), tonsillar ectopia, basilar invagination, and idiopathic intracranial hypertension [47].

Primary Central Nervous System Tumors

Incidence/Prevalence

The overall incidence of CNS tumors is 19 per 100,000 persons-years and was noted to have increased by about 3% between 2000 and 2012 [50]. Due to heterogeneity of CNS masses, incidence and prevalence of vertigo secondary to CNS tumors are unknown, though isolated vertigo or dizziness is rare.

Typical Findings in the HPI

History of present illness varies depending on the type of CNS tumor and its regional involvement, with symptoms typically being divided into general and focal. General symptoms usually cause pathology from pressure on the cerebral or spinal tissue. This mass effect may manifest as morning headaches, nausea and emesis, seizures, cognitive and personality changes. Focal symptoms include ataxic gait, impaired balance, vertigo, unspecified dizziness, vision changes, cranial nerve deficits, aphasia, and agnosia [51].

Typical Physical Exam Findings

Neurologic examination is paramount, which is variable and dependent on tumor location. Papilledema can be seen due to the mass effect. Visual field defects, other cranial nerve deficits, and focal findings may be present [51].

Typical Laboratory/Radiological Findings

When CNS mass or tumor is suspected, the next step is gadolinium-enhanced MRI. The likelihood ratios depend on the type of underlying tumor type and size. 18F-fluorodeoxyglucose (18F-FDG) positron emission tomography (PET) may have a role when primary CNS lymphoma is suspected [52].

Screening Tools

Due to heterogeneity of CNS masses, there are no screening tools.

Pitfalls/Differential Diagnosis

There is a broad differential but may be narrowed based on a patient's age, immunocompetency, and risk of peripheral malignancies with avidity for CNS metastasis. The greatest branch point is malignancy vs. infection [53].

Cerebellar Hemorrhagic or Ischemic Infarction

Incidence/Prevalence

There are approximately 600,000 strokes in the United States each year. Of these, 2–3% are cerebellar ischemic or hemorrhagic strokes [54]. Vertigo presents in 48% of patients with posterior circulation ischemia [13, p. 373].

Typical Findings in the HPI

With hemorrhagic stroke, there is usually a sudden headache with nausea, vomiting, or vertigo. This is followed by an ataxic gait and decreased level of consciousness. Ischemic infarction has an array of symptoms including nystagmus, limb ataxia, and cranial nerve deficits, but there is a significant overlap with hemorrhagic stroke symptoms, which also include vertigo, nausea, and emesis [55].

Typical Physical Exam Findings

The neurologic exam is imperative. Findings may include small and sluggish pupils, and/or gaze palsy towards the affected side. Patients can have ipsilateral limb ataxia and fall towards the side with pathology. Additionally, dysarthria, nystagmus, and sensory deficits can occur. It is crucial to have the patient ambulate, since impairments in gait are usually the earliest neurologic sign, especially with a hemorrhagic etiology [55].

Typical Laboratory/Radiological Findings

There are no specific laboratory findings, but if cerebrospinal fluid is obtained, it is usually bloody with hemorrhagic stroke [13, p. 209]. Head CT can help with assessing for hemorrhage but its sensitivity diminishes when a posterior fossa stroke is a concern. Brain MRI with DWI sequences is the imaging of choice to exclude posterior fossa strokes [56].

Screening Tools

The HINTS exam should be the primary screening tool used to assess patients presenting with vertigo where there is a concern for posterior circulation infarction. If there is a normal head impulse test, a positive test of skew, or direction-changing nystagmus then there is a 100% sensitivity and 96% specificity for infarction [57]. The Cincinnati Prehospital Stroke Scale (discussed in section "Transient Ischemic Attack" above) is also valuable for cerebral strokes, although it is insensitive for posterior fossa strokes, including cerebellar.

Pitfalls/Differential Diagnosis

All causes of central etiologies of vertigo should be considered on the differential when the HINTS exam is positive. These include vestibular migraine, multiple sclerosis, midbrain or cerebral strokes, or vertebrobasilar insufficiency [21]. Indolent symptoms that develop over weeks to months suggest a cause other than stroke since it is an acute illness. It is important to assess for gait impairment since this is usually one of the initial signs of cerebellar pathology, which would warrant neuroimaging [55].

Multiple Sclerosis

Incidence/Prevalence

Approximately 2.8 million people worldwide live with multiple sclerosis (MS) with a 2:1 ratio of females to males. The global incidence is 2.1 per 100,000 persons-year [58]. Vertigo is a rare presenting symptom, only accounting for 8% of presenting symptoms of MS [59].

Typical Findings in the HPI

Clinical course is variable with insidious or acute symptoms. Some hallmark signs and symptoms are optic neuritis, worsening of symptoms with heat (Uhthoff phenomenon), and Lhermitte's phenomenon, which is a radiating electric sensation after neck flexion. Other associated symptoms include sensory loss, weakness, bladder dysfunction, and fatigue. The clinical course is usually relapsing and remitting but can be primary or secondary progressive [60, 61].

Typical Physical Exam Findings

Physical exam findings are highly variable. Some notable findings include cranial nerve palsies, optic disc swelling, sensory impairments, limb and facial weakness, spasticity, and ataxia [61].

Typical Laboratory/Radiological Findings

Cerebrospinal fluid is notable for oligoclonal immunoglobulin IgG bands. MRI findings would include multifocal white matter lesions that are disseminated in time and space and can be seen within the brain, brainstem, and/or spinal cord [60, 61].

Screening Tools

While there are no screening assessments for the diagnosis of multiple sclerosis, there are screening assessments for *cognitive impairment* in people affected by MS. The Brief International Cognitive Assessment for Multiple Sclerosis (BICAMS) is a validated tool that evaluates information processing speed, immediate verbal recall memory, and immediate visual recall memory [62].

Pitfalls/Differential Diagnosis

The differential is wide due to the variable nature of MS as well as the extensive symptomatology that can occur. This includes stroke, neuromyelitis optica, sarcoidosis, antiphospholipid syndrome, vasculitis, B12 deficiency, and space-occupying lesions [60].

Traumatic Brain Injury

Incidence/Prevalence

There were 27 million cases of traumatic brain injury (TBI) globally in 2016. The global incidence of TBI was 369 per 100,000/year [63]. The prevalence of vertigo symptoms depends on the severity of the TBI and the time since injury. The greater the TBI severity, the higher the likelihood of vertigo. In one study of 321 patients, 23.8% of those with mild TBI reported symptoms of vertigo, 65% of those with moderate TBI reported symptoms of vertigo, and 78% with severe TBI had vertigo. The overall prevalence of vertigo dropped to 20% among the entire cohort after 6 months [64]. In another study ($n = 1255$) of subjects with mild TBI, the prevalence of nonspecific symptoms of dizziness was 28% at 2 weeks and 9% at 6 weeks [65]. Of note, the DSM classifies TBI as a mild or major neurocognitive disorder due to TBI [p. 624].

Typical Findings in the HPI

Traumatic brain injuries occur after trauma to the brain such as motor vehicle accidents, sports injuries, concussive forces (e.g., blast trauma), or rapid acceleration or deceleration. Patients usually endorse a history of loss of consciousness, amnesia, or disorientation following trauma. Headaches, vertigo, photo/phonophobia, irritability, and cognitive impairments in executive function, learning, and memory are common [pp. 625–627]. About 65% of patients with moderate to severe TBI report cognitive problems while up to 15% of mild TBI patients have persistent complaints of neurocognitive deficits [66]. Depending on the severity of the injury, other neurologic sequelae may include seizures, vision deficits, cranial nerve impairments, focal motor or peripheral sensory deficits, and sleep disturbances. Comorbid psychiatric symptoms may be present as well including depressed mood, poor concentration, sleep disturbance, and apathy [pp. 625–627].

Typical Physical and Mental Status Exam Findings

Physical exam findings vary depending on severity. Visual field defects can be seen, as well as cranial nerve abnormalities, weakness, and peripheral sensory deficits. Mental status exam findings vary as well. They include labile, inappropriate, apathetic, or dysphoric affect. Cognitive assessment can show executive function, language, attention, and/or memory impairment [pp. 626–627].

Typical Laboratory/Radiological Findings

Computed tomography and magnetic resonance imaging can be used to identify cerebral contusions or petechial, subarachnoid, and/or epidural and subdural hemorrhages depending on the location and severity of trauma [p. 627].

The Canadian CT Head Injury/Trauma Rule is a helpful tool to assess the need for head imaging. It applies to patients aged 16 and older, not on anticoagulation, with the absence of seizure after injury. There are seven criteria and if all are negative then it rules out the need for computed tomography or neurosurgical intervention [67].

Several candidate biomarkers of intracranial injury are under consideration. The Center for Disease Control and Prevention (CDC) mild traumatic brain injury (mTBI) guidance mentions the serum S-100B biomarkers with a possible role in assessing the need for head CT though it is currently not approved for clinical use in the United States [68]. The Food and Drug Administration (FDA) has approved a blood test for marketing in the United States. This test looks at the combination of two biomarkers including glial fibrillary acidic protein (GFAP) and ubiquitin C-terminal hydrolase-L1 (UCH-L1) [69]. The sensitivity and negative predictive value of the combined biomarkers are 97.6% and 99.6%, respectively, for the detection of acute intracranial injuries on head CT scan [70]. The impact of these tests on clinical practice is currently unclear but has great potential for resource constraint environments and reducing radiation exposure by eliminating unnecessary head CT scans.

Screening Tools

The Veterans Affairs Traumatic Brain Injury Clinical Reminder Screen is a four question self-assessment to screen for prior traumatic brain injuries [71]. In diagnosing head injuries in the past, the sensitivity is 72% and specificity is 54% when all four questions are answered positively. The screening questionnaire is helpful for clinicians to rule out TBI with a negative predictive value of 91–94% [72].

Pitfalls/Differential Diagnoses

Differential diagnosis includes somatic symptom disorder, factitious disorder, acute stress disorder, and posttraumatic stress disorder, which can overlap with TBI [p. 627]. Vertebrobasilar insufficiency should also be on the differential, which may present after reduced cerebral perfusion from prolonged standing or hypovolemia [21]. Another consideration is persistent postural-perceptual dizziness, which is associated with waxing and waning dizziness spells and can be from a medical or psychiatric etiology [73].

Psychiatric Conditions Presenting with Vertigo

In the DSM-5-TR, the term "dizziness" is used 26 times (with "dizzy" having two additional mentions), "vertigo" and "syncope" are each mentioned six times, "lightheadedness" is mentioned once, and there is no mention of "disequilibrium." It is worth highlighting that there are only a very small number of psychiatric diagnoses from the DSM-5-TR that have dizzy or dizziness as part of their diagnostic description or criteria: panic disorder, panic attack specifier, and inhalant intoxication, although "dizziness" is not required to diagnose these disorders. Table 5.1 highlights various conditions where dizziness, vertigo, and other associated complaints and symptoms may present.

In the DSM-5-TR, "vertigo," is more narrowly mentioned. It is essentially restricted to association with substance/medication-induced anxiety disorder and major or mild neurocognitive disorder due to traumatic brain injury. Vertigo is not part of either condition's diagnostic criteria but may be part of a patient's presentation. Onset of panic disorder after age 45 or atypical panic attack symptoms including vertigo should lead the clinician in the direction of a potential substance/medication-induced etiology. In regard to major or mild neurocognitive disorder due to traumatic brain injury, vertigo (and dizziness) are mentioned as a potential associated physical disturbance [74].

Anxiety disorder due to another medical condition in DSM-5-TR does not have vertigo or dizziness as part of the presentation, but vertigo due to another medical condition may result in this diagnosis. Any medical condition can create significant suffering and stress for a patient. Conditions with chronic vertigo can be distressing if unresponsive to therapy [75].

It is important to recognize, that most "classic" psychiatric conditions are diagnoses of exclusion, so all behavioral health clinicians need to consider a full work-up to rule out malignant etiologies.

Substance/Medication-Induced Anxiety Disorder

Incidence/Prevalence

Prevalence is unclear. General data suggests it is rare, with a 12-month prevalence of roughly 0.002% (likely to be higher in clinical populations) [p. 229]. The prevalence of vertigo is not known.

Typical Findings of the HPI

Anxiety, including panic attacks, is predominant in the clinical picture and there is evidence from the history, physical exam, or laboratory tests that the anxiety developed during or soon after starting a medication, or a substance intoxication or withdrawal. The substance or medication involved must also be capable of producing panic or anxiety symptoms. In general, intoxication with central nervous system stimulants or cannabis and withdrawal from central nervous system depressants can precipitate a panic attack but there are many different classes of specific drugs, that can precipitate the spectrum of anxiety presentations [p. 217, 228, 229]. Patients can present with concerns for feelings of choking, chest pain, nausea, dizziness or lightheadedness, palpitations, paresthesias/cold extremities, fear of losing control, or that they may die during a panic attack. For a more general anxiety presentation, there may be fatigue, restlessness, irritability, sleep disturbance, muscle tension, or concentration deficits, and may also include tinnitus and neck soreness [pp. 222–223].

Typical Findings on Physical and Mental Status Exam

The presentation depends on the substance or medication and its associated effects on the autonomic nervous system. Physical exam may reveal atypical panic attack symptoms like slurred speech, loss of bladder control, loss of balance, and loss of consciousness [p. 229]. Familiarity with classic toxidromes is important. Patient's presenting with acute toxicity with anticholinergic, sympathomimetic, and serotonergic compounds (serotonin syndrome) have tachycardia, hyperthermia, and mydriasis on examination [76]. Hyperreflexia may be present in anticholinergic and sympathomimetic toxidromes, with extreme hyperreflexia and clonus unique to serotonin syndrome [77]. Withdrawal from sedative-hypnotics and alcohol may result in anxiety and panic symptoms. Patients in withdrawal may present with mental status changes, tachycardia, hypertension, mydriasis, as well as hyperreflexia. In Wernicke's encephalopathy, the classic triad of delirium, ataxia, and oculomotor abnormalities may be seen [78].

Typical Laboratory/Radiological Findings

Laboratory findings depend on the suspected substance or medication involved. Urine drug screens and blood alcohol level (BAL) may be positive for illicit substances. For alcohol, there are numerous biomarkers that may be helpful in assessing recent or excessive drinking. One such marker is the carbohydrate-deficient transferring (CDT) that has a sensitivity of 46–90% and a specificity of 70–100% based on alcohol consumption in the prior 2-week period [79]. Combining CDT with gamma-glutamyltransferase (GGT) and mean corpuscular volume (MCV) improves the sensitivity and specificity by 88% and 95% respectively for chronic excessive drinking [80]. Other laboratory tests may be abnormal due to secondary end-organ damage such as acid-base abnormalities, acute kidney injury, liver injury, or rhabdomyolysis [76]. In case of specific syndromes such as Wernicke's encephalopathy, serum thiamine levels or red blood cell transketolase activity can confirm the diagnosis. MRI has a sensitivity and specificity of 53% and 93%, respectively. In the T2 and FLAIR sequences, MRI can show hyperintensities in the medial thalami, hypothalamus, mammillary bodies, periaqueductal area, and tectal plate [78].

Screening Tools

Laboratory testing such as urine and serum toxicology may be helpful to measure intoxication as discussed above. There are no other singular screening tools given the broad possibilities of substances and drugs.

Cultural Concepts Associated with Dizziness and Vertigo

In considering the full differential for dizziness and its subtypes, one must also consider the cultural aperture through which there can be numerous—and often incongruent—meanings attached to these terms. According to the DSM-5-TR, mental disorders are defined in relation to cultural and social norms which provide the interpretive context for the symptoms, signs, and behaviors used to make a diagnosis. Therefore, clinical assessment must consider whether an individual's presentation differs from sociocultural norms [81 p. 833].

Historically, previous versions of the DSM utilized the term, "culture-bound syndrome," when speaking about cultural psychiatry, but the DSM-5-TR has clarified and refined cultural considerations with three concepts, hoping to increase clinical utility: cultural syndrome, cultural idiom of distress, and cultural explanation or perceived cause. Readers are referred to the DSM-5-TR pages 16–17 and pages 871–874 for a lengthier explanation of the concepts in the cultural issues section of the introduction and the glossary of cultural concepts of distress. The important takeaway is that the ability to classify symptoms and conditions culturally impacts many important aspects of the clinical encounter, including symptomatology, help-seeking, treatment expectations, illness adaptation, and treatment response.

In DSM-5-TR, vertigo is only mentioned within the cultural context of nervios, or "nerves," which is a common idiom of distress among Latinos that refers to vulnerability to stressful life experiences and circumstances [82]. Although this chapter focuses specifically on vertigo, there are cultural phenomena that may present with the complaint of "dizziness." Kufungisisa ("thinking too much" in Shona) is an idiom of distress and a cultural explanation among the Shona of Zimbabwe. As a cultural explanation, it may be the underlying cause of anxiety, depression, and somatic complaints. In the context of it being an idiom of distress, kufungisisa may represent social and interpersonal difficulties. "Khyâl attacks" (khyâl cap) or "wind attacks," is a syndrome found among Cambodian people. It is defined by thoughts centered on the worry that khyâl (a windlike substance) may increase in the body—along with blood—and cause a range of symptoms such as compressing the lungs to cause shortness of breath and asphyxia; entering the cranium to cause tinnitus, dizziness, blurry vision, and a fatal syncope. Of note, there are no diagnostic criteria per se for each of these cultural concepts. The goal is to broaden the clinician's differential by highlighting the important consideration of culture in the clinical encounter. The additional cultural elements add a richer layer to the biopsychosocial formulation of our patients [83, pp. 833–837].

Nervios "Nerves"

Incidence/Prevalence

There is a prevalence of 15.5% in the general Mexican population. Women have a significantly higher prevalence (20.8%) than men (9.5%). Somatic and psychological symptoms associated with nervios have a higher prevalence among women than men [84]. Incidence and prevalence of Nervios "nerves" presenting with dizziness or vertigo is unknown [p. 835].

Typical Findings of the HPI

Findings may include emotional distress, somatic issues, and functional concerns. The most common presentation includes headaches and "brain aches" (occipital neck tension), tingling, stomach issues, sleep concerns, trembling, easy tearfulness, concentration difficulty, nervousness, irritability, and mareos (dizziness with occasional vertigo-like exacerbations) [p. 835].

Typical Findings on Physical and Mental Status Exam

Physical exam may reveal trembling and occipital muscle tension [p. 835]. The mental status exam can range in affective changes to include anxiety and depression. There may be dissociative and psychotic features expressed [p. 835].

Typical Laboratory/Radiological Findings

None.

Screening Tools

No known screening tools exist for nervios, but the patient should be screened for depressive and anxiety disorders.

Pitfalls/Differential Diagnoses

Differential diagnoses include major depressive disorder, persistent depressive disorder (dysthymia), generalized anxiety disorder, social anxiety disorder, other specified or unspecified dissociative disorder, somatic symptom disorder, and schizophrenia. There are related conditions in other cultures in North American Greeks and Sicilians, as well as Whites in Appalachia and Newfoundland [p. 835].

Kufungisisa "Thinking Too Much"

Incidence/Prevalence

Kufungisisa is experienced by up to 80% of Zimbabweans who present with a common mental disorder (mainly depressive and anxiety disorders). The estimated lifetime prevalence of common mental disorders in low- and middle-income countries is roughly 22% [85]. Incidence and prevalence of Kufungisisa presenting with dizziness or vertigo are unknown.

Typical Findings of the HPI

Kufungisisa is associated with anxiety symptoms, worry, panic, depressive symptoms, irritability, and somatic complaints. In many cultures, "thinking too much" is damaging to the mind and body and can cause specific symptoms like headache and dizziness [p. 834, 835].

Typical Findings on Physical and Mental Status Exam

Physical exam may reveal panic attack symptoms such as palpitations, tachycardia, sweating, trembling, shaking, and dyspnea [p. 834, 835]. Mental status exam may reveal ruminating on upsetting thoughts, particularly worries. Affect can present as anxious or depressed [p. 834, 835].

Typical Laboratory/Radiological Findings

None.

Screening Tools

No known screening tools exist for nervios, but the patient should be screened for depressive and anxiety disorders.

Pitfalls/Differential Diagnoses

Differential diagnoses include major depressive disorder, persistent depressive disorder (dysthymia), generalized anxiety disorder, posttraumatic stress disorder, obsessive-compulsive disorder, and persistent complex bereavement disorder. There are related conditions in other cultures described in Africa, the Caribbean, Latin America, and East Asian and Native American groups [p. 834, 835].

Khyâl Cap "Wind Attacks"

Incidence/Prevalence

Unknown.

Incidence/Prevalence of Khyâl Cap "Wind Attacks" Presenting with Dizziness

Unknown.

Typical Findings of the HPI

Common symptoms include panic attacks to include dizziness. The attacks may occur suddenly but are commonly triggered by worrisome thoughts, orthostasis from standing, odors with negative associations, and agoraphobic cues like crowded spaces as one example. These attacks usually meet panic attack criteria [p. 834].

Typical Findings on Physical and Mental Status Exam

Physical exam symptoms include those of panic attacks, such as palpitations, shortness of breath, and cold extremities [p. 834]. The mental status exam can reveal anxious affect.

Typical Laboratory/Radiological Findings

None.

Screening Tools

No known screening tools exist for Khyâl cap, but the patient should be screened for depressive disorders, anxiety disorders, and trauma spectrum disorders.

Pitfalls/Differential Diagnoses

Differential diagnoses include panic attacks, panic disorder, generalized anxiety disorder, agoraphobia, posttraumatic stress disorder, and illness anxiety disorder. There are related conditions in other cultures of Laos, Tibet, Sri Lanka, and Korea as well [p. 834].

Conclusion

As the reader can grasp by now, "dizziness" is a broad and difficult to quantify presenting symptom across medical specialties, cultures, and individual patients. For culturally discordant clinicians, the task of negotiating subjective complaints of dizziness and associated symptoms become even more challenging. While we briefly mention some of the phenomena, the prudent approach is openness and curiosity on the part of the clinician to understand the individual patient's full breadth of experiences and suffering.

To conclude, obtaining clinical utility from a chief concern of "dizziness," a term shown in this chapter to be vague and unclear in its meaning (not only from person to person, but also culture to culture, and specialty to specialty), requires differentiation into the subcategories of vertigo, syncope, or disequilibrium. As discussed, this is best accomplished by transitioning from an open-ended inquisition to more closed-ended follow-up questions that all take place in an empathic environment. Once a subcategory is identified, it allows for a narrower medical and psychiatric differential with implications for acuity of presentation that can impact patient outcomes.

Although understanding disequilibrium/lightheadedness and syncope/presyncope are crucial for a comprehensive approach to "dizziness," this chapter focused on vertigo, given its representation as the major etiological cause. As highlighted, vertigo results from direct vestibular apparatus pathology or from how the brain processes information from it, resulting in a false sense of environmental spinning/motion. Key points worth remembering are that most vertiginous cases are the result of peripheral etiologies as opposed to central, and that evaluation of vertigo by psychiatric providers should focus on ruling out medical causes including TBI, substances and medications use or withdrawal.

Although, "dizziness" can be a scary experience for patients and a daunting assessment for clinicians, following the mental model laid out in this chapter provides a framework to ensure that is not the case.

References

1. Definition of DIZZY [Internet]. [cited 2022 Feb 8]. https://www.merriam-webster.com/dictionary/dizzy.
2. Salvinelli F, Firrisi L, Casale M, Trivelli M, D'Ascanio L, Lamanna F, et al. What is vertigo? Clin Ter. 2003;154(5):341–8.
3. Post RE, Dickerson LM. Dizziness: a diagnostic approach. Am Fam Physician. 2010;82(4):361–8, 369.
4. Arthur W, Kaye GC. The pathophysiology of common causes of syncope. Postgrad Med J. 2000;76(902):750–3.
5. Vaz Garcia F. Disequilibrium and its management in elderly patients. Int Tinnitus J. 2009;15(1):83–90.
6. Bisdorff A, Bosser G, Gueguen R, Perrin P. The epidemiology of vertigo, dizziness, and unsteadiness and its links to co-morbidities. Front Neurol. 2013;4:29.
7. Hall JE, Hall ME. Cortical and brain stem control of motor function. In: Guyton AC, editor. Guyton and Hall textbook of medical physiology. 14th ed. Philadelphia, PA: Elsevier; 2021. p. 697–709.
8. Hullar TE, Zee DS, Minor LB. Evaluation of the patient with dizziness. In: Flint PW, Francis H, Haughey B, Lesperance M, Lund V, Robbins KT, et al., editors. Cummings otolaryngology: head and neck surgery. 7th ed. Philadelphia, PA: Elsevier Inc.; 2021. p. 2495–516.
9. Kim H-J, Lee J-O, Choi J-Y, Kim J-S. Etiologic distribution of dizziness and vertigo in a referral-based dizziness clinic in South Korea. J Neurol. 2020;267(8):2252–9.
10. 2017 ACC/AHA/HRS guideline for the evaluation and management of patients with syncope. a report of the American College of Cardiology/American Heart Association Task Force on Clinical Practice Guidelines and the Heart Rhythm Society | Circulation [Internet]. [cited 2022 Feb 9]. https://www.ahajournals.org/doi/10.1161/CIR.0000000000000499.
11. Muncie HL, Sirmans SM, James E. Dizziness: approach to evaluation and management. Am Fam Physician. 2017;95(3):154–62.
12. Cognitive systems [Internet]. National Institute of Mental Health (NIMH). [cited 2022 Feb 9]. https://www.nimh.nih.gov/research/research-funded-by-nimh/rdoc/constructs/cognitive-systems.
13. Simon RP, Aminoff MJ, Greenberg DA. Clinical neurology [Internet]. 2018 [cited 2022 Feb 9]. http://accessmedicine.mhmedical.com/book.aspx?bookid=2274.
14. Brandt T, Dieterich M. The dizzy patient: don't forget disorders of the central vestibular system. Nat Rev Neurol. 2017;13(6):352–62.
15. Newman-Toker DE, Edlow JA. TiTrATE: a novel, evidence-based approach to diagnosing acute dizziness and vertigo. Neurol Clin. 2015;33(3):577–99, viii.
16. Nuti D, Masini M, Mandalà M. Benign paroxysmal positional vertigo and its variants. Handb Clin Neurol. 2016;137:241–56.
17. Omron R. Peripheral vertigo. Emerg Med Clin North Am. 2019;37(1):11–28.
18. Lou Y, Cai M, Xu L, Wang Y, Zhuang L, Liu X. Efficacy of BPPV diagnosis and treatment system for benign paroxysmal positional vertigo. Am J Otolaryngol. 2020;41(3):102412.
19. Vaduva C, Estéban-Sánchez J, Sanz-Fernández R, Martín-Sanz E. Prevalence and management of post-BPPV residual symptoms. Eur Arch Oto-Rhino-Laryngol. 2018;275(6):1429–37.
20. Halker RB, Barrs DM, Wellik KE, Wingerchuk DM, Demaerschalk BM. Establishing a diagnosis of benign paroxysmal positional vertigo through the dix-hallpike and side-lying maneuvers: a critically appraised topic. Neurologist. 2008;14(3):201–4.
21. Alyono JC. Vertigo and dizziness: understanding and managing fall risk. Otolaryngol Clin N Am. 2018;51(4):725–40.
22. Wipperman J. Dizziness and vertigo. Prim Care. 2014;41(1):115–31.
23. Hain T. Dix-Hallpike test for BPPV [Internet]. Dizziness-and-balance.com. 2020 [cited 2020 Nov 25]. https://www.dizziness-and-balance.com/disorders/bppv/supine-roll.html.

24. Kim H-J, Song J-M, Zhong L, Yang X, Kim J-S. Questionnaire-based diagnosis of benign paroxysmal positional vertigo. Neurology. 2020;94(9):e942–9.
25. Bhattacharyya N, Gubbels SP, Schwartz SR, Edlow JA, El-Kashlan H, Fife T, et al. Clinical practice guideline: benign paroxysmal positional vertigo (Update). Otolaryngol Head Neck Surg. 2017;156(3_Suppl):S1–47.
26. Strupp M, Brandt T. Vestibular neuritis. Semin Neurol. 2009;29(05):509–19.
27. Goddard JC, Fayad JN. Vestibular neuritis. Otolaryngol Clin N Am. 2011;44(2):361–5.
28. Yacovino DA, Hain TC. Clinical characteristics of cervicogenic-related dizziness and vertigo. Semin Neurol. 2013;33(3):244–55.
29. Wright T. Menière's disease. BMJ Clin Evid. 2015;2015:0505.
30. Gürkov R, Pyykö I, Zou J, Kentala E. What is Menière's disease? A contemporary re-evaluation of endolymphatic hydrops. J Neurol. 2016;263:71–81.
31. Chen M, Fan Z, Zheng X, Cao F, Wang L. Risk factors of acoustic neuroma: systematic review and meta-analysis. Yonsei Med J. 2016;57(3):776–83.
32. Carlson ML, Link MJ. Vestibular schwannomas. N Engl J Med. 2021;384(14):1335–48.
33. Haque S, Hossain A, Quddus MA, Jahan MU. Role of MRI in the evaluation of acoustic schwannoma and its comparison to histopathological findings. Bangladesh Med Res Counc Bull. 2011;37(3):92–6.
34. Celebisoy N, Karapolat H, Gokcay F, Bilgen C, Ozgen G, Kirazli T, et al. Establishing a "vestibular migraine diagnosis questionnaire" and testing its validity. Neurologist. 2016;21(4):51–4.
35. Lempert T, von Brevern M. Vestibular migraine. Neurol Clin. 2019;37(4):695–706.
36. Lioutas V-A, Ivan CS, Himali JJ, Aparicio HJ, Leveille T, Romero JR, et al. Incidence of transient ischemic attack and association with long-term risk of stroke. JAMA. 2021;325(4):373–81.
37. Kleindorfer D, Panagos P, Pancioli A, Khoury J, Kissela B, Woo D, et al. Incidence and short-term prognosis of transient ischemic attack in a population-based study. Stroke. 2005;36(4):720–3.
38. Kerber KA, Brown DL, Lisabeth LD, Smith MA, Morgenstern LB. Stroke among patients with dizziness, vertigo, and imbalance in the emergency department: a population-based study. Stroke. 2006;37(10):2484–7.
39. Carrera D, Campbell BCV, Cortés J, Gorchs M, Querol M, Jiménez X, et al. Predictive value of modifications of the prehospital rapid arterial occlusion evaluation scale for large vessel occlusion in patients with acute stroke. J Stroke Cerebrovasc Dis. 2017;26(1):74–7.
40. Karatas M. Central vertigo and dizziness: epidemiology, differential diagnosis, and common causes. Neurologist. 2008;14(6):355–64.
41. Easton JD, Saver JL, Albers GW, Alberts MJ, Chaturvedi S, Feldmann E, et al. Definition and evaluation of transient ischemic attack: a scientific statement for healthcare professionals from the American Heart Association/American Stroke Association Stroke Council; Council on Cardiovascular Surgery and Anesthesia; Council on Cardiovascular Radiology and Intervention; Council on Cardiovascular Nursing; and the Interdisciplinary Council on Peripheral Vascular Disease: The American Academy of Neurology affirms the value of this statement as an educational tool for neurologists. Stroke. 2009;40(6):2276–93.
42. Brunser AM, Hoppe A, Illanes S, Díaz V, Muñoz P, Cárcamo D, et al. Accuracy of diffusion-weighted imaging in the diagnosis of stroke in patients with suspected cerebral infarct. Stroke. 2013;44(4):1169–71.
43. Kummer BR, Gialdini G, Sevush JL, Kamel H, Patsalides A, Navi BB. External validation of the Cincinnati Prehospital Stroke Severity Scale. J Stroke Cerebrovasc Dis. 2016;25(5):1270–4.
44. Simmons BB, Cirignano B, Gadegbeku AB. Transient ischemic attack: Part I. Diagnosis and evaluation. Am Fam Physician. 2012;86(6):521–6.
45. Langridge B, Phillips E, Choi D. Chiari malformation type 1: a systematic review of natural history and conservative management. World Neurosurg. 2017;104:213–9.
46. Levo H, Tapani E, Karppinen A, Kentala E. Chiari malformation in otology practice. Auris Nasus Larynx. 2010;37(1):95–9.

47. Kular S, Cascella M. Chiari I malformation. In: StatPearls [Internet]. Treasure Island, FL: StatPearls Publishing. 2021 [cited 2022 Jan 8]. http://www.ncbi.nlm.nih.gov/books/NBK554609/.
48. Kelkar AA, Yates PD. Chiari type 1 malformation presenting as an atypical benign paroxysmal positional vertigo in a 16 year old patient. Int J Otorhinolaryngol Head Neck Surg. 2017;4(1):253–5.
49. Fakhri A, Shah MN, Goyal MS. Advanced imaging of Chiari 1 malformations. Neurosurg Clin N Am. 2015;26(4):519–26.
50. Pouchieu C, Gruber A, Berteaud E, Ménégon P, Monteil P, Huchet A, et al. Increasing incidence of central nervous system (CNS) tumors (2000–2012): findings from a population based registry in Gironde (France). BMC Cancer. 2018;18(1):653.
51. Alomar SA. Clinical manifestation of central nervous system tumor. Semin Diagn Pathol. 2010;27(2):97–104.
52. Zou Y, Tong J, Leng H, Jiang J, Pan M, Chen Z. Diagnostic value of using 18F-FDG PET and PET/CT in immunocompetent patients with primary central nervous system lymphoma: a systematic review and meta-analysis. Oncotarget. 2017;8(25):41518–28.
53. Omuro A, DeAngelis LM. Glioblastoma and other malignant gliomas: a clinical review. JAMA. 2013;310(17):1842–50.
54. Kelly PJ, Stein J, Shafqat S, Eskey C, Doherty D, Chang Y, et al. Functional recovery after rehabilitation for cerebellar stroke. Stroke. 2001;32(2):530–4.
55. Sarikaya H, Steinlin M. Cerebellar stroke in adults and children. Handb Clin Neurol. 2018;155:301–12.
56. Hwang DY, Silva GS, Furie KL, Greer DM. Comparative sensitivity of computed tomography vs. magnetic resonance imaging for detecting acute posterior fossa infarct. J Emerg Med. 2012;42(5):559–65.
57. Kattah JC, Talkad AV, Wang DZ, Hsieh Y-H, Newman-Toker DE. HINTS to diagnose stroke in the acute vestibular syndrome: three-step bedside oculomotor examination more sensitive than early MRI diffusion-weighted imaging. Stroke. 2009;40(11):3504–10.
58. Walton C, King R, Rechtman L, Kaye W, Leray E, Marrie RA, et al. Rising prevalence of multiple sclerosis worldwide: insights from the Atlas of MS, third edition. Mult Scler Houndmills Basingstoke Engl. 2020;26(14):1816–21.
59. Burina A, Sinanović O, Smajlović D, Vidović M, Brkić F. Some aspects of balance disorder in patients with multiple sclerosis. Bosn J Basic Med Sci. 2008;8(1):80–5.
60. Dobson R, Giovannoni G. Multiple sclerosis - a review. Eur J Neurol. 2019;26(1):27–40.
61. Doshi A, Chataway J. Multiple sclerosis, a treatable disease. Clin Med. 2016;16(Suppl 6):s53–9.
62. Corfield F, Langdon D. A systematic review and meta-analysis of the brief cognitive assessment for multiple sclerosis (BICAMS). Neurol Ther. 2018;7(2):287–306.
63. GBD 2016 Neurology Collaborators. Global, regional, and national burden of neurological disorders, 1990–2016: a systematic analysis for the Global Burden of Disease Study 2016. Lancet Neurol. 2019;18(5):459–80.
64. Berman JM, Fredrickson JM. Vertigo after head injury—a five year follow-up. J Otolaryngol. 1978;7(3):237–45.
65. Haboubi NH, Long J, Koshy M, Ward AB. Short-term sequelae of minor head injury (6 years experience of minor head injury clinic). Disabil Rehabil. 2001;23(14):635–8.
66. Rabinowitz AR, Levin HS. Cognitive sequelae of traumatic brain injury. Psychiatr Clin North Am. 2014;37(1):1–11.
67. Stiell IG, Clement CM, Rowe BH, Schull MJ, Brison R, Cass D, et al. Comparison of the Canadian CT Head Rule and the New Orleans Criteria in patients with minor head injury. JAMA. 2005;294(12):1511–8.
68. Mild TBI pocket guide: guideline for adult patients [Internet]. Center for Disease Control, American College of Emergency Physicians. https://www.cdc.gov/traumaticbraininjury/pdf/TBI_Pocket_Card-a.pdf.

69. U.S. Food and Drug Administration. FDA authorizes marketing of first blood test to aid in the evaluation of concussion in adults. 2018. https://www.fda.gov/news-events/press-announcements/fda-authorizes-marketing-first-blood-test-aid-evaluation-concussion-adults.
70. Bazarian JJ, Biberthaler P, Welch RD, Lewis LM, Barzo P, Bogner-Flatz V, et al. Serum GFAP and UCH-L1 for prediction of absence of intracranial injuries on head CT (ALERT-TBI): a multicentre observational study. Lancet Neurol. 2018;17(9):782–9.
71. Fortier CB, Amick MM, Kenna A, Milberg WP, McGlinchey RE. Correspondence of the Boston Assessment of Traumatic Brain Injury-Lifetime (BAT-L) clinical interview and the VA TBI screen. J Head Trauma Rehabil. 2015;30(1):E1–7.
72. Pape TLB, Smith B, Babcock-Parziale J, Evans CT, Herrold AA, Phipps Maieritsch K, et al. Diagnostic accuracy of the veteran affairs' traumatic brain injury screen. Arch Phys Med Rehabil. 2018;99(7):1370–82.
73. Popkirov S, Staab JP, Stone J. Persistent postural-perceptual dizziness (PPPD): a common, characteristic and treatable cause of chronic dizziness. Pract Neurol. 2018;18(1):5–13.
74. American Psychiatric Association: Diagnostic and Statistical Manual of Mental Disorders, Fifth Edition, Text Revision. Washington, DC, American Psychiatric Association, 2022, pp 235, 242, 605.
75. Clark MR, Swartz KL. A conceptual structure and methodology for the systematic approach to the evaluation and treatment of patients with chronic dizziness. J Anxiety Disord. 2001;15(1–2):95–106.
76. Rasimas JJ, Sinclair CM. Assessment and management of toxidromes in the critical care unit. Crit Care Clin. 2017;33(3):521–41.
77. Jamshidi N, Dawson A. The hot patient: acute drug-induced hyperthermia. Aust Prescr. 2019;42(1):24–8.
78. Ota Y, Capizzano AA, Moritani T, Naganawa S, Kurokawa R, Srinivasan A. Comprehensive review of Wernicke encephalopathy: pathophysiology, clinical symptoms and imaging findings. Jpn J Radiol. 2020;38(9):809–20.
79. Andresen-Streichert H, Müller A, Glahn A, Skopp G, Sterneck M. Alcohol biomarkers in clinical and forensic contexts. Dtsch Arzteblatt Int. 2018;115(18):309–15.
80. Helander A. Biological markers in alcoholism. J Neural Transm Suppl. 2003;(66):15–32.
81. Culture and Psychiatric Diagnosis" in American Psychiatric Association: Diagnostic and Statistical Manual of Mental Disorders, Fifth Edition, Text Revision. Washington, DC, American Psychiatric Association, 2022, pp 859.
82. Culture and Psychiatric Diagnosis" in American Psychiatric Association: Diagnostic and Statistical Manual of Mental Disorders, Fifth Edition, Text Revision. Washington, DC, American Psychiatric Association, 2022, pp 877
83. American Psychiatric Association: Diagnostic and Statistical Manual of Mental Disorders, Fifth Edition, Text Revision. Washington, DC, American Psychiatric Association, 2022, pp 871–4
84. Salgado de Snyder VN, Diaz-Perez MJ, Ojeda VD. The prevalence of nervios and associated symptomatology among inhabitants of Mexican rural communities. Cult Med Psychiatry. 2000;24(4):453–70.
85. Kidia K, Machando D, Bere T, Macpherson K, Nyamayaro P, Potter L, et al. 'I was thinking too much': experiences of HIV-positive adults with common mental disorders and poor adherence to antiretroviral therapy in Zimbabwe. Tropical Med Int Health. 2015;20(7):903–13.

Memory Loss

6

Jeffrey D. Lewis, Margaret Swanberg, Emily Bien,
Jessica Porcelan, and Pamela Broderick

Introduction

Memory loss is a common complaint among patients presenting to various specialists. Patients may use the term "memory loss" to capture a wide variety of symptoms. Whereas insomnia is often shared as a primary symptom because of the perceived lack of stigma associated with sleep dysfunction (as compared to depression or anxiety), memory loss is often shared because it captures the crux of what is causing occupational or social dysfunction for a patient. A college or university student might report memory loss in relation to struggles associated with learning new material—but these memory problems could be the result of anxiety, depression, attentional difficulties, or just a lack of interest in the course material. In the patient's mind, anxiety or a lack of interest may be present, but it is the inability to *remember* the answers on the test that brings them to the clinic. As such, the standard approach is to explore for additional symptoms to determine if memory loss is simply part of a constellation of symptoms (i.e., *part* of a disorder), or the *sole* presenting symptom. While using such a review-of-systems approach is not wholly ineffective, it undermines the *richness of meaning* of what "memory loss" might be. Indeed, for each of the etiologies of memory difficulties described above, the type

J. D. Lewis (✉)
Mental Health Clinic, Wright Patterson Medical Center, Wright Patterson AFB, OH, USA

Department of Neurology, Uniformed Services University of the Health Sciences,
Bethesda, MD, USA
e-mail: Jeffrey.d.lewis@wright.edu

M. Swanberg
Lincoln Memorial University-DeBusk College of Osteopathic Medicine,
Knoxville, TN, USA
e-mail: margaret.swanberg@lmunet.edu

E. Bien · J. Porcelan · P. Broderick
Mental Health Clinic, Wright Patterson Medical Center, Wright Patterson AFB, OH, USA

E. G. Meyer et al. (eds.), *The Medical Evaluation of Psychiatric Symptoms*,
https://doi.org/10.1007/978-3-031-14372-4_6

of memory loss can be different—and determining "what type" by getting behind the general term "memory loss" will provide valuable data to a physician attempting to develop a differential diagnosis. In this chapter, we review historical and medical specialty-specific perspectives pertaining to memory loss, and outline the evaluation of memory loss symptoms with a focus on declarative memory complaints. We then methodically discuss general medical and psychiatric disorders associated with memory loss.

History of Memory Loss

Memory and memory loss have interested philosophers at least since ancient Greece, and memory constructs were advanced by Aristotle [1]. In the eighteenth century, loss of memory was classified clinically as *amnesia*, based upon the Greek word for "forgetfulness." At that time, François Boissier de Sauvages developed a systematic classification of illnesses and described various causes of amnesia including physical ailments, physical trauma, episodes of strong emotionality, and the effect of various substances [2]. Additional causes of memory loss were subsequently described, including stroke. Benjamin Franklin contributed to the amnesia literature by describing memory loss from accidental electrical shock [3]. In the 1950s, the memory impairments of H.M., a patient who lost the ability to form new memories after surgical removal of bilateral temporal lobes, were reported [4]. H.M.'s memory dysfunction was studied extensively by neuropsychologists Brenda Milner, Suzanne Corker, and others, and their discoveries were critical for the modern view of memory loss [5]. In the 1980s, the information gained by the study of H.M.'s temporal lobe lesions was integrated with results from a nonhuman primate model of amnesia to provide a more comprehensive understanding of memory function and the role of the medial temporal structures in memory formation, storage, and recall [2].

Defining Memory Loss

Memory loss is the inability to acquire, retain, or retrieve information. This information could be goal-oriented or task-relevant information that is briefly retained, concerns how to complete a previously learned skill, or includes information about experiences and facts learned in the distant past. Symptoms of memory loss may include difficulty remembering recent events, remembering the names of common objects, or maintaining conscious awareness of information briefly needed for a specific task.

Memory systems are classified by the type of information that is being processed [6]. Memory systems that involve conscious awareness are classified as *explicit*, whereas learned behaviors, such as typing a frequently used password, are classified as *implicit*. Explicit memory systems involve consciously recalled knowledge and are defined in the Research Domain Criteria (RDoC) and elsewhere as *declarative memory* [7]. Usually, patients expressing "memory loss" are referring to *declarative*

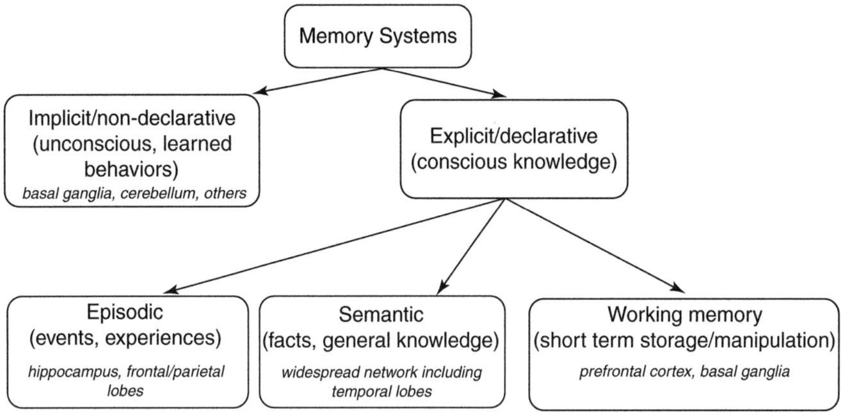

Fig. 6.1 Categories and subtypes of memory systems

memory difficulty. A patient describing declarative memory difficulty may not be able to recall what she and her spouse had for dinner the night before when asked, the recall of previously learned facts, or may recount episodes of walking from one room to another without remembering why they were going into the other room. The different categories of memory systems and subtypes are described in Fig. 6.1.

Declarative Memory Subtypes

Declarative memory systems involve consciously recalled knowledge, which may be of events (*episodic* memory), specific facts (*semantic* memory), or holding goal- or task-relevant information for a brief period (*working* memory). For purposes of this chapter, we classify these systems as subtypes of declarative memory, as all three involve the retention and processing of declarative information.

The *episodic memory subtype* of declarative memory is specific for autobiographical events that occur throughout life. It involves interactions among the frontal lobes, hippocampus, and other cortical regions, such as parietal cortex.

The *semantic memory subtype* is specific for general knowledge acquired through life, as well as the meaning of symbols and concepts. This definition is based upon the work of Tulving, who distinguished "autobiographical versus cognitive reference" in declarative memory [8]. This view has been supported by neuropsychological testing that focuses on categorical recall, such as asking how many names of animals an individual can produce in 1 min. Semantic memory, while initially considered a static collection of facts and information, may be involved in establishing meaning of somatosensory information and is dependent upon learned experience stored in episodic memory systems [9]. Semantic memory is most likely supported by a large network within the brain and includes the temporal lobes. Both semantic and episodic memory are declarative memory subtypes mutually important for learning and interpreting the meaning of new information.

Table 6.1 Relative impairment of declarative memory subtypes in various disorders

Subtypes of declarative memory likely impaired	Representative disorders
Working, episodic, and semantic	Attention-deficit/hyperactivity disorder
	Major depressive disorder
	Mild cognitive impairment (DSM-5-TR mild neurocognitive disorder)
	Mild traumatic brain injury (DSM-5-TR mild neurocognitive disorder due to traumatic brain injury)
	Obstructive sleep apnea
	Posttraumatic stress disorder
Working > episodic and semantic	Generalized anxiety disorder
	Medication/substance-induced mild neurocognitive disorder
Working, episodic, and semantic without measurable impairment	Subjective cognitive decline

The *working memory subtype* allows the brief retention of goal- or task-relevant information. It is sometimes classified separately from declarative memory but is dependent upon other declarative memory subtypes and declarative information is stored in working memory for a brief period of time. RDoC describes working memory as the construct which involves the subconstructs of active maintenance, flexible updating, control of interference from other input, and is of limited capacity [10]. Working memory subconstructs are important to consider when evaluating a memory complaint, as interference control may be impacted by psychiatric conditions such as ADHD, major depressive disorder, generalized anxiety disorder, and posttraumatic stress disorder (PTSD) [11–14]. For example, a patient with significant anxiety may be preoccupied with worries that interfere with her ability to retain a phone number she was just provided to call someone. The limited capacity of working memory decreases because of normal aging, so individuals are able to hold less information for a brief period of time, or the information is more quickly lost from working memory.

The relative involvement of the different subtypes in various general medical and psychiatric diagnoses are listed in Table 6.1. It is important to note these relative differences are general trends and not diagnostic but provide helpful additional information to guide the differential diagnosis.

Pathophysiology of Memory Loss

Memory loss occurs from the loss of function in several areas of the brain involved with encoding, storage, or retrieval of information. Episodic and semantic memory are primarily supported by the temporal lobe structures, and working memory relies on prefrontal cortex [6]. Damage from physical trauma or hypoxia, or dysfunction as the result of different substances, medications, poor sleep, or extreme emotional states, will impair memory function.

How Is Memory Loss Confused with Other Symptoms?

Memory (and its subcomponents) and learning are combined and conflated as one of several cognitive domains (complex attention, executive function, language, perceptual motor and social cognition) described in the DSM-5 and DSM-5-TR. Table 6.2 provides more nuanced clarifications between these domains. [15, 16].

While not expanded upon in this chapter, impairment of other cognitive domains beyond memory differentiates disorders that are solely *amnestic* from those involving multiple cognitive domains [16]. For example, HIV-associated neurocognitive disorder (HAND) commonly causes disturbances in memory, attention, and executive function [17]. Dysfunction in multiple cognitive domains broadens the medical differential beyond amnestic mild cognitive impairment, where just declarative memory is exclusively impaired.

Avoidance of Memory Recall

Patients may exhibit an inability to recall information that may be conscious, subconscious, or unconscious, to avoid recalling an emotionally charged event. This deficit is typically in reference to specific information, rather than a broad or general difficulty with memory function. This is particularly true in PTSD, with further elaboration in section "Posttraumatic Stress Disorder" below.

Table 6.2 Additional cognitive domains beyond "learning and memory"

Cognitive domain	Elements
Complex attention	Sustain, divide, or selectively attend to the environment
Executive function	Planning, decision-making, flexibility, and inhibition
Language	Naming, fluency, word-finding, and grammar
Perceptual motor	Coordination, ability to complete constructional tasks, and visually perceive the environment
Social cognition	Recognition of one's own emotions, insight, and the ability to perceive the emotional state of others

Memory Loss and Normal Aging

Older adults commonly complain of memory loss, with a prevalence of 50–60% in community-based samples [18]. An important consideration when assessing memory loss is distinguishing memory loss due to normal aging from pathologic or accelerated memory loss. The definition of age-related memory loss has undergone multiple iterations in terminology over time, from "benign senescent forgetfulness" defined in the 1960s, to the current terminology, "age-related cognitive decline" (ARCD) [19]. As a rule of thumb, individuals over the age of 50 normally experience difficulty recalling some information, particularly names of people or places, and other proper nouns.

In contrast to ARCD, relatively mild pathologic memory loss is currently classified as subjective cognitive decline (SCD) if objective measures do not demonstrate a deficit. In contrast, the term mild neurocognitive disorder (mild NCD) is used if the cognitive dysfunction is greater than age-matched individuals, and there are minor abnormalities demonstrated on standardized memory assessments.

Differences Among Specialties/Fields of Medicine

While the concept of memory loss is generally well understood in medicine, the presentations and settings vary among clinicians. Anesthesiologists and nurse anesthetists anticipate some memory impairment following anesthesia, but prolonged memory loss with other cognitive disturbances may cause concern for delirium or brief medication-induced neurocognitive disorder after the usual time course for anesthesia recovery. Surgeons or other proceduralists may be concerned that a peri-procedural embolic stroke has caused sudden memory loss after the patient recovers from anesthesia when symptoms exceed the usual presentation [20].

Internists, neurologists, and geriatricians typically use the term *mild cognitive impairment* (MCI) rather than mild NCD and *dementia* rather than major neurocognitive disorder. The DSM-5-TR criteria for mild NCD are similar to the criteria for MCI in the medical literature. One important distinction between MCI and mild NCD is that MCI has been almost exclusively studied in geriatric populations, while mild NCD includes conditions that may be present at any age. However, the DSM-5-TR Neurocognitive Disorders task force stated during development that mild NCD most frequently reflects what has been previously referred to as MCI, and criteria are the same or very similar depending upon the definition of MCI used for comparison [21].

Neurologists and psychiatrists approach memory loss relatively comprehensively and in a similar fashion, but the evaluation may emphasize different aspects of the patient examination. Neurologists typically emphasize the neurologic exam to evaluate other memory domains such as implicit memory. Psychiatrists usually employ the mental status exam and additional measures that comprehensively evaluate *declarative memory* and other cognitive domains while considering the various neurocognitive disorders as classified in DSM-5-TR. The psychiatric approach to memory loss includes the RDoC classification of *declarative* and *working memory* by assessing consciously recalled knowledge, and asking about diagnoses that may contribute to *working memory* difficulty such as interference control seen in ADHD [14] and PTSD [13].

Regional Differences in the Conceptualization of Memory Loss

While we could not identify any literature that assessed regional differences in the conceptualization of memory loss, differences in cultural representations of dementia have been reported. In one qualitative study of dementia patients, individuals of higher socioeconomic status expressed greater concern over their memory impairment than individuals of lower socioeconomic status [22]. Also, expectations of aging often vary by region and influence the emotional valence attached to the experience of progressive memory loss [23]. Therefore, regional differences in the conceptualization of the *significance* of the symptom likely exist.

Evaluation of the Patient with Declarative Memory Loss

Patients with a memory disorder may lack insight into the reason for an evaluation, relying upon accompanying family members to respond to questions, or communicate using vague and general language. For example, a patient may say, "Well, you know, I'm here to get checked out. I might be having a problem but it's really nothing that I'm worried about."

Patients may report forgetting conversations, appointments, or other planned events. If other cognitive domains are involved, they may show increasingly poor judgment or impulsivity. Finding their way in familiar environments, making plans or decisions, or following conversations may become challenging and overwhelming, which may lead to anxiety, irritability, and/or depression. These changes may also be noticed by clinicians or other individuals who interact with the patient. Establishing the rate of decline is important, as the differential diagnosis for sudden or rapidly progressive cognitive decline is different than for insidious, slow decline late in life.

The physical examination begins with the clinician's first introduction to the patient, in the waiting area or in the examination room. The mental status examination is conducted throughout the patient interview and includes an assessment of the patient's behavior, thought process, thought content, mood, and cognition. This can be accomplished informally during the history-taking process in a busy primary care encounter. The bedside examination of memory loss can be as simple as asking the patient to discuss current events, recount their medical history, or talk about upcoming plans for the holidays. Although this may be helpful for identifying a potential deficit in memory function, these methods of examination will likely miss memory dysfunction in high-functioning individuals and those with mild or early changes in memory function, who will require a more in-depth rating scale such as the Mini-Mental State Examination (MMSE), Montreal Cognitive Assessment (MoCA), or Saint Louis University Mental Status examination (SLUMS). These scales are described below. The individual may need even more sensitive standardized testing obtained by referral to a neuropsychologist.

The next step in the physical, neurologic, and psychiatric exam is to evaluate for signs of reversible and nonreversible conditions that may cause or contribute to memory deficits. For example, evaluation of a patient's skin may suggest recent or chronic intravenous drug use, infected decubiti, or foot infection. Abdominal evaluation may show evidence of a *caput medusae* sign suggesting portal hypertension and chronic alcoholism [24]. An enlarged thyroid may suggest thyroid pathology, and carotid bruits or murmurs suggest cerebrovascular disease.

A patient who frequently becomes tearful during the history and exam or gives up easily during the cognitive exam may be suggestive of underlying major depressive disorder as the etiology of the memory complaint, which is an important finding, as treating depressive disorder effectively will improve memory-related symptoms in most depressed patients.

A neurologic examination may demonstrate restricted vertical gaze suggestive of progressive supranuclear palsy [25], or a distal symmetric polyneuropathy suggestive of a cobalamin deficiency. Referring the patient to a neurologist for further work-up is warranted if a primary neurologic disorder is suspected based on physical exam findings.

Rating Scales for Memory Loss

If patients, and more importantly family members and/or caregivers, are concerned about their memory function, standardized measures should be completed during the encounter, as a general rule. If the clinician has a concern about memory performance, a referral for standardized neuropsychological testing should be considered.

There are multiple quick-to-administer cognitive rating scales available to the primary care provider for the assessment of memory function such as the Mini-Cog [26], Memory Impairment Screen (MIS) [27], and General Practitioner Assessment of Cognition (GPCOG). However, the three most commonly employed in the clinical setting are the MMSE [28], MoCA [29], and the SLUMS [30]. Each of these instruments has strengths and weaknesses, as discussed in Table 6.3.

Table 6.3 Commonly used measures to rate severity of memory loss

Cognitive measure	Time to complete (min)	Type of memory tested	Clinical significance
Montreal Cognitive Assessment (MoCA)	10–12	Working memory, episodic memory	Well validated Expanded language and executive function testing Better for detecting Mild Neurocognitive Disorder Useful when other cognitive domains are affected, e.g., visuospatial problems when someone describes difficulty driving
Mini-mental state examination (MMSE)	7–8	Working memory, episodic memory	Well validated Frequently used Can be done without use of form Better for detection of major neurocognitive disorder Particularly useful when the patient describes a language difficulty
Saint Louis University Mental Status Examination (SLUMS)	7	Working memory, episodic memory	Well validated Freely available online Developed specifically for mild and major neurocognitive disorder Multiple attempts until patient learns word list Cutoff scores vary based on patient education level Useful when more severe impairment is suspected
Mini-cog	< 3	Episodic memory	Quick to perform Minimal education effect Mainly tests memory Limited use in mild neurocognitive disorder; better for detection of dementia Useful when time is limited
Memory impairment screen (MIS)	< 3	Episodic memory	Quick to perform Only assesses memory No education effects Useful when language appears to be affected, and available in picture version
General Practitioner Assessment of Cognition (GPCOG)	4 for interviewer 2 for caregiver	Episodic memory	Not language or culturally influenced Online version Includes caregiver interview, so provides useful collateral information

Differential Diagnosis for Memory Loss

A comprehensive history, physical exam, and rating scale score are key elements required to formulate the differential diagnosis. Many general medical and psychiatric diagnoses may contribute to memory impairment. It is important to note that these conditions do not necessarily occur in isolation, and comorbid

Table 6.4 General differential diagnosis for cognitive decline. For a comprehensive list, see Ref. [31]

General etiological classification	Disorder (examples)
Traumatic	Traumatic brain injury, hemorrhage/hematoma
Inflammation/infection	HIV, HSV, Lyme disease, subacute/chronic meningitis, neurosyphilis, sarcoidosis
Neoplastic	Limbic encephalitis, tumor, lymphoma
Metabolic	Renal disease, hepatic encephalopathy, vitamin deficiency (e.g., thiamine, niacin, cyanocobalamin, cholecalciferol), thyroid disease
Vascular	Infarction, vascular dementia, cerebral amyloid angiopathy
Autoimmune	Steroid-responsive encephalopathy syndrome, systemic lupus erythematosus, polyarteritis nodosa
Medications or substances	Alcohol, heroin, cocaine, lead, or mercury exposure
Demyelinating diseases	Multiple sclerosis, acute disseminated encephalomyelitis, leukodystrophy
Neurodegenerative disorders	Alzheimer's disease, frontotemporal dementia, Parkinson's disease, Lewy body disease, Huntington's disease

HIV human immunodeficiency virus; *HAS* herpes simplex virus

psychiatric conditions occur in patients with memory disturbance with a systemic medical etiology. Table 6.4 provides a broad differential for multi-domain cognitive impairment of which a declarative memory impairment may be the presenting complaint.

Neurocognitive Disorders

The systematic approach to evaluating declarative memory deficits is difficult using the DSM-5-TR classification system. The criteria for mild and major neurocognitive disorders are based upon severity and impact of dysfunction, and do not describe declarative memory loss. In addition, the relative weight of each cognitive domain is equal, limiting the specificity of the diagnosis. For instance, memory, executive function, and visuospatial deficits in early Alzheimer's disease and the perceptual motor and executive dysfunction deficits in early Parkinson's disease may meet the criteria for either mild or major neurocognitive disorder, and a specific medical diagnosis is required to differentiate the two diagnoses. This is true for most specifiers, including Alzheimer's disease, frontotemporal lobar degeneration, Lewy body disease, vascular disease traumatic brain injury, HIV infection, prion disease, Parkinson's disease, and Huntington's disease.

Three neurocognitive disorders that tend to present early with declarative memory complaints are unspecified mild neurocognitive disorder, medication-induced neurocognitive disorder, and mild neurocognitive disorder due to traumatic brain injury. These and several other neurocognitive disorders are described in this chapter. mild NCD due to a traumatic brain injury is limited by the requirement for cognitive dysfunction, which is relatively transient compared to other symptoms such as headache or insomnia that tend to persist in mild traumatic brain injury.

Subjective Cognitive Decline (SCD)

Subjective cognitive decline is memory loss beyond ARCD and before it is detected on objective measures of impairment, such as neuropsychological testing. In 2014, an international consortium established the research criteria for SCD [32], and SCD is recognized by the National Institute on Aging–Alzheimer's Association [33]. SCD is particularly common in individuals who are more introspective, with higher levels of formal education, and currently or previously high-functioning as professionals. Identifying SCD is important, as individuals with SCD are at higher risk of dementia when compared to the general population [18]. Additionally, risk factors such as advanced age, lower baseline MMSE scores, and APOEε4 status in individuals with SCD are more likely to experience more rapid cognitive decline [34]. SCD is not included in the DSM-5-TR, which seems appropriate as SCD by definition does not cause significant impairment in function.

Prevalence of SCD

According to the Centers for Disease Control and Prevention, approximately 11.1% of adults experience SCD, and prevalence increases with increasing age [35].

Typical Findings in the Presenting Symptoms for SCD

Essentially all patients with SCD describe declarative memory loss. In the earliest form of SCD, patients may simply note the need for compensatory strategies for worsened memory. The use of these strategies is sufficient for others to notice memory loss, by definition [32].

Typical Physical Exam Findings in SCD

There are no specific physical exam findings for SCD, although it is important to complete a detailed physical exam to evaluate for mild NCD.

Rating Scales for SCD

There are no rating scales specific for SCD, but scores on the rating scales for mild NCD detailed previously are in the normal range.

Pitfalls/Differential Diagnosis

The most important aspect of the evaluation is to distinguish SCD from ARCD and mild NCD. One distinguishing feature is that informants (such as close family members) may express concern in cases of mild NCD. Another distinguishing feature is the rate of decline, and individuals with SCD are more likely to notice a deterioration in memory function faster than their peers of similar age. As assessment modalities such as advanced neuroimaging become clinically available, distinguishing SCD, ARCD, and mild NCD will become more objective [36].

Mild Neurocognitive Disorder (mild NCD)

The diagnostic criteria for mild NCD by DSM-5-TR include modest decline in cognitive function as noted by the patient, informant, or clinician with minimal functional impairment, that is preferably documented by standardized testing or clinical assessment [15]. mild NCD most commonly involves the single domain of memory but may involve multiple cognitive domains. mild NCD may improve, remain unchanged, or progress to a major neurocognitive disorder. Those diagnosed with mild NCD who do return to normal cognition have a higher risk of progressing to major neurocognitive disorder than those who have never been diagnosed with mild NCD. As per the US Preventative Services Task Force, approximately 2.4–5.5 million people in the US have dementia [37].

Incidence/Prevalence of mild NCD

There is limited data on the incidence and prevalence of mild NCD, and most epidemiologic studies use MCI criteria. Because mild NCD criteria are more stringent than MCI as mild NCD requires functional impairment, prevalence of mild NCD is likely lower than MCI [38]. The estimated prevalence of MCI ranges from 6.7% to 25.2%, with percentages increasing every 5 years from age 60 to 84 [39].

Incidence/Prevalence of mild NCD Presenting with Memory Loss

In a systematic review, the incidence of MCI with memory impairment in patients presenting with a complaint of memory loss was between 9.9 and 46.4 per 1000 person-years for *amnestic*, or *single* cognitive domain (memory), and between 28 and 36.3 per 1000 person-years for *multiple* cognitive domains [40]. Prevalence of MCI increased with increasing age, with prevalence of 6.7% for ages 60–64, 8.4% for ages 65–69, 10.1% for ages 70–74, 14.8% for ages 75–79, and 25.2% for ages 80–84. Compared to MCI involving other cognitive domains, MCI involving memory only has a higher incidence rate for individuals of older age and single marital status, and a decreased rate for individuals with a higher education level [39]. Presumably, the same pattern exists for mild NCD.

Typical Findings in the Presenting Symptoms for mild NCD

There are no specific features on physical exam for mild NCD. It is recommended that the clinician evaluate the patient for sensory or motor deficits, symptoms of thyroid disease, vitamin B12 deficiency, and infectious illnesses including insect-borne and sexually transmitted infections.

Typical Laboratory/Radiological Findings for mild NCD

There are no specific laboratory or radiological findings for mild NCD, and one of the criticisms of mild NCD as a diagnostic construct is that biomarkers are not included in the diagnostic criteria [21].

Pitfalls/Differential Diagnoses for mild NCD

Mild neurocognitive disorder has many etiologies. Since normal age-related memory decline and subjective cognitive decline are considerations, completing an appropriate screening instrument to determine the degree of objective memory impairment is important. Next, ask about recent history of mild traumatic brain injury from a fall or motor vehicle accident, sleep disorders (including sleep-disordered breathing, sleep-stage disorders, or abnormal movement disorders), or accompanying major depressive disorder (MDD) is important. More details about screening for these disorders can be found in chapters and are also included below. The past medical history is important for consideration of additional causes of neurocognitive dysfunction such as HIV or uncommon secondary causes such as systemic lupus erythematosus.

Delirium is another possible etiology of memory loss and should be considered when evaluating patients for possible mild NCD. The DSM-5-TR Neurocognitive Disorders Workgroup separated delirium from major and mild neurocognitive disorders because delirium symptom severity waxes and wanes and so cannot be classified as major or mild. The waxing and waning character due to impaired attention is an important consideration when working to distinguish delirium from mild NCD [41].

Delirium is especially common in the elderly. While attention is the primary cognitive domain affected in delirium, memory deficits can persist following recovery and are often one of the last symptoms to resolve. One longitudinal study of 173 geriatric patients found persistent memory deficits in approximately 50% of participants, and memory deficits persisting a mean of 45 days [42].

Medication-Induced Neurocognitive Disorder

Certain classes of medications may cause cognitive impairment, particularly in older adults. Medication side effects are generally reversible following medication discontinuation; however, chronic use may lead to irreversible cognitive effects. Medications that may cause cognitive impairment include benzodiazepines, nonbenzodiazepine sedative hypnotics, opioids, and proton-pump inhibitors. Anticholinergic medications are particularly problematic, including antihistamines and antimuscarinics (e.g., bladder antispasmodics), as well as psychotropic medications, such as first- and second-generation antipsychotics and tricyclic antidepressants. Anticonvulsant medications and lithium are problematic due to drug-drug interactions that can lead to decreased alertness or concentration, among other problems.

Incidence/Prevalence

The incidence of medication-induced cognitive impairment is unknown; however, the utilization of several classes of medication known to cause this impairment have increased in recent years. From 1990 to 2011, the estimated prevalence of anticholinergic use in the United Kingdom increased from 49.6% to 64.3% among individuals aged 65 or older [43]. Notably, both urologic medications such as oxybutynin and antidepressant medications such as tricyclic antidepressants (TCAs) and paroxetine have led to an increase of potent anticholinergic medications being prescribed to the elderly population [43]. Additionally, from 2015 to 2016, 30.6 million US adults reported using benzodiazepines, with 17.2% of overall use being benzodiazepine misuse [44].

Incidence/Prevalence of Diagnosis of Medication-Induced Neurocognitive Disorder Presenting with Memory Loss

The incidence of medication-induced neurocognitive disorder presenting with symptoms of memory loss is unknown. When comparing adults 65 years of age and older without anticholinergic medication exposure to those who were exposed to at least three anticholinergic medications for 90 days or more, the odds ratio was 2.73 for having MCI and 0.43 for having dementia [45]. Additionally, reduced working memory and recent memory performance have been found to be significantly reduced for current benzodiazepine users [46]. Many negative effects on memory persisted even after users had discontinued benzodiazepine use and remained abstinent [46]. In a 2012 study, benzodiazepines and non-benzodiazepines sedative hypnotics were shown to induce both amnestic and non-amnestic cognitive impairment, whereas first-generation antihistamines and TCAs induced deficits in attention and information processing [16].

Typical Symptoms of Medication-Induced Neurocognitive Disorder Presenting with Memory Loss

Patients initially experience increasing difficulty sustaining attention and awareness soon after starting a medication, and the symptoms usually wax and wane. These characteristics, along with other cognitive dysfunction, often initially meet the criteria for acute delirium rather than a medication-Induced mild neurocognitive disorder, as attention is the primary cognitive domain affected by subsequent poor registration of information into memory. When symptoms persist and cognitive function remains lower than at baseline, patients (and usually caregivers) may present with a concern for mild or major neurocognitive disorder.

Typical Physical Exam Findings of Medication-Induced Neurocognitive Disorder Presenting with Memory Loss

The physical exam and mental status exam may show signs and symptoms of cognitive impairment, memory loss, and other side effects specific to the medication in question. For example, anticholinergic medications may cause dizziness, unsteadiness, slurred speech, urinary retention, constipation, dry mouth, and blurred vision.

Typical Laboratory/Radiological Findings

There are no specific laboratory or radiological findings for medication-induced neurocognitive disorder. The following work-up is recommended:

- Basic metabolic panel.
- Serum levels of medications that have been shown to cause impairment at high serum concentrations (e.g., antiseizure medications, TCAs).
- Computed tomography of the head (Head CT) without contrast if the patient demonstrates focal abnormalities on neurologic exam or does not improve with time.
- EKG for long QRS or QTc associated with medications such as TCAs or antipsychotics.

Assessment Measures

Two tools that identify medications that may be contributing to a medication-induced neurocognitive disorder are the Beers criteria and Screening Tool of Older Persons' Prescriptions (STOPP) criteria. While not specific to memory loss, these tools help identify medications that cause a patient's cognitive dysfunction.

The Beers Criteria lists medications that are potentially inappropriate for all older adults, older adults with certain medical conditions, those to use with caution in older adults, those causing potential drug-drug interactions, and those that should be avoided or dose adjusted in patients with poor renal function [47]. The list of medications that meet Beers Criteria as potentially inappropriate for older adults is updated regularly by the American Geriatrics Society [47]. The sensitivity is 60.6% and specificity is 73.9% [48–50]. The STOPP criteria are also used to identify potentially inappropriate medications in older adults [51]. The sensitivity and specificity for STOPP criteria are 53.4% and 80.2%, respectively [48].

Pitfalls/Differential Diagnoses

Clinical factors that may contribute to the failure to identify a medication-induced neurocognitive disorder include the presence of memory loss, receiving an inadequate history and/or medication reconciliation, and nondisclosed over-the-counter or nonprescription medication use. As discussed above, delirium is an important consideration in differential diagnosis.

Substance-Induced Neurocognitive Disorder

The DSM-5-TR categorizes substance-induced memory impairment within the general category of substance/medication-induced major or mild neurocognitive disorder. One of the diagnostic criteria is persistence of symptoms beyond intoxication or acute withdrawal. Declarative memory deficits are commonly associated with severe alcohol use disorder, particularly in patients with poor nutrition (e.g., Korsakoff's syndrome). Declarative and working memory systems are impaired in cannabis and stimulant use disorders as well [52, 53].

Incidence/Prevalence

Alcohol use disorder is the most common substance use disorder, and the most likely disorder to manifest with memory disturbances. Prevalence of alcohol use disorder of any severity was approximately 13.9%, and lifetime prevalence is approximately 29.1% of respondents in the National Epidemiologic Survey on Alcohol and Related Conditions III [54].

Incidence/Prevalence of Substance-Induced Neurocognitive Disorder Presenting with Memory Loss

The number of patients presenting with memory complaints due to an underlying substance use disorder is unknown. However, cognitive impairment was found to be present in approximately one-third of patients presenting for substance abuse treatment [55].

Typical Presenting Symptoms of Substance-Induced Neurocognitive Disorder

Patients presenting with memory impairment due to alcohol or other substances may demonstrate executive function deficits and appear malnourished. Utilization of laboratory evaluation including aspartate aminotransferase (AST), alanine aminotransferase (ALT), carbohydrate deficient transferrin (CDT), phosphatidylethanol (Peth), and gamma-glutamyl transferase (GGT) is recommended to screen for use of alcohol and other substances.

Rating Scales for Substance-Induced Neurocognitive Disorder

The following rating scales are recommended for evaluation of alcohol and other substance use disorders that may be contributing to mild NCD:

- Alcohol Use Disorders Identification Test (AUDIT) cutoff of 3 (sensitivity 81%, specificity 95%, PPV 66.7%) [56]
- Drug Abuse Screening Test (DAST-20) cutoff of 5 (sensitivity 96%, specificity 79%, PPV 73%, NPV 97%) [57]

Pitfalls/Differential Diagnosis of Substance-Induced Neurocognitive Disorder

Patient may underreport or conceal their use of alcohol or substances. Seeking collateral information is recommended to inquire about a patient's recent use of alcohol or substances, history of alcohol or substance use, and recent behaviors that may indicate current use.

Another consideration in the differential diagnosis is substance-induced delirium. As previously mentioned, memory impairment can be the last symptom to resolve in delirium. The time course of the illness and the presence of waxing and waning symptoms is a helpful differentiating characteristics.

Mild Neurocognitive Disorder Due to Traumatic Brain Injury (mild NCD-TBI)

Traumatic brain injury (TBI) occurs when an external force on the head affects the function or structure of the brain. This may lead to transient or permanent cognitive dysfunction. In addition to cognitive disturbance, several additional symptoms may occur, such as headache, nausea and/or vomiting, dizziness, mood changes, photophobia, phonophobia, and disturbed sleep that are not included in the diagnostic criteria of mild neurocognitive disorder-TBI therefore limiting the utility of the DSM-5-TR diagnosis. There is an increasing recognition of oculomotor dysfunction following concussion, so asking about difficulty watching fast-paced sports or video games on a screen can be helpful [58].

Individuals who meet diagnostic criteria for mild neurocognitive disorder-TBI are a specific subset of TBI patients with impaired cognition and reduced function that persists after the acute period following injury. The majority of traumatic brain injuries are classified as mild traumatic brain injury (mTBI) by clinical criteria as listed in the Department of Veterans Affairs/Department of Defense Clinical Practice Guideline (VA/DoD CPG) for Management and Rehabilitation of Mild Traumatic Brain Injury, available at https://www.healthquality.va.gov/guidelines/Rehab/mtbi/. mTBI usually causes a transient mild neurocognitive disorder. Individuals with more severe injury are likely to experience more protracted symptoms and may meet the criteria for major neurocognitive disorder. This chapter emphasizes mTBI and mild neurocognitive disorder-TBI because individuals with more severe injuries are usually seen and treated in acute care settings.

The criteria for classification of mTBI in the VA/DoD CPG include a loss of consciousness ranging from 0 to 30 min, an alteration of consciousness lasting 1 min to 24 h, posttraumatic amnesia from 0 to 1 day, and normal neuroimaging. The criteria for mild neurocognitive disorder-TBI in the DSM-5-TR do not include duration of loss of consciousness or posttraumatic amnesia but include disorientation, confusion, or neurologic signs such as seizure or neuroimaging abnormalities as additional criteria. Therefore, mild neurocognitive disorder-TBI may represent a more impaired patient population than mTBI.

The anticipated recovery of memory disturbance following mTBI is improvement over days to weeks. However, if memory disturbance lasts longer than a month, then comorbid diagnoses, such as depression or anxiety, should be considered.

Incidence/Prevalence of mild NCD-TBI

The incidence of mild neurocognitive disorder-TBI is unknown. However, the incidence of mild TBI who seek acute care is approximately 0.5% of people in the United States [59]. Globally, it has been estimated that over 0.3% of people suffer a mTBI every year [60].

Incidence/Prevalence of mild neurocognitive disorder-TBI Presenting with Memory Loss

While estimates vary widely and are limited by recall or attribution biases, approximately 15% of patients with mild TBI will have persistent symptoms of cognitive impairment and post-concussion syndrome. However, this percentage is likely a significant underestimation, particularly in cases with cooccurring psychiatric disorders [61]. The cognitive impairment most frequently, although not exclusively, is memory loss [61].

Typical Presenting Symptoms in mild neurocognitive disorder-TBI

Patients may present acutely with a variety of symptoms, although many do not meet the criteria for mild neurocognitive disorder-TBI that emphasize cognitive disturbance, as previously discussed.

Typical Physical Exam Findings

The physical, neurologic, and mental status examination in the acute phase of injury may demonstrate a variety of signs. The patient's level of arousal or level of consciousness may be depressed. Short-term episodic memory may be limited, although long-term episodic memory is usually intact. The patient may also be disoriented, unable to focus cognitively, repeat the same answers, be slow to answer questions or follow instructions, and may be emotionally volatile. Vestibulo-ocular testing may show abnormalities such as receded near point of convergence, but this is not diagnostic of concussion and can be seen in several conditions [62].

Typical Laboratory/Radiological Findings

Mild neurocognitive disorder-TBI and mTBI are clinical diagnoses ideally based upon a witnessed traumatic event, although patients presenting with a memory complaint are typically in the subacute or chronic phase and the evaluation is typically limited by self-report. By definition, neuroimaging is normal in mTBI and serum biomarkers are limited in utility to the first hours following an injury. The presence of neuroimaging abnormalities such as subdural hematoma, traumatic subarachnoid hemorrhage is included in mild NCD-TBI criteria, however.

Assessment Tools

By DSM-5-TR criteria, individuals with a history of mTBI with objective memory impairment that is relatively mild are classified as mild NCD-TBI. The screening tests used for unspecified mild NCD described above may be useful in the subacute to chronic phase of injury. However, validation studies for these instruments in mild NCD-TBI are limited. Additionally, several sideline assessment instruments are available for the immediate assessment of mild NCD-TBI and are listed in Table 6.5. According to American Academy of Neurology clinical practice guidelines, no instrument used for sideline assessment is superior to other instruments but is helpful in characterizing initial symptoms [63].

Pitfalls/Differential Diagnoses

Following mTBI/mild NCD-TBI, patients may present immediately, or days to weeks after the traumatic event. Chronic traumatic encephalopathy should be considered if the patient has a history of multiple head injuries over time with persistent and worsening deficits and behavioral disturbance. Additionally, PTSD should always be considered in patients with a persistent deficit months after a traumatic

Table 6.5 Screening tools available for the sideline assessment following a sports-related acute mTBI. For details, see Ref. [64]

Sideline assessment tool	Sensitivity	Specificity	PPV
Standardized Assessment of Concussion (SAC)	0.94	0.76	
Sport Concussion Assessment Tool (SCAT) 3	0.83–0.96	0.81–0.91	
Balancing Error Scoring System (BESS)	0.34–0.71	0.87	
King-Devick Test (KDT)	0.86–0.98	0.90–0.96	0.89
Post-Concussion Symptom Scale (PCSS)	0.47–0.72	0.79–0.92	

PPV positive predictive value

event. Observing the patient during the interview, (particularly their affect while the traumatic event is described) and the symptom's impact on present functioning, can help the provider assess for psychiatric comorbidity.

Obstructive Sleep Apnea

Disturbed sleep may cause working and declarative memory dysfunction [65]. Obstructive sleep apnea (OSA) is a sleep-related respiratory disorder characterized by five or more recurring events per hour of sleep when partial or complete obstruction of the upper airway impedes airflow. OSA can also be diagnosed by the presence of 15 or more obstructive respiratory events per hour of sleep, even without reported sleep symptoms. Frequent apneic or hypopneic episodes interfere with restorative sleep and disrupt blood oxygenation, both of which impact brain function. The reader is referred to Chap. 4 for further discussion.

Incidence/Prevalence of Obstructive Sleep Apnea

The prevalence of OSA is approximately 10–17% for men and 3–9% for women in the US population. From 2000 to 2020, there has been a substantial increase in the prevalence of OSA [66]. Worldwide, approximately 936 million people have mild to moderate OSA [67].

Incidence/Prevalence of OSA Presenting with Memory Loss

The incidence of OSA presenting with a complaint of memory loss is unknown. However, in a pooled prospective study analyzing over 200,000 adults, there was a 26% likelihood of cognitive impairment, including dementia, in those with chronic sleep-disordered breathing [68]. Specifically, deficits in delayed long-term visual and verbal memory have been identified in individuals with OSA [69].

Typical Presenting Symptoms

Patients present with complaints of daytime sleepiness, sleep fragmentation, morning headaches, awakenings from gasping or choking, nocturia, and dry mouth. Additionally, their bed partners may report that the patient snores loudly and has interrupted breathing during sleep.

Typical Physical Exam Findings

The physical exam may show a large neck or waist circumference, crowded oropharyngeal airway, obesity, and systemic hypertension.

Typical Laboratory/Radiological Findings:

While there is no specific routine laboratory testing for OSA, plasma cysteine has shown promise as a potential biomarker, although this is not currently used in clinical settings [70]. For evaluation of OSA, radiographic imaging of the upper airway is not routinely performed. Polysomnography (PSG) performed in laboratory is the gold standard diagnostic test for OSA.

Rating Scales for OSA

In a systematic review and meta-analysis, the STOP-Bang questionnaire had a sensitivity of 90% for any OSA, and 96% for severe OSA. NPV were 46% and 90%, respectively [71]. Of note, studies in the general population are limited, as most research on OSA screening tools has been conducted in patients referred to a sleep clinic [72]. Therefore, screening tools such as STOP-Bang may be useful, but patients clearly endorsing clinical symptoms consistent with OSA should be referred to a sleep specialist for possible PSG if available. See Chap. 4 for more details.

Pitfalls/Differential Diagnoses for Memory Loss Due to a Sleep Disorder

Excessive daytime somnolence is also a symptom of other, non-OSA conditions, including narcolepsy, central sleep apnea, periodic limb movement disorder, and restless leg syndrome, and circadian-rhythm sleep disorders. Psychiatric conditions among the differential diagnoses include depression and panic attacks.

Psychiatric Differential for Memory Loss

Several psychiatric disorders (including many *not* listed as neurocognitive disorders in DSM-5-TR may present with declarative memory loss. It is important to anticipate that patients may initially reject the notion of a psychiatric condition causing their memory problems. In these cases, providing psychoeducation, exploring possible mental health stigma, and developing therapeutic rapport, potentially over several visits, are all imperative components of the patient's treatment plan. While a general medical practitioner may be well-practiced in treating many psychiatric conditions, a referral to a psychiatrist for medication evaluation and to either a psychiatrist, psychologist, or other behavioral therapists for evidence-based psychotherapy interventions may be warranted.

Major Depressive Disorder (MDD)

Clinicians treating major depressive disorder (MDD) are likely to focus on depressive symptoms, and may not appreciate the associated cognitive impairment, including poor memory, that occurs as part of the pathophysiology of MDD. A meta-analysis of depressive symptomatology demonstrated moderate cognitive deficits in memory, attention, and executive function, such as multitasking [73]. MDD impairs episodic memory storage more than the retrieval, which can be assessed by using cues or triggers during the assessment [6]. Therefore, individuals with MDD usually have little difficulty with memories prior to the onset of the depressive episode [74, 75]. Individuals with depressive disorder classified as mild or moderate by DSM-5-TR criteria usually experience subjective memory impairment that is not observed on objective measures. MDD-related memory deficits typically improve or resolve with successful treatment. Thus, it is recommended to reevaluate cognitive impairment following treatment of MDD, before considering a referral for additional cognitive evaluation.

The term "pseudodementia" has been used in the past to describe memory impairment from MDD. This term can be confusing to patients and physicians who may assume the patient is embellishing symptoms or malingering. Therefore, a term such as "neurocognitive dysfunction due to depressive disorder" is preferred.

Incidence/Prevalence of MDD

Prevalence data for MDD, according to the National Institute of Mental Health website for health statistics, shows that approximately 7.1% of all US adults experienced one major depressive episode, and 4.5% of all adults experienced severe impairment from depression [37].

Incidence/Prevalence of MDD Presenting with Memory Loss

Estimates of the prevalence of cognitive impairment in MDD vary from 4% to 21% and are more frequent in psychiatric inpatients [74, 75]. In the DSM-5-TR criteria for MDD, cognitive dysfunction is characterized as diminished ability to think or concentrate, or indecisiveness occurring nearly every day [76]. Many patients with MDD report a concern about their memory out of fear of having dementia. It is recommended that the clinician consider the patient's premorbid cognitive functioning and evaluate for other symptoms of depression when considering MDD in the differential diagnosis for memory loss. This is particularly important for indecisiveness, which can also be a symptom of obsessive-compulsive disorder or anxiety disorder.

Typical Findings in the Presenting Symptoms for MDD

Patients with memory disturbance secondary to MDD will typically endorse other symptoms to include loss of interest, sleep disturbance, change in appetite, psychomotor retardation or agitation, feelings of hopelessness or worthlessness, excessive guilt, low energy, loss of libido, and thoughts of death or suicide. It is important to remember that diagnostic criteria for MDD are met when >5 of the abovementioned symptoms are present for at least 2 weeks, with one necessarily being irritable mood or loss of interest and thus a patient may meet MDD criteria *without* endorsing feeling depressed. In some cultures and subpopulations, depressed mood is less likely to be openly discussed, but other signs and symptoms of MDD may be evident, such as somatic complaints and changes in behavior [77].

Rating Scales for MDD

Patients with memory deficits due to MDD often show poor effort when asked to perform a cognitive task and/or may give up easily during screening evaluations. For example, a depressed patient may respond repeatedly with, "I don't know," or "I can't," when asked to remember words for a rating scale. If MDD is suspected, the Patient Health Questionnaire-9 (PHQ-9) is recommended, with positive predictive value (PPV) at 59% in an unselected primary care population, increasing to 85–90% in populations with a higher prevalence of MDD, such as a psychiatric outpatient population [78]. Another tool that can be used as part of a structured interview is the Hamilton Depression Rating Scale (HAM-D). In a study of dementia patients, a score of 13 or greater on the HAM-D provided a PPV of 76% and NPV of 86% for diagnosing depression [79].

Pitfalls/Differential Diagnosis

As MDD may cooccur with mild NCD, it is recommended that if a patient's memory does not improve after a full clinical trial of antidepressant treatment and symptom resolution, a separate etiology of the memory deficit should be revisited. It is also important to remember that MDD later in life doubles one's risk of later developing dementia (or major neurocognitive disorder in the DSM) thus aggressive treatment of MDD to remission of symptoms is recommended in the elderly population [80].

Generalized Anxiety Disorder

Identifying anxiety in patients presenting with poor memory or concentration can be tricky due to the great variety of clinical presentations. It is often telling to inquire what patients think about when they are not engaged in an activity and their mind is not occupied. Patients with anxiety will typically respond that their thoughts are "racing" while scrutinizing past events or potential negative outcomes yet to come. Patients experiencing somatic symptoms of anxiety may worry and ruminate about physical symptoms and fear medical conditions they believe they may have. In short, patients with anxiety experience negative, anxiety-provoking thoughts when their mind is left to its own devices.

Anxiety disorders most often impair capacity of working memory. Implicit memory may also be impaired by anxiety, while explicit memory is typically preserved [81–83]. Therefore, it is recommended that clinicians directly inquire about working memory difficulties when an anxiety disorder is suspected.

Diagnostic features of GAD, per DSM-5-TR criteria, include excessive anxiety and worry about several events or activities, as well as difficulty controlling worry, and/or difficulty concentrating or "mind going blank." Patients may experience or interpret symptoms of difficulty concentrating or their mind going blank as memory loss and present with this complaint [84].

Incidence/Prevalence of GAD

According to US government statistics, approximately 2.7% of adults have had GAD in the past year, and 5.7% of adults will experience GAD within their lifetime [37].

Prevalence of Memory Loss in GAD

There is limited data on the prevalence of memory loss associated with GAD. It is suggested that the prevalence of cognitive impairment in GAD is like that of MDD, in which 19% experience cognitive impairment. Although GAD and MDD may have a similar associated cognitive impairment, typically the impairment is less severe with GAD [74].

Typical Presenting Symptoms

The presentation of patients with GAD can vary greatly due to differences in symptoms, as well as variable patient insight into their symptoms. The hallmark symptoms of GAD include excessive and uncontrollable worry, as well as poor concentration. However, many patients also experience physical symptoms of anxiety, such as rapid heart rate, shaking, sweating, dizziness, blurred vision, and shortness of breath. Patients may also present with other associated anxiety symptoms, such as irritability, sleep disturbance, restlessness, inability to relax, and poor memory. Still other patients may complain of somatic symptoms, such as stomach pain or upset, headaches, or muscle tension, without endorsing worry or feelings of anxiety. Additionally, individuals with limited insight into their anxiety may believe their symptoms are purely physical in nature and evidence of a feared medical condition.

Rating Scales for Anxiety

The Generalized Anxiety Disorder 7-Item (GAD-7) is recommended for evaluation of anxiety symptoms. A GAD-7 score of 10 or higher has PPV of 29%, NPV of 99% in primary care samples [85].

Pitfalls/Differential Diagnosis

Anxiety may be the cause of a patient's memory complaint, or anxiety may be comorbid with another medical etiology of cognitive impairment. For example, anxiety as a symptom is common prior to the onset of major neurocognitive disorder [86]. Additionally, anxiety may worsen the outcome in patients with subjective memory complaints. Patients with SCD who express worry about their memory loss are more likely to progress to mild NCD. The risk is further elevated if the patient's memory impairment is endorsed by a collateral source, such as a family member [34]. In these cases, further evaluation of the memory complaint is recommended to avoid a missed medical cause.

Posttraumatic Stress Disorder (PTSD)

Post traumatic stress disorder (PTSD) may impact memory function through multiple mechanisms. Memory of traumatic events is encoded and recalled differently than memories of non-traumatic events. Portions of traumatic memories are often excessively preserved and difficult to extinguish, so-called burned in one's memory, while other portions are hazy or absent entirely. This phenomenon is thought to be because of stress hormones, such as glucocorticoids on the hippocampus and epinephrine on the prefrontal cortex [87, 88]. The impact of traumatic memory is characteristic of PTSD to such a degree that one of the core diagnostic PTSD criteria is recurrent, involuntary, and intrusive distressing memories of the traumatic event.

Some symptoms of PTSD mimic declarative memory deficits but are likely due to other emotional factors. Actively avoiding distressing memories associated with the event is a criterion for the diagnosis in DSM-5-TR. Another criterion is the inability to remember an important event independent of factors such as head injury or substances. The cause of the deficit in the latter case is due to dissociative amnesia specific to the trauma, rather than a generalized impairment in declarative memory function.

Disturbances in multiple cognitive domains have been demonstrated in PTSD, including working and verbal memory [89]. The working memory deficit associated with PTSD is thought to result from impairment of interference control mechanisms related to aberrant stress hormones [90].

Incidence/Prevalence of PTSD

According to the National Comorbidity Survey Replication survey results, the annual incidence of PTSD in US adults is 3.6%, with a lifetime prevalence of 6.8% [37].

Incidence/Prevalence of PTSD Presenting with Memory Loss

Prevalence data of cognitive symptoms of PTSD is limited, and it is confounded by differences in subjective cognitive complaints, that are frequent in individuals with PTSD, and objective cognitive deficits of neuropsychological testing [91].

Typical Findings in Presenting Symptoms of PTSD

Patients with PTSD often initially present with symptoms seemingly unrelated to trauma. Patients typically do not readily disclose their trauma history and may suffer from PTSD symptoms for years without seeking treatment. Patients may present for evaluation due to the negative effects of their symptoms on their relationships or occupational functioning. Presenting symptoms commonly include sleep disturbance, irritability or anger, poor memory or concentration, anxiety, depressed mood, or suicidal ideation. Behavioral problems, sometimes leading to legal issues, and substance or alcohol misuse are also commonly reported.

Memory difficulty is often a presenting complaint of PTSD. Careful evaluation of the time course of the patient's memory impairment may reveal a precipitating event, which may be traumatic in nature. A useful screening question for trauma is, "Can you recall any situation or event in your past that most people would consider traumatic?" It is important to note that trauma is subjective, and responses to this question will likely elicit a variety of responses, only some of which meet PTSD criterion A for trauma. Additional exploration of the patient's experiences is necessary to differentiate trauma meeting PTSD criteria from other more normative stressful events or bereavement. PTSD-related memory impairment is typically experienced as a consistent, baseline level, with periods of exacerbation related to PTSD triggers. A discussion of what seems to make a patient's memory problems worse may identify triggers related to potential trauma thus putting PTSD on the differential diagnosis.

Rating Scale for PTSD

The PTSD Checklist for DSM-5-TR (PCL-5) with a cutoff score of 31–33 was found to have sensitivity of 0.69, specificity of 0.69, and PPV of 0.81 in a validation study conducted on veterans [92]. This scale asks one direct question about memory impairment and one about avoiding memories related to the stressful experience.

Pitfalls/Differential Diagnosis

PTSD is commonly comorbid with other psychiatric conditions, such as alcohol or substance use disorders, ADHD, and depressive disorders. In some military populations and occupations with greater likelihood of head trauma, mild NCD-TBI should also be considered and assessed. It is also important to recognize that most individuals exposed to trauma do *not* develop PTSD [93]. Acute stress disorder is the appropriate diagnosis for PTSD symptoms that occur within 3 days to 1 month following a traumatic event and are common in the immediate aftermath of trauma. Fortunately, acute stress disorder symptoms usually dissipate within 1 month and with nonmedical supportive interventions, although psychopharmacology may be indicated to help to improve sleep; symptoms persisting after 30 days warrant a rediagnosis as PTSD.

Attention Deficit Hyperactivity Disorder (ADHD)

The DSM-5-TR criteria for ADHD are composed of three symptom clusters: inattention, hyperactivity, and impulsivity. The inattentive symptoms of ADHD include forgetfulness in daily activities, and, thus, poor memory is a common complaint. In ADHD, the interference control mechanism in working memory is impaired, and working memory deficits are common [94, 95]. Additionally, meta-analyses demonstrated that ADHD is associated with other declarative memory deficits [96].

The duration of symptoms is an important factor when considering the ADHD diagnosis. Diagnostic criteria for ADHD include the onset of symptoms prior to age 7 thus ADHD is unlikely if symptom onset is in adulthood. It is also important to recognize that ADHD symptoms may change with age, with inattentive symptoms most often persisting into adulthood, while hyperactivity symptoms may improve or remit in adulthood. As ADHD has a strong hereditary competence, a history of ADHD may be present in a review of family psychiatric history. Specific questions regarding ADHD or treatment with stimulant medication in family members, including the patient's children, is important.

Incidence/Prevalence in Adults

Among US adults, the annual prevalence of adult ADHD is estimated at 4.4% [97], and lifetime prevalence in adults is estimated at 8.1% [98]. ADHD is roughly twice as prevalent in males than in females.

Incidence/Prevalence of ADHD Presenting with Memory Loss

Although specific numbers are unknown, poor memory is a common presenting symptom in patients with ADHD. Forgetfulness is a key diagnostic criterion as working memory is dependent on attention.

Typical Findings in Presenting Symptoms

Patients with ADHD typically present with symptoms of poor concentration, poor organization, difficulty with task completion, distractibility, difficulty with academic pursuits or reading comprehension, and forgetfulness, often manifested as frequently misplacing or losing important items. Patients have a history of poor academic performance in grade school or academic underachievement, incongruent with their intelligence. Patients will often present when their ADHD symptoms are uncovered or exacerbated by a change in occupational or academic demands, specifically when there are greater administrative or multitasking responsibilities. Inattentive symptoms can also be exacerbated by stress or sleep deprivation.

An important line of inquiry is to ask about what improves a patient's concentration or memory. Behaviors which improve attention, including needing a quiet location away from distraction, engaging in a physical activity while studying or reading (such as pacing/listening to music), or having a robust response to caffeine, all point towards ADHD as an etiology. Interestingly, patients with ADHD do not have difficulty paying attention to or remembering things that interest them or describe that they can be "hyperattentive" in these areas. For example, a patient may remember many facts and details about a favorite sport, but they may not remember other things, such as appointments or deadlines. Collateral information from those close to the patient is also helpful when assessing for ADHD, as others may notice symptoms the patient may not.

Mental status examination findings suggestive of ADHD include difficulty sustaining attention during the interview (looking around the room, appearing to pay poor attention to the conversation, especially during extended discussion), interrupting or responding before the clinician is finished talking, or excessive fidgeting.

Assessment Tools

There are no reliable tools to assess for ADHD. The gold standard for diagnosing ADHD is a clinical interview by an experiencing mental health professional, with collateral history. Contrary to popular belief, neuropsychological testing is not needed or recommended to diagnose ADHD. While neuropsychological testing is useful for identifying specific learning disorder and neurocognitive disorders, it has limited sensitivity and specificity for ADHD.

Pitfalls/Differential Diagnosis

Conditions that may appear similar in presentation to ADHD include substance abuse, mild NCD-TBI, and anxiety. Reviewing the time course of symptoms is helpful to rule out ADHD if symptom onset is in adulthood. Poor concentration due to anxiety versus ADHD is often challenging to tease apart. Patients with ADHD and anxiety may both report "racing" thoughts, but patients with ADHD will typically report random thoughts about many things, rather than negative and anxiety-provoking thoughts.

Conclusion

When writing this chapter, we faced the challenging task of integrating general medical, neurologic, and psychiatric diagnoses that are sometimes incompletely described, or not described at all, in the DSM-5-TR. We have tried to draw upon the relative strengths of several different classification systems to aid the clinician treating a patient complaining of memory loss.

The symptom of memory loss, although seemingly straightforward, can be difficult. Evaluation of a complaint of memory loss requires careful listening and observing to fully understand exactly what the patient is experiencing, and what their informant is witnessing. The differential diagnosis is broad and includes what is classically subdivided into primary medical, neurologic, and psychiatric practice domains.

While there are several subtypes of memory, each with its own unique anatomic networks and symptom clusters, this chapter focuses on declarative memory as it is the most common type of memory loss complaint seen in the general clinical setting. When presented with a patient, or their informant, concerned about "memory loss" the clinician needs to learn the following:

1. What exactly does the patient mean by "memory loss?" Is this truly related to a deficit in a memory system or some other cognitive system, such as attention, concentration, language, or another cognitive domain?
2. What type of memory loss is the patient experiencing? Is it *episodic*, *semantic*, or *working* as defined above?
3. What is the underlying etiology?

When considering underlying etiology, the clinician must wrestle with differences between DSM-5-TR classification and diagnostic terminology employed in the neurologic or primary care setting. Classification in the DSM-5-TR limits diagnoses to either major or mild neurocognitive disorder, while terms such as dementia, mild cognitive impairment, or subjective cognitive decline are commonly utilized by other clinicians to describe the same or similar memory impairment.

For an accurate diagnosis to explain the memory loss, the clinician must determine the specific memory-related symptom, take a detailed history, perform a physical examination, complete an appropriate screening tool, order targeted laboratory studies, and initiate a management plan. By taking a methodical approach, the clinician can usually achieve the goal of providing the correct diagnosis, optimizing treatment, and improving the patient's quality of life.

References

1. Howes MB. Human memory: structures and images. Thousand Oaks, CA: SAGE Publications, Inc.; 2007.
2. Squire LR, Wixted JT. The cognitive neuroscience of human memory since H.M. Annu Rev Neurosci. 2011;34:259–88.

3. Langer KG. The history of amnesia-a review. Curr Neurol Neurosci Rep. 2021;21(8):40.
4. Scoville WB, Milner B. Loss of recent memory after bilateral hippocampal lesions. J Neurol Neurosurg Psyschiatry. 1957;12(1):103–13.
5. Eichenbaum H. What H.M. taught us. J Cogn Neurosci. 2013;25(1):14–21.
6. Budson AE, Price BH. Memory dysfunction. N Engl J Med. 2005;352(7):692–9.
7. National Institute of Mental Health. Declarative memory. 2021. https://www.nimh.nih.gov/research/research-funded-by-nimh/rdoc/constructs/declarative-memory.
8. Tulving E. Episodic and semantic memory. In: Tulving E, Donaldson W, editors. Organization of memory, I. Cambridge, MA: Academic Press; 1972. p. 381–403.
9. Kumar AA. Semantic memory: a review of methods, models, and current challenges. Psychon Bull Rev. 2021;28(1):40–80.
10. National Institute of Mental Health. Working memory. 2021. https://www.nimh.nih.gov/research/research-funded-by-nimh/rdoc/constructs/working-memory.shtml.
11. Moran TP. Anxiety and working memory capacity: a meta-analysis and narrative review. Psychol Bull. 2016;142(8):831–64.
12. Demeyer I, et al. Rumination mediates the relationship between impaired cognitive control for emotional information and depressive symptoms: a prospective study in remitted depressed adults. Behav Res Ther. 2012;50(5):292–7.
13. Aupperle RL, et al. Executive function and PTSD: disengaging from trauma. Neuropharmacology. 2012;62(2):686–94.
14. van Mourik R, Oosterlaan J, Sergeant JA. The Stroop revisited: a meta-analysis of interference control in AD/HD. J Child Psychol Psychiatry. 2005;46(2):150–65.
15. "Neurocognitive Disorders", American Psychiatric Association: Diagnostic and Statistical Manual of Mental Disorders, Fifth Edition, Text Revision. Washington, DC, American Psychiatric Association, 2022.
16. Tannenbaum C, et al. A systematic review of amnestic and non-amnestic mild cognitive impairment induced by anticholinergic, antihistamine, GABAergic and opioid drugs. Drugs Aging. 2012;29(8):639–58.
17. Antinori A, et al. Updated research nosology for HIV-associated neurocognitive disorders. Neurology. 2007;69(18):1789–99.
18. Mendonca MD, Alves L, Bugalho P. From subjective cognitive complaints to dementia: who is at risk?: a systematic review. Am J Alzheimers Dis Other Dement. 2016;31(2):105–14.
19. Golomb J, Kluger A, Ferris SH. Mild cognitive impairment: historical development and summary of research. Dialogues Clin Neurosci. 2004;6(4):351–67.
20. Laible M, et al. Peri-procedural silent cerebral infarcts after left atrial appendage occlusion. Eur J Neurol. 2017;24(1):53–7.
21. Stokin GB, et al. Mild neurocognitive disorder: an old wine in a new bottle. Harv Rev Psychiatry. 2015;23(5):368–76.
22. Hulko W. From 'not a big deal' to 'hellish': experiences of older people with dementia. J Aging Stud. 2008;23(3):131–44.
23. Hillman A, Latimer J. Cultural representations of dementia. PLoS Med. 2017;14(3):e1002274.
24. Yang PM, Chen DS. Images in clinical medicine. Caput medusae. N Engl J Med. 2005;353(21):e19.
25. Ali F, Josephs K. The diagnosis of progressive supranuclear palsy: current opinions and challenges. Expert Rev Neurother. 2018;18(7):603–16.
26. Lorentz WJ, Scanlan JM, Borson S. Brief screening tests for dementia. Can J Psychiatr. 2002;47(8):723–33.
27. Kuslansky G, et al. Screening for Alzheimer's disease: the memory impairment screen versus the conventional three-word memory test. J Am Geriatr Soc. 2002;50(6):1086–91.
28. Folstein MF, Folstein SE, McHugh PR. "Mini-mental state". A practical method for grading the cognitive state of patients for the clinician. J Psychiatr Res. 1975;12(3):189–98.
29. Nasreddine ZS, et al. The Montreal Cognitive Assessment, MoCA: a brief screening tool for mild cognitive impairment. J Am Geriatr Soc. 2005;53(4):695–9.

30. Tariq SH, et al. Comparison of the Saint Louis University mental status examination and the mini-mental state examination for detecting dementia and mild neurocognitive disorder—a pilot study. Am J Geriatr Psychiatry. 2006;14(11):900–10.
31. Dickerson BC, Atri A. Dementia : comprehensive principles and practice. Oxford, NY: Oxford University Press; 2014. xx, 666 pages
32. Jessen F, et al. A conceptual framework for research on subjective cognitive decline in preclinical Alzheimer's disease. Alzheimers Dement. 2014;10(6):844–52.
33. Sperling RA, et al. Toward defining the preclinical stages of Alzheimer's disease: recommendations from the National Institute on Aging-Alzheimer's Association workgroups on diagnostic guidelines for Alzheimer's disease. Alzheimers Dement. 2011;7(3):280–92.
34. Slot RER, et al. Subjective cognitive decline and rates of incident Alzheimer's disease and non-Alzheimer's disease dementia. Alzheimers Dement. 2019;15(3):465–76.
35. CDC. Subjective cognitive decline-a public health issue. 2021. https://www.cdc.gov/aging/data/subjective-cognitive-decline-brief.html.
36. Hedden T, Gabrieli JD. Insights into the ageing mind: a view from cognitive neuroscience. Nat Rev Neurosci. 2004;5(2):87–96.
37. National Institute of Mental Health. Mental health information. 2021 [cited 2021 10/11/2021]. https://www.nimh.nih.gov/health/statistics.
38. Lopez-Anton R, et al. Mild cognitive impairment diagnosed with the new DSM-5 criteria: prevalence and associations with non-cognitive psychopathology. Acta Psychiatr Scand. 2015;131(1):29–39.
39. Petersen RC, et al. Practice guideline update summary: Mild cognitive impairment: report of the guideline development, dissemination, and implementation Subcommittee of the American Academy of Neurology. Neurology. 2018;90(3):126–35.
40. Luck T, et al. Incidence of mild cognitive impairment: a systematic review. Dement Geriatr Cogn Disord. 2010;29(2):164–75.
41. Ganguli M, et al. Classification of neurocognitive disorders in DSM-5: a work in progress. Am J Geriatr Psychiatry. 2011;19(3):205–10.
42. Rockwood K. The occurrence and duration of symptoms in elderly patients with delirium. J Gerontol. 1993;48(4):M162–6.
43. Grossi CM, et al. Increasing prevalence of anticholinergic medication use in older people in England over 20 years: cognitive function and ageing study I and II. BMC Geriatr. 2020;20(1):267.
44. Maust DT, Lin LA, Blow FC. Benzodiazepine use and misuse among adults in the United States. Psychiatr Serv. 2019;70(2):97–106.
45. Cai X, et al. Long-term anticholinergic use and the aging brain. Alzheimers Dement. 2013;9(4):377–85.
46. Crowe SF, Stranks EK. The residual medium and long-term cognitive effects of benzodiazepine use: an updated meta-analysis. Arch Clin Neuropsychol. 2018;33(7):901–11.
47. By the 2019 American Geriatrics Society Beers Criteria Update Expert Panel. American Geriatrics Society 2019 updated AGS Beers Criteria(R) for potentially inappropriate medication use in older adults. J Am Geriatr Soc. 2019;67(4):674–94.
48. Brown JD, et al. Predictive validity of the Beers and Screening Tool of Older persons' Potentially Inappropriate Prescriptions (STOPP) criteria to detect adverse drug events, hospitalizations, and emergency department visits in the United States. J Am Geriatr Soc. 2016;64(1):22–30.
49. American Geriatrics Society Beers Criteria Update Expert Panel. American Geriatrics Society updated Beers Criteria for potentially inappropriate medication use in older adults. J Am Geriatr Soc. 2012;60(4):616–31.
50. Moriarty F, et al. Comparing potentially inappropriate prescribing tools and their association with patient outcomes. J Am Geriatr Soc. 2020;68(3):526–34.
51. O'Mahony D. STOPP/START criteria for potentially inappropriate medications/potential prescribing omissions in older people: origin and progress. Expert Rev Clin Pharmacol. 2020;13(1):15–22.

52. Potvin S, et al. Cognitive deficits in individuals with methamphetamine use disorder: a meta-analysis. Addict Behav. 2018;80:154–60.
53. Broyd SJ, et al. Acute and chronic effects of cannabinoids on human cognition-a systematic review. Biol Psychiatry. 2016;79(7):557–67.
54. Grant BF, et al. Epidemiology of DSM-5 alcohol use disorder: results from the National Epidemiologic Survey on Alcohol and Related Conditions III. JAMA Psychiat. 2015;72(8):757–66.
55. Bruijnen C, et al. Prevalence of cognitive impairment in patients with substance use disorder. Drug Alcohol Rev. 2019;38(4):435–42.
56. Gomez A, et al. Diagnostic usefulness of brief versions of Alcohol Use Disorders Identification Test (AUDIT) for detecting hazardous drinkers in primary care settings. J Stud Alcohol. 2005;66(2):305–8.
57. Gavin DR, Ross HE, Skinner HA. Diagnostic validity of the drug abuse screening test in the assessment of DSM-III drug disorders. Br J Addict. 1989;84(3):301–7.
58. Broglio SP, et al. Current and emerging rehabilitation for concussion: a review of the evidence. Clin Sports Med. 2015;34(2):213–31.
59. Bazarian JJ, et al. Mild traumatic brain injury in the United States, 1998–2000. Brain Inj. 2005;19(2):85–91.
60. Gardner RC, Yaffe K. Epidemiology of mild traumatic brain injury and neurodegenerative disease. Mol Cell Neurosci. 2015;66(Pt B):75–80.
61. McInnes K, et al. Mild traumatic brain injury (mTBI) and chronic cognitive impairment: a scoping review. PLoS One. 2017;12(4):e0174847.
62. Raghuram A, et al. Postconcussion: receded near point of convergence is not diagnostic of convergence insufficiency. Am J Ophthalmol. 2019;206:235–44.
63. Giza CC, et al. Summary of evidence-based guideline update: evaluation and management of concussion in sports: report of the guideline development Subcommittee of the American Academy of neurology. Neurology. 2013;80(24):2250–7.
64. Yue JK, et al. Sideline concussion assessment: the current state of the art. Neurosurgery. 2020;87(3):466–75.
65. Delhikar N, et al. Autobiographical memory from different life stages in individuals with obstructive sleep apnea. J Int Neuropsychol Soc. 2019;25(3):266–74.
66. Peppard PE, et al. Increased prevalence of sleep-disordered breathing in adults. Am J Epidemiol. 2013;177(9):1006–14.
67. Benjafield AV, et al. Estimation of the global prevalence and burden of obstructive sleep apnoea: a literature-based analysis. Lancet Respir Med. 2019;7(8):687–98.
68. Leng Y, et al. Association of sleep-disordered breathing with cognitive function and risk of cognitive impairment: a systematic review and meta-analysis. JAMA Neurol. 2017;74(10):1237–45.
69. Bucks RS, Olaithe M, Eastwood P. Neurocognitive function in obstructive sleep apnoea: a meta-review. Respirology. 2013;18(1):61–70.
70. Cintra F, et al. Cysteine: a potential biomarker for obstructive sleep apnea. Chest. 2011;139(2):246–52.
71. Nagappa M, et al. Validation of the STOP-Bang questionnaire as a screening tool for obstructive sleep apnea among different populations: a systematic review and meta-analysis. PLoS One. 2015;10(12):e0143697.
72. Chiu HY, et al. Diagnostic accuracy of the Berlin Questionnaire, STOP-BANG, STOP, and Epworth sleepiness scale in detecting obstructive sleep apnea: a bivariate meta-analysis. Sleep Med Rev. 2017;36:57–70.
73. Rock PL, et al. Cognitive impairment in depression: a systematic review and meta-analysis. Psychol Med. 2014;44(10):2029–40.
74. Gualtieri CT, Morgan DW. The frequency of cognitive impairment in patients with anxiety, depression, and bipolar disorder: an unaccounted source of variance in clinical trials. J Clin Psychiatry. 2008;69(7):1122–30.
75. Douglas KM, et al. Prevalence of cognitive impairment in major depression and bipolar disorder. Bipolar Disord. 2018;20(3):260–74.

76. "Depressive Disorders", American Psychiatric Association: Diagnostic and Statistical Manual of Mental Disorders, Fifth Edition, Text Revision. Washington, DC, American Psychiatric Association, 2022, p. 183.
77. Kerr LK, Kerr LD Jr. Screening tools for depression in primary care: the effects of culture, gender, and somatic symptoms on the detection of depression. West J Med. 2001;175(5):349–52.
78. Wittkampf KA, et al. Diagnostic accuracy of the mood module of the Patient Health Questionnaire: a systematic review. Gen Hosp Psychiatry. 2007;29(5):388–95.
79. Naarding P, et al. Disease-specific properties of the Rating Scale for Depression in patients with stroke, Alzheimer's dementia, and Parkinson's disease. J Neuropsychiatry Clin Neurosci. 2002;14(3):329–34.
80. Cherbuin N, Kim S, Anstey KJ. Dementia risk estimates associated with measures of depression: a systematic review and meta-analysis. BMJ Open. 2015;5(12):e008853.
81. Vytal KE, et al. The complex interaction between anxiety and cognition: insight from spatial and verbal working memory. Front Hum Neurosci. 2013;7:93.
82. Berggren N. Anxiety and apprehension in visual working memory performance: no change to capacity, but poorer distractor filtering. Anxiety Stress Coping. 2020;33(3):299–310.
83. Coles ME, Heimberg RG. Memory biases in the anxiety disorders: current status. Clin Psychol Rev. 2002;22(4):587–627.
84. "Anxiety Disorders", American Psychiatric Association: Diagnostic and Statistical Manual of Mental Disorders, Fifth Edition, Text Revision. Washington, DC, American Psychiatric Association, 2022, pp. 250–251.
85. Spitzer RL, et al. A brief measure for assessing generalized anxiety disorder: the GAD-7. Arch Intern Med. 2006;166(10):1092–7.
86. Gulpers B, et al. Anxiety as a predictor for cognitive decline and dementia: a systematic review and meta-analysis. Am J Geriatr Psychiatry. 2016;24(10):823–42.
87. Wingenfeld K, Wolf OT. Stress, memory, and the hippocampus. Front Neurol Neurosci. 2014;34:109–20.
88. Arnsten AF. Stress impairs prefrontal cortical function in rats and monkeys: role of dopamine D1 and norepinephrine alpha-1 receptor mechanisms. Prog Brain Res. 2000;126:183–92.
89. Scott JC, et al. A quantitative meta-analysis of neurocognitive functioning in posttraumatic stress disorder. Psychol Bull. 2015;141(1):105–40.
90. Swick D, et al. Dissociation between working memory performance and proactive interference control in post-traumatic stress disorder. Neuropsychologia. 2017;96:111–21.
91. O'Neil ME, et al. Objective cognitive impairment and subjective cognitive problems in veterans initiating psychotherapy for posttraumatic stress disorder: an exploratory study. Appl Neuropsychol Adult. 2019;26(3):247–54.
92. ADHD, American Psychiatric Association: Diagnostic and Statistical Manual of Mental Disorders, Fifth Edition, Text Revision. Washington, DC, American Psychiatric Association, 2022.
93. Breslau, N. The Epidemiology of Trauma, PTSD, and Other Posttrauma Disorders. Trauma, Violence, & Abuse. 2009;10(3):198–210. https://doi.org/10.1177/1524838009334448.
94. Musser ED, Raiker JS Jr. Attention-deficit/hyperactivity disorder: an integrated developmental psychopathology and Research Domain Criteria (RDoC) approach. Compr Psychiatry. 2019;90:65–72.
95. "Attention-Deficit/Hyperactivity Disorder" in American Psychiatric Association: Diagnostic and Statistical Manual of Mental Disorders, Fifth Edition, Text Revision. Washington, DC, American Psychiatric Association, 2022, pp 68–75.
96. Skodzik T, Holling H, Pedersen A. Long-term memory performance in adult ADHD. J Atten Disord. 2017;21(4):267–83.
97. Kessler RC, et al. The prevalence and correlates of adult ADHD in the United States: results from the National Comorbidity Survey Replication. Am J Psychiatry. 2006;163(4):716–23.
98. Kessler RC, et al. Lifetime prevalence and age-of-onset distributions of DSM-IV disorders in the National Comorbidity Survey Replication. Arch Gen Psychiatry. 2005;62(6):593–602.

Concentration

7

Michaela A. Marziale, Hongjing Cao, and James A. Bourgeois

Introduction

"I can't concentrate" is a common chief complaint. This compliant can present solitarily or be associated with many other symptoms. An initial clinical challenge is figuring out what the patient means by "concentrate." To help the clinician know how to clarify such a complaint more accurately, we discuss the clinical definition of "concentration" and how to differentiate it from the often-confused (though related) concept of "attention."

Definition of Concentration

The verb *concentration* is from the assimilated form of Latin *com* which means "with, together." Merriam Webster defines concentration as the objective to "bring or direct toward a common center or objective" [1]. This more familiar definition derives from the 1860s meaning to concentrate the mind or mental powers. Concentration has two elements, the ability to *focus on pertinent stimuli*, and the ability to *disregard*

M. A. Marziale (✉)
Department of Psychiatry, Baylor Scott and White Health, Central Texas Division, Temple, TX, USA
e-mail: Michaela.Marziale@BSWHealth.org

H. Cao
Department of Psychiatry, MedStar Georgetown University Hospital, Washington, DC, USA
e-mail: Hongjing.cao@medstar.net

J. A. Bourgeois
Department of Psychiatry and Behavioral Sciences, University of California, Davis, Sacramento, CA, USA
e-mail: jbourgeois@ucdavis.edu

E. G. Meyer et al. (eds.), *The Medical Evaluation of Psychiatric Symptoms*, https://doi.org/10.1007/978-3-031-14372-4_7

irrelevant stimuli [2]. Although this seems relatively straightforward, things become more complicated when one tries to delineate *concentration* from *attention*.

How Is Concentration Confused or Conflated with Other Symptoms?

Attention is a broad concept that includes a range of behaviors, including automatic auditory behaviors and visual orientation stimuli, as well as the capacity to integrate multiple stimuli at the same time or alternate back and forth between stimuli [2]. Types of attention include Voluntary Attention, Focused Attention, Divided Attention, Alternating Attention, and Sustained Attention (Fig. 7.1) [2]. *Concentration* is dependent on intact Attention, and is best conceptualized as *Sustained Attention* [2]. Sustained Attention is the ability to focus on a stimulus over a period of time, even when stimulus is not continuous [2]. This represents a basic attentional function that determines the effectiveness of the "higher" aspects of attention (selective and divided) and cognitive capacity [2]. Therefore, when a patient complains of "poor concentration," they are most likely referring to difficulties with sustained attention. Although this may seem to be a relatively semantic point, it becomes important when trying to pinpoint exactly what the chief complaint is and how that relates to different clinical syndromes. Furthermore, it brings into question the precision of using "attention" vs "concentration" in diagnostic criteria for different psychiatric disorders.

Levels of Attention

- Voluntary Attention
- Focused Attention
- Divided Attention
- Sustained Attention (Concentration)
- Alternating attention [2]

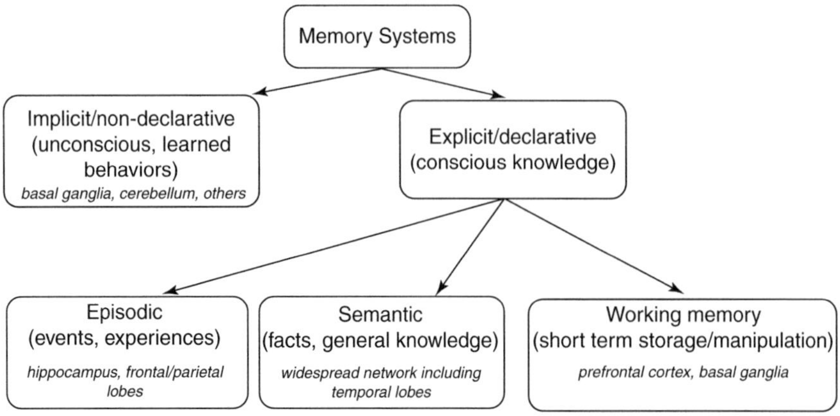

Fig. 7.1 Schematic representation of various levels of attention [2]

Paradigms, Models, and Important Brain Regions

In 1948, Norman Mackworth was the first researcher to use an experimental device called the *Mackworth Clock* to study sustained attention. This research was born out of World War II when the Royal Air Force was evaluating the optimal length of time to have airborne radar operators on anti-submarine patrol watching radar screens in order to maintain accuracy [3]. This research on sustained attention eventually developed into a scientific discipline by the human factors research community [4]. An initial review by Posner & Peterson looking at the neural foundation of attention defined three components of attention: (1) *orienting* to sensation, (2) *recognition* of signal processing, and (3) *altering*, which included long and short (<1 s) time intervals [5].

Important brain regions involved in concentration include the Default Mode Network (DMN), Frontal-Parietal Control Network, and Dorsal Attention Network. The DMN is active when one does not have a specific task to focus on and is associated with mind-wandering. The Frontal-Parietal Control Network is associated with executive and attentional control; the effects of arousal in this network are thought to impact concentration via locus coeruleus-norepinephrine (LE-NE) neuromodulation. Lastly, the Dorsal Attention Network is associated with attentional control [6, 7].

There are currently five different neurocognitive models of sustained attention [4, 6]. The first, the *Arousal Model*, focuses on the importance of physiologic arousal in sustained attention. A major player in arousal is the LC-NE neuromodulation in the frontoparietal control regions [4]. It is thought that at moderate levels of activity, these projections decrease responses to irrelevant stimuli and augment neural responses to important stimuli [4]. This, in turn, strengthens pertinent "task-related" processing and reduces background noise [4]. Next, the *Attentional Allocation Model* describes arousal as the baseline amount of attentional resources, but performance on a task is also dependent on how that resource is allocated [4]. Interestingly, patients diagnosed with obsessive-compulsive disorder (OCD) and attention deficit hyperactivity disorder (ADHD) report higher rates of unintentional mind-wandering [7]. *Resource-Control Theory* argues that cognitive control is vital in sustained attention [4]. It makes this assertion based on the concept that off-task thoughts can be intentional or unintentional [4, 6]. In this model, mind-wandering is the default state, and there is a perpetual bias for resources to be directed to that state [4]. It predicts that frontal-parietal and dorsal attention networks (attentional control) should change with, and be inversely related to, sustained attention performance [4, 6]. The *Opportunity Cost Model* attempts to explain why default states are preferred [4]. It suggests that the price of cognitive control is a negotiation between current mental activity relative to the value of other mental activities [4]. Lastly, the *Information Processing Perspective* looks at what it means for attention to be allocated to a particular task [4]. Recent studies by Esterman et al. show increased communication of stimulus information between attentional networks and DMN during rewarded trials [4].

Highlight Differences Among Specialties/Fields of Medicine

It is important to note that in other fields, Sustained Attention and Vigilance are used interchangeably. This is because researchers use the term (vigilance) to describe an ability to sustain attention to a task for a period of time, whereas clinicians use this term more specifically in reference to potential threats [8].

Delineate Subtypes/Variants of the Symptom

Focused Attention (Selective Attention): This is the ability to ignore irrelevant stimuli and focus on a specific or chosen target [2].

Divided Attention: This can be thought of as "working memory." It is the ability to integrate multiple stimuli simultaneously, or attend to more than one task "keeping information from multiple stimuli or tasks 'on-line' and responding appropriately to several operations of a task simultaneously" [2].

Rapid Alternating Attention: This is the capability to quickly shift focus between/among stimuli/tasks [2].

DSM-5-TR and RDoC Conceptualizations

Concentration is mentioned in the DSM-5-TR numerous times. More specifically, it is mentioned in relation to depressive disorders (MDD, dysthymia, and premenstrual dysphoric disorder), generalized anxiety disorder, bipolar disorder, PTSD, TBI, acute stress disorder, dissociative identity disorder, sleep disorders (insomnia, normal sleep variation, hyper-somnolence disorder, and nightmare disorder), stimulant use disorder, and attenuated psychosis syndrome [9].

Sustained Attention is explicitly mentioned in the DSM-5-TR in relation to ADHD, with the diagnostic criteria stating "Often has difficulty sustaining attention in tasks or play activities," caffeine withdrawal: "Caffeine abstinence has been shown to be associated with impaired behavioral and cognitive performance (e.g., sustained attention)," and delirium in reference to attentional domains in Criterion A [9].

Interestingly, *Concentration* is not specifically included in the diagnostic criteria for diagnoses such as ADHD and delirium. This is likely because conditions with poor attention at the core of the diagnosis, such as ADHD and delirium (poor attention plus arousal), do not list poor *Concentration* as a symptom simply because they lack *all* attentional processes, including sustained attention. In contrast, conditions such as generalized anxiety and depressive disorder maintain attentional processes, but these patients struggle with the maintenance of attention over a period of time.

The Research Domain Criteria (RDoC) do not list *Concentration* as a construct or sub-construct; rather, *Attention* is listed as a construct. RDoC defines attention as "a range of processes that regulate access to capacity-limited systems, such as awareness, higher perceptual processes, and motor action (10). The concepts of capacity limitation and competition are inherent to the concepts of selective and divided attention" [10]. *Sustained Attention* is mentioned in the section "Paradigms, Models, and Important Brain Regions" as described as "target detection tasks in the absence of competition" [10].

A Psychiatric Differential for Poor Concentration

Bipolar Disorders

There is strong evidence that bipolar disorder is associated with impairments in sustained attention. It has also been reported that individuals with bipolar disorder have deficits in sustained attention during mania, remission, and in first-degree relatives [11].

Incidence/Prevalence

Epidemiological studies have suggested a lifetime prevalence of about 1% for bipolar I disorder in the general population. A large cross sectional survey of 11 countries found that the overall lifetime prevalence of bipolar spectrum disorders was 2.4%, with a prevalence of 0.6% for bipolar I disorder and 0.4% for bipolar II disorder. First-episode bipolar I disorder with mania has an annual incidence of around 5 per 100,000 population and peak incidence occurs between 21 and 25 years [12].

Typical Findings of HPI

A patient with bipolar I disorder may present in either a manic or depressive episode. Patients with bipolar II disorder or cyclothymic disorder may present in either a hypomanic or depressive episode. If the patient presents in a manic episode, they may state they feel a decreased need for sleep coupled with an elevated or expansive mood. The interviewer may also notice that they are excessively talkative, grandiose, or have a flight of ideas. These symptoms need to persist for at least 1 week; otherwise, they may be indicative of a hypomanic episode where the symptoms must be present for 4 days. If the patient presents in a depressive episode, they may describe their mood as hopeless or down, and endorse difficulties with interest, feelings of guilt, low energy, poor concentration, poor sleep, decreased appetite, and suicidal ideation [9].

Typical Findings on Physical Exam and Mental Status Exam

In a manic episode, the patient may have pressured speech, which is of loud volume, and/or has an increased rate. Affect may be elevated, expansive, euphoric, irritable, or labile. The patient may be grandiose and have racing or tangential thoughts. The patient could also present with depressive symptoms simultaneously, which is referred to as a mixed episode. In a hypomanic episode, the patient will present in a manner similar to a manic episode, but less extreme in magnitude with more overlap with normal function [9].

Patients with a major depressive episode may endorse low mood, hopelessness, appear dysphoric and/or blunted, tearful, have poor eye contact, and withdrawn. Children may present with symptoms of irritability or acting out [9].

Typical Laboratory/Radiological Findings

Rule out substance-induced disorders with toxicology. Hyperthyroid states may present with behavioral symptoms consistent with mania or hypomania; thyroid hormones are elevated and TSH is correspondingly suppressed.

Unipolar Depressive Disorders

"Findings in unipolar depression indicate possible impairment in [sustained attention] which may subside in partially and completely remitted patients," in contrast to bipolar depression [11].

Incidence/Prevalence

It has been estimated that in the United States, the 12-month prevalence of unipolar major depression is about 10% and the lifetime prevalence is 21% [13].

Typical Findings of HPI

As mentioned above, a patient experiencing a depressive episode may describe their mood as down or hopeless. In addition to this, they may endorse difficulties with interest, feelings of guilt, low energy, poor concentration, poor sleep, decreased appetite, and suicidal ideation. These symptoms must be present for at least 2 weeks to meet the criteria for a major depressive episode [9].

Typical Findings on Physical Exam and Mental Status Exam

Patients with a major depressive episode may endorse low mood, hopelessness, appear dysphoric and/or blunted, tearful, have poor eye contact, and withdrawn. Children may present with symptoms of irritability or acting out [9].

Typical Laboratory/Radiological Findings

Rule out substance-induced depressive disorder with toxicology. Rule out hypothyroidism with TSH and thyroid hormones (TSH is elevated in compensatory response to low thyroid hormones).

Generalized Anxiety Disorder

Studies have shown an association between trait anxiety and decreased frontal-thalamo-striatal connectivity, pointing toward a link between trait anxiety and poor frontal control of attention, even when there are no external distractors. Contrary to trait anxiety, worry was not associated with reduced frontal-striatal-thalamo connectivity. Both trait anxiety and worry were associated with greater DLPFC-precuneus and DLPFC-posterior cingulate connectivity, suggestive of increased off-task thought [14].

Incidence/Prevalence

According to the NIMH, an estimated 2.7% of US adults had generalized anxiety disorder, with a higher prevalence in women. It is estimated that 5.7% of adults in the United States will experience generalized anxiety disorder at some point in their lives [15].

Typical Findings of HPI

A patient with generalized anxiety disorder will present with complaints of immoderate anxiety or worry for at least 6 months. They may also describe feeling "edgy," "keyed up," irritable, or easily fatigued. The patient may complain about difficulties with concentration and "going blank" at times due to their high, basal levels of anxiety [9].

Typical Findings on Physical Exam and Mental Status Exam

They may have an increased heart rate or elevated blood pressure when reflecting on stressful events/situations. The patient experiences enhanced perspiration (clammy hands, axillary sweating). The patient may demonstrate worry about numerous things (including somatic complaints). This may manifest in the patient describing their thoughts as moving too fast, or they may complain of their mind "going blank" when put "on the spot." Some patients may even describe their thought process or come off at times as being somewhat circumstantial. This thought process may be interfering with their sleep. The interviewer may also notice an increased rate of speech when the patient is talking about something anxiety-provoking; this needs to be clearly distinguished from pressured speech in mania [9].

Typical Laboratory/Radiological Findings

Patients experiencing excessive anxiety should receive a basic metabolic panel, CBC, TSH, and UDS. In addition to this, as patients with anxiety will sometimes have somatic complaints (nausea/vomiting, stomach upset, constipation/diarrhea, headache) a targeted general medical workup should be performed to rule out "medical" causes of these symptoms.

Posttraumatic Stress Disorder/Acute Stress Disorder

A 1998 study showed that patients with PTSD when compared to controls "responded similarly to identified targets on a sustained attention and vigilance task"; however, "the PTSD sample responded to significantly more distractor items" which could point toward an inability to "inhibit responses to irrelevant information" [16]. The researchers hypothesize that this disinhibited performance could be connected to dysregulated arousal in patients with PTSD [16].

Incidence/Prevalence

As per the VA, the lifetime prevalence of PTSD among adult Americans is estimated to be 6.8% [17]. According to the DSM-5-TR, the prevalence of acute stress disorder following traumatic events ranges from 6% to50%, with higher rates reported following an assault, while the prevalence of PTSD following traumatic events including rape, combat, captivity, and politically motivated internment and genocide range from 33% to more than 50% [9]. Lifetime PTSD risk in the general population at age 75 is 9% in the US [9].

Typical Findings of HPI

The patient will have been exposed to either actual or threatened death, injury, or violence. This may result in the patient experiencing mood changes, flashbacks, nightmares, hypervigilance, or avoidance behaviors. For the diagnosis of PTSD, these symptoms must be present for at least 1 month, whereas if it is less than 1 month the diagnosis is acute stress disorder [9].

Typical Findings on Physical Exam and Mental Status Exam

The patient may demonstrate increased vigilance, exaggerated startle response, and arousal when recounting the traumatic experience. Affect may be dysphoric, anxious, or tearful [9].

Typical Laboratory/Radiological Findings

Rule out comorbid substance use disorder with toxicology.

Delirium

Delirium is a neuropsychiatric condition that occurs in the setting of acute illness or substance intoxication/withdrawal. The patient presents with a disturbance in consciousness, and reduced ability to focus, shift, or sustain attention [9]. This is a subacute change from baseline and fluctuates, and is associated with additional cognitive disturbance (e.g., amnesia, disorientation, aphasia, psychosis, or visuospatial disturbance).

Complicating the assessment of delirium, it may present with symptoms that are subsyndromal for the full DSM-5-TR criteria and/or attenuated form, which is common upon (incomplete) recovery from an explicit episode of full spectrum delirium attributable to an acute illness. While attentional difficulties are the key symptom of delirium, subsyndromal delirium can result in difficulties with concentration. Common clinical examples of subsyndromal delirium include mild hyperglycemia/hypoglycemia in diabetes mellitus, where the patient may have unimpaired level or arousal, normal sleep/wake cycle, and absence of psychotic symptoms or frank cognitive impairment (e.g., normal range MoCA score) but have clinically significant complaints of poor concentration and task accomplishment, which may dominate the clinical presentation. Another common example is corticosteroid-associated psychiatric side effects, where patients receiving corticosteroids in excess of 40 mg per day of prednisone equivalents may present with sleep disturbance, poor attention and concentration, and distractibility, but be subsyndromal for a delirium episode per se. The same can be seen with toxicity from immunomodulating agents such as macrolide calcineurin inhibitors (e.g., tacrolimus) with a subsyndromal delirium presentation.

Attenuated delirium is a residual state following recovery from a frank delirium episode. Patients typically no longer manifest psychotic symptoms, grossly impaired cognitive function on formal cognitive assessment, or significant sleep-wake disturbances, but will have a persistent (even for many months) and functionally limiting experience of impaired (compared to baseline) attention and concentration often with other cognitive complaints. While there are no specific, validated psychopharmacological interventions for this attenuated delirium state, it could easily be misattributed as a comorbid depressive or anxiety disorder, or attributed to PTSD for the major illness, trauma, or surgical procedure that generated the episode of delirium in the first place.

Incidence/Prevalence

At admission to the hospital, about 11–25% of elderly patients will have delirium, and 29–31% of hospitalized elderly patients will develop delirium during their stay [18]. According to the DSM-5-TR [9], the community prevalence of delirium is 1–2% overall but 14% in patients over 85 years. Given that hospitalization is a common context of delirium presentation, more meaningful prevalence figures for delirium include 10–30% of ED patients, 15–53% in older patients postoperatively, and 70–87% of patients in intensive care.

Typical Findings of HPI

A typical illness narrative for delirium would be an elderly patient with an acute change in attention, cognition, and/or other mental function who was found to have a UTI, other infectious diseases, or metabolic decompensation. This acute change in mental status could be anything from confusion to visual hallucinations, with prominent deficits in arousal, attention, and concentration. Delirium can affect any patient, though the elderly and/or premorbid cognitively impaired are at greater risk [18, 19]. If possible, try to speak with a relative who knows the patient, and try to get an idea of baseline function and education.

Typical Findings on Physical Exam and Mental Status Exam

The patient may present as very active with restlessness/agitation, hallucinating, and requiring constant nurse attention. This is the typical delirium patient that would receive a psychiatric consultation in the hospital. It is important to also be on the lookout for hypoactive delirium patients, who are often missed because they are not disruptive to the hospital setting/staff. A helpful tool is the Confusion Assessment Method (CAM) which uses four questions to screen for the presence of delirium in a medical/surgical setting. The CAM-ICU is a similar version adapted for the ICU setting. One can also use the MoCA to trend the patient's progress during the hospital stay. Another quick assessment is to have the patient recite the months of the year backward; successful recitation of the reversed months to "July" or onward makes delirium unlikely [18–21].

Typical Laboratory/Radiological Findings

CBC, CMP, TSH, UDS, UA, serum HCG, BUN, Serum Cr, vitamins B12 and D, Folate, Thiamine, TSH, free T3/T4, CT head, and CXR. While the laboratory and neuroimaging findings are not specific for the delirium syndrome per se, they are indicated to search for underlying systemic medical disturbances leading to delirium. EEG typically shows bilateral diffuse slowing [22].

Dementia/Major Neurocognitive Disorder

major neurocognitive disorder (MNCD) (formerly dementia) is a series of neurodegenerative and/or vascular diseases that are typically insidious in onset, relatively steadily progressive (although there are some exceptions, e.g., post-CVA major neurocognitive disorder, which can be acute onset but thereafter relatively static), leading to impairments in multiple areas of brain function. The formal DSM-5-TR criteria for MNCD include a significant cognitive decline in one or more major cognitive domains (e.g., complex attention, executive function, learning and memory, language, perceptual-motor, social cognition) with demonstrated impairment in cognitive performance on formal assessment, not solely due to delirium [9]. Major neurocognitive disorder exists on a functional continuum with mild neurocognitive disorder (formerly mild cognitive impairment), which exhibits many domains of similar cognitive symptoms, but *without* meaningful functional impairment. It is not unusual for a patient to come to clinical attention in the major neurocognitive disorder phase; retrospectively, he/she will typically have previously experienced mild neurocognitive disorder that escaped formal clinical ascertainment.

As MNCD, by definition, affects many areas of CNS function, one of the major sources of symptoms is commonly decreased sustained attention/concentration. This is both subjectively noted by the patient and affirmed by formal neurocognitive assessment. The patient (or often, the patient's confederates) may complain that the patient is cognitively inefficient (e.g., reading material several times, still leading to impaired understanding), losing focus while writing or speaking, and the like.

Incidence/Prevalence

Prevalence of MNCD varies by patient age and specific illness subtype. The prevalence of all dementia subtypes is estimated to range from 1% to 2% at age 65 to 30% at age 85 [9]. In a similar vein, the prevalence of mild neurocognitive disorder is estimated as 2–10% at age 65, increasing to 5–25% by age 85.

Typical Findings on HPI

History may be subtle, and often the patient's confederates will have more salient observations, as dementia patients may be poor self-observers. Patients will be described as forgetful, inefficient, losing objects and papers, exhibiting poor judgment while driving or in social situations, making unusual errors in speech, reading, writing, or mathematics. Patients may withdraw from formerly treasured activities that have a high cognitive demand (e.g., reading, playing or listening to music, writing, operating a computer, or other electronics).

Typical Findings on Physical and Mental Status Examination

Overall physical appearance may be unremarkable, though patients with MNCD attributable to other CNS illnesses (e.g., Huntington's disease, Parkinson's disease, multiple sclerosis) will exhibit the motor signs typical of these illnesses. Patients often show varying degrees of poor self-care (e.g., poor hygiene and grooming), poor nutritional status with weight loss and wasting due to poor po intake, and may appear fatigued due to poor or irregular sleep.

Mental status examination findings can be variable, although there is (by definition) decreased cognitive function on formal cognitive examination (e.g., <26 on the MoCA or <24 on the MMSE). The emotional state can be quite varied. Patients may appear pleasant, as if unaware of or nonperturbed by their cognitive impaired, or "pleasantly perplexed" (showing a quizzical affect), or, conversely, may be excessively depressed/distressed, even catastrophizing and exaggerating their manifest cognitive deficits. Effort on examination may be similarly varied; patients may persist with multiple erroneous responses to a single exam query or may give up at the first sign of inefficiency. Exam items requiring sustained effort (e.g., recall memory, serial subtractions, list generation) may be much more problematic than other tasks which are more "cognitively reflexive" (e.g., naming of objects, picture identification, orientation). Patients may do particularly poorly on tasks demanding cognitive flexibility and organization (e.g., abstraction, list generation, sequencing of past US presidents, knowledge of salient historical events).

Typical Laboratory and Neuroimaging Findings

In most MNCD/dementia syndromes, there are no specific confirmatory laboratory values or neuroimaging findings. However, since some systemic medical conditions, if corrected, may be considered to be reversible dementia syndromes, they should be screened for. These include hypothyroidism (TSH), hypoparathyroidism (Ca^+ and PTH), vitamin D deficiency (vitamin D level), Wernicke's encephalopathy (thiamine level), inflammatory vasculitis (ESR), and substance abuse (toxicology and alcohol level). Neuroimaging should be obtained; cortical dementias such as Alzheimer's disease will show prominent cortical atrophy while vascular disease will also have white matter disease and/or evidence of past CVAs.

Traumatic Brain Injury

Traumatic brain injury may have a variegated presentation, depending on the severity of injury and time since traumatic injury. With more severe TBI, the acute presentation may include diffuse axonal injury and comorbid delirium, which may take a long time to clear to leave a residual deficit state. Milder TBI will not have any neuroimaging findings and not be associated with delirium syndrome at the time of presentation. Some cases of TBI will have multiple cognitive deficits that meet the criteria for major neurocognitive disorder and should be managed as other dementia syndromes.

Milder TBI in the post-acute residual state will not meet diagnostic criteria for dementia syndrome. These milder residual cases often include a clinical triad of sleep disturbance, depressive disorder, and attentional/concentration deficits; some patients may primarily experience one of these three symptom clusters. The patient with attentional/concentration problems may resemble adult residual ADHD clinically, but will not have a childhood ADHD history. The formal DSM-5-TR criteria for major or mild NCD due to TBI require that the patient meets the diagnostic criteria for one of these syndromes, with at least one of the following having occurred as a result of the acute CNS injury: loss of consciousness, posttraumatic amnesia, disorientation/confusion, or neurological signs [9].

Incidence/Prevalence

The prevalence of TBI in general population is estimated at 2%. The prevalence among hospitalized patients is increased, especially following falls, vehicular accidents, assault, and sports injuries [9].

Typical Findings on HPI

The patient will report a history of head trauma or "concussion," which may have occurred in a variety of contexts, e.g., sports injury, industrial accident, motor vehicle accident, combat injury. While at some loss of consciousness is common, mild TBI may result in only fleeting loss of consciousness. More severe TBI will often lead to hospitalization for observation and mental status monitoring. It is not unusual for other physical trauma to be the cause of clinical attention, with comorbid mild TBI relatively overlooked. The initial peri-TBI period (if severe enough) may lead to a delirium presentation. After recovery from delirium (which may take several weeks), the patient may then experience a period characterized by depressed mood with neurovegetative signs (which may independently meet diagnostic criteria for a major depressive episode), sleep disturbance (which may be punctuated by nightmares of the injury leading to TBI and may be part of a constellation of comorbid PTSD), and/or attentional deficits which may be reported as "poor concentration." These lingering psychiatric symptoms a month or later after initial TBI may be the nidus of clinical attention [23].

Typical Findings on Physical and Mental Status Examination

The general physical examination on TBI is nonspecific, though there may be lingering stigmata of comorbid physical injuries cooccurring with TBI. Mental status examination may be variable, depending on the persistent psychiatric sequelae of TBI. Severe TBI sufficient to result in a chronic post-TBI dementia syndrome will have mental status findings common in MNCD/dementia, e.g., cognitive impairment on formal cognitive testing, word-finding difficulties, aphasia, dysarthric or otherwise impaired speech, and vacant/"vacuous"/perplexed affect.

Milder post-TBI patients may have mental status findings consistent with the prevailing psychiatric sequelae. Patients may exhibit dysphoric, blunted, or tearful affect with soft, slow, hesitant speech if they have a primarily depressed condition. Patients may exhibit poor memory and concentration on formal cognitive assessment and impersistence in tasks requiring sustained mental effort (e.g., recall memory, list generation).

Typical Laboratory and Neuroimaging Findings

There are no pathognomonic laboratory findings in post-TBI conditions. Neuroimaging findings are variable; mild TBI may have normal neuroimaging both acutely and chronically; more severe TBI may lead to areas of encephalomalacia in the areas and/or blunt or penetrating trauma. Cases that initially presented with diffuse axonal injury are generally reversible; months after initial presentation, neuroimaging may revert to normal or nonspecific findings.

Attention Deficit Hyperactivity Disorder

ADHD is a childhood-onset neurodevelopmental disorder that by definition features abnormally poor attention (compared to same-aged peers) that leads to impaired function and development. Although ADHD affects several attentional domains, patients may initially present complaining of poor concentration because of an inability to maintain attention over time. The more classic presentation is combined inattention and motor hyperactivity/impulsivity [9]. Patients may not experience motor hyperactivity, which is classified as a predominantly inattentive presentation [9].

Incidence/Prevalence

According to a study done by the WHO, across 20 upper, middle, and low-income countries the mean worldwide prevalence was about 2.8% [24]. According to the CDC in 2016, the number of children ever diagnosed with ADHD was 6.1 million (9.4%). Boys are more likely than girls to be diagnosed with this condition at 12.9% vs. 5.6% [25].

Typical Findings of HPI

The patient must demonstrate a persistent pattern of inattention and/or hyperactivity-impulsivity that interferes with their everyday functioning or development. This may manifest as an aversion to mentally demanding tasks, forgetting instructions, or impulsivity. These children may throw tantrums during major transitions, but this is secondary to poor self-control rather than rigidity [2, 26]. It is also important to remain vigilant for children with ADHD inattentive type, as these children may go unnoticed until later school grades, as they are not being overtly disruptive during class.

Typical Findings on Physical Exam and Mental Status Exam

The patient may appear to be "all over the place" during the interview (crawling around on the floor, "running on a motor"), although inattentive children may not appear this way during the interview and may only describe being forgetful.

Typical Laboratory/Radiological Findings

Rule out substance-induced conditions with toxicology, and obtain basic labs (CBC, CMP), vitamin B9 (folate), vitamin B12, and vitamin D.

Autism/Autism Spectrum Disorder

attention deficit hyperactivity disorder (ADHD) and autism spectrum disorder (ASD) are often comorbid and share difficulties in sustained attention [24]. Studies have shown that boys with both ADHD and ASD have difficulties in fronto–striato–parietal activation and default mode suppression. ADHD shows more DLPFC dysfunction, whereas ASD shows more specific fronto–striato–cerebellar dysregulation [26].

Incidence/Prevalence

According to the CDC 1 in 54 children has been identified with ASD. It is four times more common in boys compared to girls. In 2016, the combined prevalence per 1000 children was 18.5 [27].

Typical Findings of HPI

In contrast with ADHD, the patient may display social disengagement, isolation, and indifference to facial and tonal communication cues. Children with ASD may display tantrums because of the inability to tolerate change from the expected course of events [26, 28].

Typical Findings on Physical Exam and Mental Status Exam

As stated above, the child may not appear to be socially engaged or pick up on common social cues. They may have tantrums or a disproportionate reaction to something being changed or not going as expected.

Typical Laboratory/Radiological Findings

Basic labs (CBC, CMP), vitamin B9 (folate), vitamin B12, and vitamin D. Genetics testing is confirmatory in specific genetic syndromes associated with autism (e.g., *FMR1* in fragile X syndrome).

A Systemic Medical Differential for Poor Concentration

As "poor concentration" may be a ubiquitous symptom present in a wide range of systemic medical conditions, an exhaustive list of conditions presenting with this symptom is not possible. As such, the authors have chosen a representative series of conditions wherein impaired concentration may be an important (though not exclusive) symptom at the time of clinical presentation.

Autoimmune Conditions

Systemic Lupus Erythematosus

Systemic lupus erythematosus (SLE) or colloquially "lupus" is a variegated rheumatologic illness affecting multiple organ systems with an autoimmune etiology. While an initial presentation of lupus with only CNS symptoms is relatively infrequent, the psychiatrist may see an established SLE patient with an acute flare of illness primarily affecting the CNS with a chief complaint of decreased concentration. The presumed mechanism of CNS lupus is autoimmune inflammation affecting the neurons and perivascular tissues in the brain called neuropsychiatric SLE (NPSLE) [29]. As the entire brain may be affected by this disease process, essentially any psychiatric complaint may be experienced by the patient. The subacute to acute presentation of NPSLE may present as a full delirium syndrome, or isolated psychiatric symptoms subsyndromal for delirium. Complicating assessment and classification, pharmacological interventions for lupus may have their own psychiatric side effects, even if their effect on systemic lupus improves other physical symptoms. This is well illustrated by a known lupus patient who is treated for a flare of SLE with high-dose corticosteroids, which lead to primarily psychiatric side effects, such as poor concentration.

Incidence/Prevalence

Based on national data from 2003 to 2008, the prevalence of SLE was estimated to be 102.94 per 100,000 people [30].

Typical Findings on HPI

It is infrequent for SLE to initially present with solely CNS symptoms, and more unlikely to present as solely "decreased concentration." Inasmuch as SLE may present in a fashion overlapping with a MDD episode, the patient may experience impaired concentration as one of the cardinal depressive symptoms. SLE is among the systemic illnesses to consider in a case of "atypical psychotic disorder."

More likely, a known patient with SLE may present with a range of CNS complaints, among them "decreased concentration." The physician must then consider if the acutely presenting psychiatric symptom(s) are referable to an acute flare of lupus illness and/or the consequence of immunomodulating therapy for lupus (e.g., corticosteroids).

Typical Findings on Physical and Mental Status Examination

The physical examination may reveal the classic malar rash of SLE, other dermatologic findings, or rheumatologic findings. Isolated CNS lupus may not have notable systemic medical examination findings. CNS lupus may have a wide range of motor, sensory, cognitive, mood, and/or attentional findings. On examination, patients may have dysphoric, tearful, or melancholic affect, cognitive impairment on formal cognitive assessment, or other findings of cognitive impairment. Some acutely decompensated patients may have full spectrum delirium.

Typical Laboratory and Neuroimaging Findings

Inflammatory markers (e.g., antinuclear antibodies, anti-extractable nuclear antigen antibodies, anti-double stranded DNA antibodies) will typically be abnormal [31]. Neuroimaging may reveal vascular disease and/or cerebral cortex involvement but can be unremarkable.

Multiple Sclerosis

Multiple sclerosis is a chronic, variably progressive demyelinating disease of presumed autoimmune origin, with T cell mediated inflammation against myelin [32]. It typically affects young to middle-aged patients, with a female predominance. Illness course is quite variable, and some patients experience prolonged periods of relative stability. Patients often present with optic neuritis, myelitis, or brainstem signs [32]. Although MS is a clinical diagnosis, additional findings of CSF oligoclonal bands and/or elevated IgG index and positive MRI are confirmatory [32]. Serial MRI is used for disease progression monitoring [33]. As much of the CNS may be affected, essentially any psychiatric syndrome (including dementia syndromes) may be experienced along with a wide variety of motor and sensory impairments. Depressive disorders are common in multiple sclerosis (sometimes as the *forme fruste* of the illness, antedating any motor or sensory symptoms); as such impaired concentration may be experienced by the patient as a part of the series of symptoms of a MS-associated depressive episode. As with SLE, the use of immunomodulating agents (notably corticosteroids) to treat acute illness flares in MS may lead to corticosteroid-associated psychiatric side effects, including poor concentration, among other symptoms [32, 34].

Incidence/Prevalence

Prevalence has been estimated to range from 39.9 to 191.2 per 100,000 [35, 36]. Incidence has been estimated to be as high as 7.3 per 100,000 [36].

Typical Findings on HPI

A patient later definitively diagnosed with MS may initially present with a rather typical-appearing MDD episode, with poor concentration commonly included among the range of major depressive symptoms. Alternatively, patients may present with a primary appearance of cognitive impairment; poor concentration may be present in this context as well.

In the case of an established MS patient, an acute flare of illness may be heralded by primarily psychiatric symptoms, which could well include a prominent complaint of poor concentration.

Typical Findings on Physical and Mental Status Examination

Physical examination in MS is variable. Early in the illness, physical examination findings might be mild and/or nonspecific. With the progression of illness, optic neuritis, internuclear ophthalmoplegia, ataxia, sensory deficits, weakness, inability to ambulate, and other neurologic signs may dominate the picture. The mental status exam will depend on the psychiatric syndrome. Patients may have exam findings consistent with a major depressive episode, dementia, or more focal finding of poor concentration.

Typical Laboratory and Neuroimaging Findings

Most routine laboratory findings can be nonspecific. CSF studies may reveal lymphocytosis, increased protein, increased IgG index, and/or oligoclonal bands [32]. Neuroimaging is typically abnormal, especially in periventricular, deep white matter, cerebellum, and spinal cord [33]. With severe, progressive disease cortical and cerebellar atrophy may be seen [37].

Normal Aging

It is important to emphasize that not all clinical complaints of "poor concentration" will necessarily reflect "illness" per se but may better be understood as "normative" or "on the spectrum of normal experience." This is well illustrated by the common experience of an internal sense of some decrease in cognitive "acuity" with aging, which patients may both experience and report to clinicians as "decreased concentration," leading to clinical inquiry to ascertain the veracity and possible medical explanations of this understandable clinical concern. The subjective sense of poor concentration attributable to normal aging may be of greater concern to the patient than is manifest in actual, discernable functional impairment or objective examination findings.

Incidence/Prevalence

In a 2019 profile of older Americans, it was reported that over the past decade, the population age 65 years and older increased from 38.8 million in 2008 to 52.4 million in 2018. The number of Americans age 45–65 years increased by 7% between 2008 and 2018 [38].

Typical Findings of HPI

The patient may complain of memory and concentration decline in terms of becoming more forgetful. It will be important to rule out depressive disorders and major or mild neurocognitive disorder (formerly dementia). If this is normal aging, studies have shown they will report memory deterioration but there will not be evidence of this on testing compared to those who are depressed or demented [39].

Typical Findings on Physical Exam and Mental Status Exam

Memory/concentration complaints correlate poorly with memory performance in "normal" elderly groups. In contrast to this, memory complaints seem to have a significant correlation in patients with depressive symptoms [39].

Sensitivity, Specificity, and PPV

A meta-analysis from 2016 showed that the MoCA (Montreal Cognitive Assessment) was better at detecting mild cognitive impairment in patients over 60 years of age compared to the MiniMental State Examination (MMSE). The study showed using a cut-off of 24/25 for the MoCA gave a sensitivity of 80.48% and a specificity of 81.19%, whereas the MMSE using a cut-off of 27/28 gave a 66.34% sensitivity and a 72.94% specificity [39].

Typical Laboratory/Radiological Findings

Normal Aging is a diagnosis of exclusion. Obtain basic laboratory tests (CBC, BMP), TSH, vitamin B9 (folate), vitamin B12, vitamin D, UA, neuroimaging, depression screen, dementia screen, and rule out substance induced (alcohol, benzodiazepines, barbiturates, anticholinergic medicines) with toxicology. This laboratory workup overlaps significantly with a standard delirium assessment.

Immunological Conditions

Allergic Rhinitis

There has been evidence to suggest that patients with seasonal allergic rhinitis show alterations in attentional control and must recruit higher cognitive control while symptomatic. Furthermore, performance changes secondary to allergies appeared to be related to IgE levels and mood, rather than subjective symptom complaints. Reduction in information processing in sustained attention tasks was associated with total IgE levels [40].

Incidence/Prevalence

AR affects an estimated 20–40 million people in the USA. The incidence of seasonal AR is estimated to be 20%, perennial rhinitis 40%, and mixed 40% [41].

Typical Findings of HPI

The patient could present with complaints of rhinorrhea, sneezing, itching, nasal obstruction, post-nasal drip (sore throat), smell dysfunction, and cough. In addition to these common symptoms, the patient could describe reduced physical and mental capacity, feeling slowed down, or foggy/fatigued. Difficulty with concentration or adaptation [40, 42, 43].

Typical Findings on Physical Exam and Mental Status Exam

Common physical exam findings include allergic "shiners," pale blue edematous nasal mucosa, clear rhinorrhea, "cobblestoning" of the posterior pharynx, or tympanic membranes that show retraction or fluid accumulation. Studies show that symptoms of allergic rhinitis are not predictive. When history and physical are taken together there does not seem to be significant inter-rater variability, whereas physical examination alone appears to have pronounced inter-rater variability. The only exception to this was in one study where the detection of polyps showed almost perfect inter-rater reliability ($k = 0.952$) [40, 42, 43].

Typical Laboratory/Radiological Findings

Basic laboratory studies are typically normal. Allergy skin testing is not necessary for initial diagnosis.

Endocrine Conditions

Diabetes Mellitus Type 1

Diabetes mellitus type I (commonly referred to as insulin-dependent diabetes mellitus) refers to juvenile onset diabetes mellitus, with a subacute to acute onset and reliance on insulin from illness onset for glycemic control. It is important to emphasize that many cases of diabetes mellitus type II (adult onset) will eventually require insulin therapy if oral antidiabetic agents are ultimately unsuccessful at managing glycemic control. Diabetic patients are prone to complaints of poor concentration attributable to hyperglycemic or hypoglycemic episodes at any time during illness course. With longer standing diabetes mellitus leading to chronic vascular complications, these patients are prone to cerebrovascular disease that may separately lead to cognitive complaints attributable to vascular cognitive impairment as well [44–47].

Incidence/Prevalence

Based on a US survey done in 2016 and 2017 among adults 20 years and older, the estimated prevalence of diabetes mellitus type 1 (DM1) was 0.5% [44].

Typical Findings of HPI

For adults with DM1, diabetic ketoacidosis may be the presenting symptom in one-fourth of the cases [48]. Compared to in children, symptoms of hyperglycemia such as polyuria, polydipsia, and fatigue may last longer in adults prior to diagnosis [45].

Typical Findings of Physical Exam and Mental Status Exam

Impaired sustained attention was found in patients with DM1 based on the sustained attention to response task (SART) reaction time [37]. Patients with DM1 have also been found to have reduced psychomotor and information processing speed [44, 45].

Typical Laboratory/Radiological Findings

Diabetes mellitus (type 1 or 2) is diagnosed with lab findings of ONE of the following: fasting glucose ≥126 mg/dL more than one time, random plasma glucose ≥200 mg/dL with classic symptoms of hyperglycemia, plasma glucose ≥200 mg/dL 2 h after glucose load in oral glucose tolerance test, HgbA1C ≥6.5% [48].

Hypothyroidism

Hypothyroidism can affect multiple organs including the CNS system. It has been noted that cognitive dysfunction occurs in a majority of patients with overt hypothyroidism (66–90%) [49]. Hypothyroidism is one well-known cause of reversible dementia; patients with this condition may experience poor concentration among many other cognitive complaints at the time of clinical presentation [50].

Incidence/Prevalence

Based on data from 1999 to 2002, it was shown that the prevalence of hypothyroidism in the US was 3.7% [51].

Typical Findings of HPI

Though clinical manifestations of hypothyroidism can vary from asymptomatic to life-threatening illnesses, the most common complaints are fatigue, cold intolerance, weight gain, constipation, voice change, and dry skin [52].

Typical Findings of Physical Exam and Mental Status Exam

On the physical exam, there may be goiter, bradycardia, diastolic hypertension, and delayed relaxation of deep tendon reflexes [53]. There may be cognitive changes on the mental status exam. The most common cognitive symptoms are slowed processing speed, poor sustained attention, and impaired short-term memory [54, 55].

Typical Laboratory/Radiological Findings

Hypothyroidism is confirmed with an elevated TSH and decreased free thyroxine levels [52]. Other laboratory abnormalities include hyponatremia, increased creatinine, hyperlipidemia, and increased plasma homocysteine [56–59].

Sensory Failure (Hearing Loss/Visual Loss)

Hearing Loss

Studies have shown that age-related hearing loss leads to an altered cognitive strategy in sustained attention tasks, resulting in decreased response efficiency for similar accuracy compared to controls. It has been suggested that patients with age-related hearing loss have poorer neuronal arousal but maintained top-down attentional control allowing them to maintain this accuracy. This may manifest as a slower rate of cognitive decline based on conventional visually based neuropsychological instruments, and more sensitive tasks may need to be implemented in order to detect cognitive decline at earlier stages [60].

Incidence/Prevalence

The prevalence of hearing loss increases with age. It is estimated that 43% of person ages 65–84 suffer from hearing loss. The World Health Organization estimates that in 2025 there will be 1.2 billion people over 60 years old worldwide, with more than 500 million people who will suffer significant hearing impairment from presbycusis [61].

Typical Findings of HPI

Initially, patients will have problems with high frequencies, and over time mid-low frequencies associated with speech will become involved. High frequencies tend to carry consonants therefore patients will report being able to hear when someone is speaking but not being able to understand what that person is saying, these symptoms are exacerbated by background noise.

Typical Findings of Physical Exam and Mental Status Exam

Examination of the ear should be normal, and other causes of hearing loss should be ruled out (e.g., cerumen impaction, tumors, perforation). Whispered voice test can be helpful, stand at arm's length behind the patient, rub the tragus of the ear not being tested to occlude hearing from that ear, and whisper a short sequence of letters/numbers and ask the patient to repeat them. Weber and Rinne Tests can be helpful in delineating conductive vs sensorineural hearing loss. On mental status examination, patients may endorse issues with concentration as they are experiencing a "cognitive overload" trying to listen and interpret sounds/what is being said to them.

Typical Laboratory/Radiological Findings

An audiogram is a standardized audiometric test that assesses the ability of the patient to hear tones and understand words.

Visual Loss

It has been suggested that children with a visual impairment have difficulties with concentration, and are more likely to be diagnosed with ADHD [61, 62]. Studies have shown that children with visual impairment may have issues processing information utilizing the visual attentional system. This causes impaired development of attentional mechanisms leading to difficulties with coordination of the oculomotor system which is expressed as symptoms of ADHD [62].

Incidence/Prevalence

In 2015, more than 174,000 US children ages 3–5 years old were visually impaired. By 2060 it is predicted the number of children ages 3–5 years old with visual impairment will increase by 26% [63].

Typical Findings on HPI

The patient may complain of blurry/fuzzy vision, headache, and visual fatigue. Parents/teachers may also report that the patient is fidgeting or having difficulties with concentration in class.

Typical Findings on Physical Exam and Mental Status Exam

An eye exam should be carried out, and any abnormalities should be noted. The exam should include observation of external structures, pupils, visual fields, visual acuity (hand-held chart/Snellen Chart), extraocular movements and cranial nerves, and lastly utilization of an ophthalmoscope to assess the fundus. On the mental status exam, the patient may demonstrate symptoms typical of ADHD: poor concentration and hyperactivity.

Typical Laboratory/Radiological Findings

If abnormalities on the physical exam are noted, referral to an ophthalmologist or optometrist may be appropriate for further testing and treatment.

Insomnia

Incidence/Prevalence

Insomnia is a ubiquitous complaint in primary care where it is among the most common causes for primary care visits. As such, insomnia can be conceptualized as an isolated symptom or a full spectrum DSM-5-TR disorder. Common presentations include difficulties in sleep onset/maintenance, though other associated symptoms (e.g., poor memory, decreased concentration, fatigue, irritability) may present as a constellation. Insomnia has an incidence of 28.1% in persons with comorbid conditions, 10.9% in those without [64]. One study estimates that 25% of Americans experience acute insomnia each year and 75% of those recover without chronic sleep issues [65].

Typical Findings of HPI

Typical complaints include trouble falling, staying asleep, or waking up too early. There must also be daytime impairment. Symptoms of daytime impairment include fatigue, poor concentration, difficulty with social/professional/educational activities, mood disturbance, daytime sleepiness, decreased motivation, decreased energy, increased accidents, behavior disturbance like hyperactivity, impulsivity, aggression, and worrying about sleep [66].

Typical Findings on Physical Exam and Mental Status Exam

Usually normal but can find hypertension, excessive oropharyngeal tissue (in cases of OSA), lower extremity swelling (in heart failure), and abnormal mental status (in dementia) [66].

Typical Laboratory/Radiological Findings

Routine screening labs are not indicated. Diagnosis is mainly clinical. Sleep diary and self-report screening tools (e.g., Pittsburgh Sleep Quality Index, Sleep problems questionnaire) can help characterize symptoms. If suspecting obstructive sleep apnea or circadian sleep-wake rhythm disorder, can obtain polysomnography or actigraphy, respectively.

Obstructive Sleep Apnea (OSA)

Incidence/Prevalence

Twenty-seven percent among males 30–70 years old.

Twelve percent among females 30–70 years old [67].

Typical Findings of HPI

Typically, patients have symptoms of daytime sleepiness or snoring, gasping, and choking during sleep. These symptoms are usually detected incidentally or during preventative visits [68].

Typical Findings on Physical Exam and Mental Status Exam

Obesity, crowded oropharyngeal pathway, large neck and/or waist circumference, hypertension, heart failure, pulmonary hypertension (less common) [67, 68].

Typical Laboratory/Radiological Findings

Polysomnography is the gold standard to diagnose OSA. OSA is confirmed if there are ≥5 obstructive respiratory events per hour of sleep along with symptoms/comorbidities or if there are ≥15 events regardless of the presence of symptoms/comorbidities [68].

Cardiovascular Conditions

Post-Stroke Fatigue

Stroke survivors often complain of loss of energy and difficulties in concentration. A recent study detailed that subtle cognitive deficits from a stroke may be initially compensated for with greater cognitive effort, but over time that effort results in fatigue ultimately resulting in poorer performance on sustained attention tasks. Interestingly, this same study showed that controls benefited from practice, whereas patients who had suffered a stroke did not. They postulate that this may be due to diminished learning ability secondary to the cost of cognitive compensation [69].

Incidence/Prevalence

Acute fatigue after a stroke can last up to 6 months, whereas chronic fatigue can persist in 40% of patients after 2 years [70]. Up to 40% of stroke survivors report it as their worst symptom [70]. Post-stroke fatigue has an estimated prevalence ranging from 25% to 85% [70].

Typical Findings of HPI

Patients will typically present with a complaint of fatigue/difficulty concentrating while performing cognitively demanding tasks over time. Clinicians can use the Fatigue Severity Scale to reliably diagnose PSF [70].

Typical Findings of Physical Exam and Mental Status

Residual motor weakness or sensory deficit from prior stroke. Complaints or poor energy, concentration, and fatigue.

Typical Laboratory/Radiological Findings

CMP, CBC, TSH.

Neurodegenerative Conditions

Parkinson's Disease

Parkinson's disease is a classic disease of the substantia nigra with classic "pill-rolling" tremor, postural and gait instability, profound bradykinesia, blunted "masked" facies, depressive disorder, psychosis, and dementia [71]. Onset is usually insidious in middle-aged with progression that can be relatively slow. It is regarded as a classic "neuropsychiatric" disease in that the majority of patients experience "neurologic" and "psychiatric" symptoms/syndromes in variable sequence across sometimes decades of illness. Prominent among Parkinson's disease psychiatric manifestations are depressive episodes and dementia syndromes (which are often comorbid); either a depressive episode or dementia syndrome, particularly early in the syndromal course, may present with "decreased concentration" as a major psychiatric complaint. Of great importance to psychiatrists, patients often experience psychotic symptoms as a consequence of dopaminergic medications used to reverse the underlying insidious dopamine deficiency in Parkinson's disease. Dopaminergic agents used for this purpose may result in an excess of dopamine thus leading to psychotic symptoms [71–73].

Incidence/Prevalence

Incidence of PD is 1–2 per 1000. The prevalence of PD increases with age, and for those above 60 years, the prevalence of PD is 1% [74].

Typical Findings on HPI

Though the first presentation of Parkinson's disease could be a depressive or dementia syndrome, the more common presentation is that of an established Parkinson's disease patient who later presents with a depressive and/or dementia syndrome. The motor symptoms reported in Parkinson's disease include bradykinesia, rest tremor (often "pill-rolling"), and rigidity [71].

Typical Findings on Physical and Mental Status Examination

The classic findings of Parkinson's disease are nearly pathognomonic, including stooped posture, pill-rolling hand tremor, bradykinesia, masked and blunted facies, bradyphrenia, dysphonic and/or dysarthric speech, depressed mood, and cognitive impairment [71, 75]. Depending on the stage of disease, patients may have an incomplete range of these classic symptoms. Patients with comorbid depressive illness have blunted, dysphoric affect, may have suicidality, and cognitive impairment on formal assessment. As the depressive and dementia symptoms are so often comorbid, it can be very difficult to completely separate them. As patients typically have decreased motor function already, they may manifest a "melancholic" appearance relatively early in the depressive episode. Dementia in Parkinson's disease is a "subcortical" dementia, with motor slowing, higher likelihood of comorbid depressive disorders, and cognitive deficits such as delayed recall that can be helped by "cueing" by the examiner.

Typical Laboratory and Neuroimaging Findings

There are no classic laboratory findings in Parkinson's disease, though, as they experience a neurodegenerative illness, they should be regarded as "delirium prone" and thus have a thorough workup for reversible causes of delirium. Neuroimaging will reveal atrophy in subcortical and cortical structures, with notable atrophy of the substantia nigra.

Conclusion

Concentration, or the maintenance of sustained attention, is a critically important mental function, upon which many other mental functions are intimately dependent. As such, concentration deficits (both subjectively experienced and objectively ascertained) may be attributable to a wide range of psychiatric and systemic illnesses. The complaint of poor concentration therefore requires active and simultaneous consideration of both CNS and systemic causes at all times. Many patients will have multiple attributable causes of poor concentration. The authors have presented a wide range (though not exhaustive) of common psychiatric illnesses that may have poor concentration as a cardinal feature. In many of these illnesses, other psychiatric signs are equally prominent. Accurate psychiatric diagnosis requires full elucidation of the various other psychiatric symptoms cooccurring with the concerns of poor concentration. Full clinical evaluation, including standardized cognitive assessment, is needed for accurate attribution. Many patients will have psychiatric comorbid illnesses and/or simultaneous psychiatric and systemic illnesses that have an additive, even synergistic, effect on the experience of poor concentration. An integrated and inclusive approach to illness workup and attribution of poor concentration to the often multiple relevant contributing factors is necessary for optimal clinical understanding, diagnosis, and clinical intervention.

References

1. Merriam-Webster. Concentrate. Merriam-Webster.com dictionary. n.d. https://www.merriam-webster.com/dictionary/concentrate. Accessed 23 May 2021.
2. Schoenberg MR, Scott JG, editors. The little black book of neuropsychology: a syndrome-based approach. Dordrecht: Springer; 2011. p. 149–58.

3. Mackworth NH. The breakdown of vigilance during prolonged visual search. Q J Exp Psychol. 1948;1(1):6–21. https://doi.org/10.1080/17470214808416738.
4. Esterman M, Rothlein D. Models of sustained attention. Curr Opin Psychol. 2019;29:174–80. https://doi.org/10.1016/j.copsyc.2019.03.005.
5. Posner MI, Petersen SE. The attention system of the human brain. Annu Rev Neurosci. 1990;13:25–42.
6. Fortenbaugh FC, Degutis J, Esterman M. Recent theoretical, neural, and clinical advances in sustained attention research. Ann N Y Acad Sci. 2017;1396(1):70–91. https://doi.org/10.1111/nyas.13318.
7. Seli P, Risko EF, Smilek D, Schacter DL. Mind-wandering with and without intention. Trends Cogn Sci. 2017;20(8):605–17. https://doi.org/10.1016/j.tics.2016.05.010.
8. Oken BS, Sakinsky MC, Elsas SM. Vigilance, alertness, or sustained attention: physiological basis and measurement. Clin Neurophysiol. 2006;117(9):1885–901. https://doi.org/10.1016/j.clinph.2006.01.017.
9. American Psychiatric Association. Diagnostic and statistical manual of mental disorders. 5th ed., text rev. Washington, DC: American Psychiatric Association; 2022.
10. Research domain criteria. National Institute of Mental Health. https://www.nimh.nih.gov/research/research-funded-by-nimh/rdoc/constructs/attention.
11. Maalouf FT, Klein C, Clark L, Sahakian BJ, LaBarbara EJ, Versace A, Hassel S, Almeida JRC, Phillips ML. Impaired sustained attention and executive dysfunction: bipolar disorder versus depression-specific markers of affective disorders. Neuropsychologia. 2010;48(6):1862–8. https://doi.org/10.1016/j.neuropsychologia.2010.02.015.
12. Rowland TA, Marwaha S. Epidemiology and risk factors for bipolar disorder. Therap Adv Psychopharm. 2018;8:251. https://doi.org/10.1177/2045125318769235.
13. Hasin DS, Sarvet AL, Meyers JL, Saha TD, Ruan WJ, Stohl M, Grant BF. Epidemiology of adult DSM-5 major depressive disorder and its specifiers in the United States. JAMA Psychiat. 2018;75(4):336.
14. Forster S, Elizalde N, Castle E, Bishop SJ. Unraveling the anxious mind: anxiety, worry, and frontal engagement in sustained attention versus off-tast processing. Cerebr Cortex. 2013;25(3):609–18. https://doi.org/10.1093/cercor/bht248.
15. Prevalence of generalized anxiety disorder among adults. National Institute of Mental Health. https://www.nimh.nih.gov/health/statistics/generalized-anxiety-disorder#:~:text=An%20estimated%202.7%25%20of%20U.S.,than%20for%20males%20(1.9%25).
16. Vasterling JJ, Constans JI, Brailey K, Sutker PB. Attention and memory dysfunction in posttraumatic stress disorder. Neuropsychology. 1998;12(1):125–33. https://doi.org/10.1037/0894-4105.12.1.125.
17. Gradus J. Epidemiology of PTSD. National center for post-traumatic stress disorder. Department of Veterans Affairs; 2000.
18. Vasilevskis EE, Han JH, Hughes CG, Ely EW. Epidemiology and risk factors for delirium across hospital settings. Best Pract Res Clin Anaesthesiol. 2012;26(3):277–87.
19. O'Regan NA, Ryan DJ, Boland E, Connolly W, McGlade C, Leonard M, Clare J, Eustace JA, Meagher D, Timmons S. Attention! A good bedside test for delirium? J Neurol Neurosurg Psychiatry. 2014;85:1122–31.
20. Marra A, Jackson JC, Ely EW, Graves AJ, Schnelle JF, Robert DS, Wilson A, Han JH. Focusing on inattention: the diagnostic accuracy of brief measures of inattention for detecting delirium. J Hosp Med. 2018;13(8):551–7. https://doi.org/10.12788/jhm.2943.
21. Culley DJ, Snayd M, Baxter MG, Xie Z, Lee IH, Rudolph J, Inouye SK, Marcantonio ER, Crosby G. Systemic inflammation impairs attention and cognitive flexibility but not associative learning in aged rats: possible implications for delirium. Front Aging Neurosci. 2014;6:107. https://doi.org/10.3389/fnagi.2014.00107.

22. Flicker L, Logiudice D, Carlin JB, Ames D. The predictive value of dementia screening instruments in clinical populations. Int J Geriatr Psychiatry. 1998;12(2). https://doi.org/10.1002/(SICI)1099-1166(199702)12:2<203::AID-GPS603>3.0.CO;2-W.
23. Wang KK, Yang Z, Zhu T, Shi Y, Rubenstein R, Tyndall JA, Manley GT. An update on diagnostic and prognostic biomarkers for traumatic brain injury. Expert Rev Mol Diagn. 2018;18(2):165–80. https://doi.org/10.1080/14737159.2018.1428089.
24. The descriptive epidemiology of DSM-IV adult ADHD in the World Health Organization World Mental Health Surveys. Atten Defic Hyperact Disord. 2017;9(1):47–65. https://doi.org/10.1007/s12402-016-0208-3.
25. Attention-Deficit/Hyperactivity Disorder. Center for Disease Control and Prevention. 2020. https://www.cdc.gov/ncbddd/adhd/data.html#:~:text=Millions%20of%20US%20children%20have,children%20aged%206%E2%80%9311%20years.
26. Christakou A, Murphy CM, Chantiluke K, Cubillo AI, Smith AB, Giampietro V, Daly E, Ecker C, Robertson D, Murphy DG, Rubia K. Disorder-specific functional abnormalities during sustained attention in youth with attention deficit hyperactivity disorder (ADHD) and with autism. Mol Psychiatry. 2013;18(2):236–44. https://doi.org/10.1038/mp.2011.
27. Autism spectrum disorder. National Institute of Mental Health. 2020. https://www.nimh.nih.gov/health/statistics/autism-spectrum-disorder-asd#:~:text=Prevalence%20of%20ASD,-Prevalence%20data%20for&text=Across%20the%20CDC%20surveillance%20sites,all%20racial%20and%20ethnic%20groups.
28. Garretson HB, Fein D, Waterhouse L. Sustained attention in children with autism. J Autism Dev Disord. 1990;20(1):101–14. https://doi.org/10.1007/BF02206860.
29. Fanouriakis A, Tziolos N, Bertsias G, Boumpas DT. Update on the diagnosis and management of systemic lupus erythematosus. Ann Rheum Dis. 2021;80:14–25. https://doi.org/10.1136/annrheumdis-2020-218272.
30. Furst DE, Clarke AE, Fernandes AW, Bancroft T, Greth W, Iorga SR. Incidence and prevalence of adult systemic lupus erythematosus in a large US managed-care population. Lupus. 2013;22(1):99–105.
31. Liu CC, Ahearn JM. The search for lupus biomarkers. Best Pract Res Clin Rheumatol. 2009;23:507–23. https://doi.org/10.1016/j.berh.2009.01.008.
32. Garg N, Smith TW. An update on immunopathogenesis, diagnosis, and treatment of multiple sclerosis. Brain Behav. 2015;5(9):e00362. https://doi.org/10.1002/brb3.362.
33. Igra MS, Paling D, Wattjes MP, Connolly DJA, Hoggard N. Multiple sclerosis update: use of MRI for early diagnosis, disease monitoring, and assessment of treatment related complications. Br J Radiol. 2017;90:20160721. https://doi.org/10.1259/bjr.20160721.
34. Lakin L, Davis BE, Binns CC, Currie KM, Rensel MR. Comprehensive approach to management of multiple sclerosis: addressing invisible symptoms – a narrative review. Neurol Ther. 2021;10:75. https://doi.org/10.1007/s40120-021-00239-2.
35. Howard J, Trevick S, Younger DS. Epidemiology of multiple sclerosis. Neurol Clin. 2016;34(4):919–39. https://doi.org/10.1016/j.ncl.2016.06.016. Epub 2016 Aug 18. PMID: 27720001
36. Mayr WT, Pittock SJ, McClelland RL, Jorgensen NW, Noseworthy JH, Rodriguez M. Incidence and prevalence of multiple sclerosis in Olmsted County, Minnesota, 1985–2000. Neurology. 2003;61:1373–7.
37. Kaunzner UW, Gauthier SA. MRI in the assessment and monitoring of multiple sclerosis: an update on best practice. Ther Adv Neurol Disord. 2017;10:247–61. https://doi.org/10.1177/1756285617708911.
38. 2019 Profile of older Americans. The Administration for community living, an operating division of the U.S. Department of health and human services. 2020. https://acl.gov/sites/default/files/Aging%20and%20Disability%20in%20America/2019ProfileOlderAmericans508.pdf.

39. Schofield P, Marder K, Dooneief G, Jacobs DM, Sano M, Stern Y. Association of subjective memory complaints with subsequent cognitive decline in community-dwelling elderly individuals with baseline cognitive impairment. Am J Psychiatry. 1997;154:609–15.
40. Trikojat K, Buske-Kirschbaum A, Schmitt J, Plessow F. Altered performance in attention tasks in patients with seasonal allergic rhinitis: seasonal dependency and association with disease characteristics. Psychol Med. 2015;45(6):1289–99. https://doi.org/10.1017/S0033291714002384.
41. Settipane RA. Demographics and epidemiology of allergic and nonallergic rhinitis. Allergy Asthma Proc. 2001;22(4):185–9.
42. Eren E, Aktas A, Arslanoglu KA, Ciger E, Ozkul Y, Onal K, Katilmus H. Diagnosis of allergic rhinitis: inter-rater reliability and predictive value of nasal endoscopic examination: a prospective observational study. J Otolaryngol. 2012;38(6):481–6.
43. Raza SN, Yousuf K, Small P, Frenkiel S. Diagnosing allergic rhinitis: effectiveness of the physical examination in comparison to conventional skin testing. J Otolaryngol. 2011;40(5):407–12.
44. Merger SR, Leslie RD, Boehm BO. The broad clinical phenotype of type 1 diabetes at presentation. Diabet Med. 2013;30(2):170–8.
45. van Dijk M, Donga E, van Schie MK, Lammers GJ, van Zwet EW, Corssmit EP, et al. Impaired sustained attention in adult patients with type 1 diabetes is related to diabetes per se. Diabetes Metab Res Rev. 2014;30(2):132–9.
46. Kodl CT, Seaquist ER. Cognitive dysfunction and diabetes mellitus. Endocr Rev. 2008;29(4):494–511.
47. Brands AM, Biessels GJ, de Haan EH, Kappelle LJ, Kessels RP. The effects of type 1 diabetes on cognitive performance: a meta-analysis. Diabetes Care. 2005;28(3):726–35.
48. American Diabetes Association. Standards of medical Care in diabetes 2011. Diabetes Care. 2011;34:S11.
49. Leigh H, Kramer SI. The psychiatric manifestations of endocrine disease. Adv Intern Med. 1984;29:413–45.
50. Annerbo S, Lokk J. A clinical review of the association of thyroid stimulating hormone and cognitive impairment. ISNR Endocrinol. 2013;2013:856017., 6 pages. https://doi.org/10.1155/2013/856017.
51. Aoki Y, Belin RM, Clickner R, Jeffries R, Phillips L, Mahaffey KR. Serum TSH and total T4 in the United States population and their association with participant characteristics: National Health and Nutrition Examination Survey (NHANES 1999–2002). Thyroid. 2007;17(12):1211–23.
52. Chaker L, Bianco AC, Jonklaas J, Peeters RP. Hypothyroidism. Lancet (London, England). 2017;390(10101):1550–62. https://doi.org/10.1016/S0140-6736(17)30703-1.
53. McDermott MT. Hypothyroidism. Ann Intern Med. 2009;151(11):ITC6-1.
54. Haupt M, Kurz A. Reversibility of dementia in hypothyroidism. Z Gesamte Inn Med. 1993;48(12):609–13.
55. Osterweil D, Syndulko K, Cohen SN, Pettier-Jennings PD, Hershman JM, Cummings JL, et al. Cognitive function in non-demented older adults with hypothyroidism. J Am Geriatr Soc. 1992;40(4):325–35.
56. Schrier RW. Body water homeostasis: clinical disorders of urinary dilution and concentration. J Am Soc Nephrol. 2006;17(7):1820–32.
57. Kreisman SH, Hennessey JV. Consistent reversible elevations of serum creatinine levels in severe hypothyroidism. Arch Intern Med. 1999;159(1):79–82.
58. O'Brien T, Dinneen SF, O'Brien PC, Palumbo PJ. Hyperlipidemia in patients with primary and secondary hypothyroidism. Mayo Clin Proc. 1993;68(9):860–6.
59. Hussein WI, Green R, Jacobsen DW, Faiman C. Normalization of hyperhomocysteinemia with L-thyroxine in hypothyroidism. Ann Intern Med. 1999;131(5):348–51.
60. Loughrey DG, Mihelji E, Lawlor BA. Age-related hearing loss associated with altered response efficiency and variability on a visual sustained attention task. Aging Neuropsychol Cogn. 2021;28:1–25. https://doi.org/10.1080/13825585.2019.1704.

61. Deafness and hearing loss. The World Health Organization. 2020. https://www.who.int/news-room/fact-sheets/detail/deafness-and-hearing-loss.
62. DeCarlo DK, Bowman E, Monroe C, Kline R, McGwin G, Owsley C. Prevalence of attention-deficit/hyperactivity disorder among children with vision impairment. J AAPOS. 2014;18(1):10–4.
63. Borsting E, Rouse M, Chu R. Measuring ADHD behaviors in children with symptomatic accommodative dysfunction or convergence insufficiency: a preliminary study. Clin Res. 2005;76(10):588–92.
64. Varma R, Tarczy-Hornoch K, Jiang X. Visual impairment in preschool children in the United States. JAMA Ophthalmol. 2017;135(6):610–6. https://doi.org/10.1001/jamaophthalmol.2017.1021.
65. Bhaskar A, Hemavathy D, Prasad S. Prevalence of chronic insomnia in adult patients and its correlation with medical comorbidities. J Family Med Prim Care. 2016;5(4):780–4.
66. Gencarelli A, Khader W, Morales KS, Vargas I, Koss J. 1 in 4 Americans develop insomnia. Penn Medicine News; 2018.
67. Bonnet MH, Arand DL. Evaluation and diagnosis of insomnia in adults. In: Benca R, editor. UpToDate. Waltham, MA: UpToDate; 2020.
68. Peppard PE, Young T, Barnet JH, Palta M, Hagen EW, Hla KM. Increased prevalence of sleep-disordered breathing in adults. Am J Epidemiol. 2013;177(9):1006–14.
69. Kline LR. Clinical presentation and diagnosis of obstructive sleep apnea in adults. In: Collop N, Finlay G, editors. UpToDate. Waltham, MA: UpToDate; 2020.
70. Ulrichsen KM, Alnaes D, Richard G, Sanders AM, Dorum ES, Ihle-Hansen H, Pedersen ML, Tornas S, Nordvik JE, Westlye LT. Dissecting the cognitive phenotype of post-stroke fatigue using computerized assessment and computational modeling of sustained attention. Eur J Neurosci. 2020;52:3228–845. https://doi.org/10.1111/ejn.14861.
71. Paciaroni M, Acciarresi M. Poststroke fatigue. Stroke. 2019;50:1927–33.
72. Kobylecki C. Update on the diagnosis and management of Parkinson's disease. R Coll Physicians. 2020. https://doi.org/10.7861/clinmed.2020.0220.
73. Narayanan NS, Rodnitzky RL, Ergun U. Prefrontal dopamine signaling and cognitive symptoms of Parkinson's disease. Rev Neurosci. 2013;24(3):267–78. https://doi.org/10.1515/revneuro-2013-0004.
74. Sun C, Armstrong MJ. Treatment of Parkinson's disease with cognitive impairment: current approaches and future directions. Behav Sci. 2021;11:54. https://doi.org/10.3390/bs11040054.
75. Tysnes O-B, Storstein A. Epidemiology of Parkinson's disease. J Neural Transm. 2017;124(8):901–5.

Muscle Tension

8

Kyle Hodges and James A. Bourgeois

Introduction to and Definition of Muscle Tension

For us to focus on this page, our eye ciliary muscles must contract to modulate the shape of the crystalline lens while our head and neck muscles steadily flex to support our cranium. Hands must fly to coffee mugs back and forth, usually imperceptibly. Fingers clutched around a steering wheel in traffic with toes ready to ride the accelerator down to the floor. This activity is well-tolerated temporarily but minutes soon turn into hours. Our hardworking muscles begin to fatigue and carry a feeling of tension. We might begin to grab at a sore spot in our neck or rub our eyes to help soothe ache and strain. Such **muscle tension** is the notable perception that a muscle or group of muscles are contracted and felt to be taut or tight, causing discomfort [1, 2].

The above is an example of muscle tension that is **musculoskeletal** in origin, but many other forms of muscle tension exist. This is due to potentially contributing processes such as **histologic** (inflammation/abnormal development causing the perception of tension), **neuromuscular** (problems with the brain, spinal cord, nerve, neuromuscular junction, or muscle itself), **neurochemical** (muscle tension affected by biochemical signaling including neurotransmitters or pharmacodynamic), and **psychological** (hyperadrenergic state associated with anxiety).

K. Hodges (✉)
Department of Psychiatry, Baylor Scott and White Health, Central Texas Division, Temple, TX, USA
e-mail: Kyle.Hodges@BSWHealth.org

J. A. Bourgeois
Department of Psychiatry and Behavioral Sciences, University of California, Davis, Sacramento, CA, USA
e-mail: jbourgeois@ucdavis.edu

E. G. Meyer et al. (eds.), *The Medical Evaluation of Psychiatric Symptoms*,
https://doi.org/10.1007/978-3-031-14372-4_8

Since muscle tension is both a *cause* and a *sequala* of different diagnoses, this creates more opportunities for confusion between both patient and clinician trying to describe symptoms related to muscle tension. Of note, the term "muscle tension" is interchangeably used with "muscle tightness" [1, 2]. However, the perception and complaint of muscle tension is colloquially and commonly confused with other terms, including muscle rigidity, muscle pain (myalgia), muscle spasm/cramps, and others. Such confusion allows for a potential mismatch of symptoms, diagnoses, and treatment, which can be harmful to the patient.

Historical Definitions of Muscle Tension

According to Cram et al., muscle tension, as well as pain and dysfunction, can be viewed through the lens of a four-factor theory of ***histologic*** (tissue-related), ***psychologic*** (emotional), ***sensory motor*** (movement), and ***biomechanical*** (postural) components [3]. This four-factor theory takes into account the factors that generate muscle tension and helps to provide a physiological explanation. For example, a patient with Duchenne muscular dystrophy experiences abnormal muscle tension at a histologic (tissue-related) level. On the other hand, when seen through a psychological lens, a patient with generalized anxiety disorder may develop muscle tension secondary to an increased adrenergic state associated with anxiety. The other three factors may also be at play, but one could miss a case of generalized anxiety disorder if muscle tension was the only explored symptom during the interview, and other associated symptoms (e.g., constant worry, insomnia) were not explored in further detail.

In this line of thinking, muscle tension poses a "the chicken or the egg?" problem, as it is possible that one patient may experience "primary" muscle tension as a physical symptom *first*, and then later develop anxiety in response to this symptom, as opposed to a patient who is *initially* anxious and develops *subsequent* muscle tension because of a hyperadrenergic state. Thus, muscle tension in the psychiatric realm remains an important, but poorly understood, symptom. To illustrate this, a study by Sainsbury and Gibson on symptoms reported by patients with known anxiety disorders, a "feeling of tension" was mostly described as a "feeling of tightness," as if muscles (are) taut, "stiffness of the muscles," "being cramped," and "unable to relax my body." However, besides the majority of patients describing tension as something experienced *exclusively* in their muscles, approximately 25% of patients experienced it *solely* as a mental state, using phrases such as "on edge," "keyed up," "over alert all the time," and "jittery and unable to settle" [4].

Anatomy, Physiology, and Pathophysiology of Muscle Tension

From an anatomical perspective, the muscles of the human body were designed to contract and relax to allow movement (skeletal muscle), digest food and excrete waste (smooth muscle), as well as deliver oxygen and vital nutrients throughout the body with rhythmic pumping (cardiac muscle). For the purposes of this chapter, muscle tension is something perceived within *skeletal* muscle, which is comprised of several muscle fibers. A motor unit, defined a single motor neuron and all the muscle fibers it innervates, triggers the contraction of skeletal muscle fibers via signaling from a motor neuron found within the ventral spinal cord or a cranial nerve with motor function. Muscle fibers and the axons of the nerves that supply them communicate via the neuromuscular junction, where neurotransmitters such as acetylcholine are released and bind to acetylcholine receptors in response to axon potentials [5].

Skeletal muscles contain many **sensory mechanisms** including muscle spindles, Golgi tendon organs, Ruffini nuclei, and free nerve endings, which sense local pain and metabolic disturbances such as too much (lactic) acid or excess internal pressure due to external trauma, swelling, congestion, or edema [5]. These mechanisms, working in concert with the CNS, coordinate the perception that a muscle is tight/contracted.

As mentioned, a variety of **neurotransmitters** are implicated in the regulation of skeletal muscle contractions and thus muscle tension. While this list is by no means exhaustive, particular focus is given to acetylcholine, norepinephrine, and serotonin.

Acetylcholine is a neurotransmitter found in the central nervous system, autonomic ganglia, and the neuromuscular junction. Acetylcholine acts both on *muscarinic* and *nicotinic* receptors and is broken down by an enzyme called acetylcholinesterase. *Muscarinic* receptors (M1-M5) are found in the brain (playing a role in learning and memory) and also form part of the parasympathetic nervous system that helps with the regulation of secretions (both in the bronchial tree and the gastrointestinal tract), heart rate, pupillary response, and urination. *Nicotinic* receptors are located in muscle fibers at neuromuscular junctions and autonomic ganglia for both the sympathetic and parasympathetic nervous systems. Acetylcholine binding to nicotinic receptors is essential for voluntary muscle contraction, while muscarinic receptor activity plays a role in modulating synaptic function [6].

Anticholinergic refers to blocking the action of the neurotransmitter acetylcholine at *muscarinic* receptors, but not at *nicotinic* receptors. Anticholinergic medication such as benztropine or first-generation antihistamines with anticholinergic properties (diphenhydramine) are commonly used to treat involuntarily muscle movements, EPS, and dystonic reactions that result from antipsychotic use [7]. On the other hand, acetylcholinesterase inhibitors such as donepezil (commonly used for neurocognitive disorders like dementia) or pyridostigmine (used to treat Myasthenia Gravis) result in increased levels of acetylcholine at both nicotinic and muscarinic receptors. During a cholinergic crisis, when there is too much acetylcholine acting at nicotinic receptors, muscle fasciculations and respiratory weakness can be clinically observed [6].

Norepinephrine (NE), produced by the locus coeruleus in the brainstem, heavily regulates the sympathetic nervous system and also plays a significant role in muscle tension. Brainstem noradrenergic cell discharge activity is tightly coupled with state-dependent changes in muscle activity and muscle contraction. Stimulants like cocaine and methamphetamines increase noradrenergic activity and some antidepressants are at least partially noradrenergic in their mode of action. In rats, norepinephrine controls motor neuron activity by modulating glutamatergic excitation and that $\alpha 1$-adrenoceptor stimulation on motor neurons increases glutamate-dependent muscle twitch activity in REM sleep [8, 9]. Further, loss of noradrenergic cell activity in REM sleep and cataplexy reduces glutamate-mediated sensorimotor reflexes during these states [10, 11].

Serotonergic neurons, originating from the midline raphe nuclei, also project widely throughout the CNS to play an integral part in the regulation of wakefulness, affective behavior, feeding behavior, thermoregulation, and motor tone [12]. As a quick and easy rule, serotonin receptors are found in the brain, gut, and muscle tissue. Most antidepressants are at least partially serotonergic in their action and increase its neurotransmission. In the periphery, serotonin (5-HT) assists in the regulation of vascular tone and gastrointestinal motility. In the spinal cord, serotonin (5-HT) plays a critical role in modulating motor activity, where the moderate synaptic release of serotonin (5-HT) onto motor neurons enhances motor activity via activation of 5-HT2 receptors. Excessive muscle tone, hyperthermia, and hyperactive bowel sounds are clinically evidenced in patients experiencing serotonin syndrome, a condition which occurs when there is excess serotonin in the body [13].

Beyond these intrinsic processes, humans are placed under different **biomechanical** conditions and/or **psychological stressors** which may cause their muscles to contract excessively and/or for prolonged periods of time, leading to increased muscle tension and impairment. For example, a person sitting at a desk in their office and concentrating for several hours will begin to experience increased tension in the muscles of their neck and shoulders (e.g., trapezius, deltoid, and rhomboid muscles) as well as those surrounding the eyes (e.g., orbicularis oculi muscles). Tension and pain from migraine headaches may increase. A man working for a moving company places repeated enormous amounts of strain in short bursts on his muscles as he lifts throughout the day. Later, he "pulls a muscle" and cannot work for a month. Paired with a lack of simple physical therapy exercises to reduce daily muscle tension in the muscles, many are at risk of developing problems related to increased levels of muscle tension [14]. Worries and stressors throughout the day may also compound the tension experienced in these muscles. This comes as no surprise, as muscle tension is a complex psychophysiological phenomenon which has been shown to have a specifically strong correlation with pathological worry [15].

Separating Muscle Tension from Other Symptoms

As discussed in the previous sections, "muscle tension" can be a somatic or psychological sensation that can manifest in different ways. Somatically, muscle tension may be reported as soreness, stiffness, cramps, tightness, or an uncomfortable overall sensation in certain muscle patterns. Psychologically, muscle tension may be reported with concomitant anxiety and a sensation that a person's body feels "on edge," "keyed up," "hyperalert all of the time," an inability to relax one's body, and/or feeling "jittery and unable to settle." While muscle tension may involve a range of somatic symptoms, there are other important pathologies that must be considered when muscle tension is implicated.

Muscle cramp Muscle cramps are defined as a continuous, involuntary, painful, and localized contraction of an entire muscle group, individual single muscle, or select muscle fibers. Palpation of the affected area will usually reveal the presence of a "knot," which is a collection of contracted muscle tissue. When the cramp continues to remain contracted and painful, it may be referred to as a "muscle spasm" or that the patient "pulled a muscle." The differential for muscle cramps is broad but there are common etiologies. For instance, it is quite common in the primary care setting to see a patient complaining of lumbar back pain after lifting a heavy box or object. The affected paraspinal lumbar muscles are usually tender to palpation and feel "knotted." In the absence of neurological deficits and with a negative straight leg raise (a physical exam maneuver for assessing radiculopathy due to a herniated disc), this would be classified as an acute lumbar paraspinal muscle spasm.

Muscle cramps are also common during or after exercise, during which oxygen demand outweighs supply and a buildup of lactic acid in the muscles causes them to feel achy. Cramping may be normal or can be due to underlying pathology. For instance, **claudication**, a sign of peripheral vascular disease, is painful cramping of the lower extremities induced by exercise and occurs from occlusion of the arteries supplying muscles of the lower extremities. This is commonly seen in long-term tobacco smokers.

Lastly, several known electrolyte abnormalities can cause muscle cramps, including but not limited to: hyponatremia, hypokalemia, and hypocalcemia. Hypocalcemia may manifest in muscle cramping and twitching in the form of **Chvostek's sign** (twitching of the facial muscles in response to tapping near the facial nerve). In addition, **Trousseau's sign** is a carpopedal spasm caused by inflating the blood-pressure cuff to a level above systolic pressure for 3 min. Both signs are observed during times of hypocalcemia and have been associated with postoperative complication of total thyroidectomy and/or parathyroidectomy [16].

Dystonia Dystonia is classified as a movement disorder characterized by sustained or intermittent muscle contractions causing abnormal, often repetitive, movements, postures, or both. Dystonia is a dynamic disorder that changes in severity, depending upon activity and posture. Included is a table of common dystonia conditions [17] (Table 8.1).

Table 8.1 Types of Dystonia

Writer's Dystonia	Cervical Dystonia (Spasmodic Torticollis)	Blepharospasm
Task-specific hand dystonia that involves the hand and arm and is present only during the action of writing.	Most common isolated focal dystonia that affects the muscles of the neck and shoulders. It may appear as horizontal turning of the head (torticollis), lateral tilt of the neck (laterocollis), flexion of the head (anterocollis), or extension of the head (retrocollis).	Focal dystonia involves the orbicularis oculi muscles and other periocular muscles, including the procerus and corrugator muscles. Clinical manifestations include increased blinking and spasms of involuntary eye closure.

Commonly seen in emergency psychiatric settings, a patient receiving high-potency neuroleptic medication may develop an **acute dystonic reaction** (a form of EPS) characterized by painful contractions of the various muscles (of importance include the muscles of the eyes, neck, jaw, and even larynx). Potentially a life-threatening emergency, this reaction results from D2 receptor blockade in the nigrostriatal pathway and subsequent alterations in acetylcholine concentrations.

Myopathies/Myositis Myopathies can be distinguished from muscle tension primarily by the presence of weakness and decreased strength in the muscles. Myopathies are neuromuscular disorders in which there is dysfunction of the muscle fibers, for instance as a result of inflammation seen in conditions of myositis. Muscle tension may be implicated in myopathies, as some of the other symptoms of myopathy can include muscle cramps, stiffness, and spasm. Myopathies can be inherited (e.g., muscular dystrophies) or acquired (e.g., polymyalgia rheumatica, idiopathic inflammatory myopathy) [18].

Variants of Muscle Tension Complaints Based on Medical Specialty Context

Internal medicine/Family medicine: Muscle tension in the setting of a primary care setting may be attributed to a variety of underlying medical causes. Such conditions that cause bothersome muscle tension may be worked up due to metabolic derangements (e.g., hypokalemia, hypocalcemia), because of an inflammatory process either autoimmune in origin (e.g., myositis, dermatomyositis), due to medication (e.g., myalgias attributable to statins/HMG-CoA reductase inhibitors), or a result of injury (e.g., lumbar muscle spasm). If the tension is in the back muscles, spasm due to injury may be attributed.

Neurology: Patients who have suffered a stroke may develop spasticity in the affected muscles. These muscles exhibit increased tone and eventually become atrophied due to lack of use. In addition to hyperreflexia, clonus may also be elicited upon physical exam. There are several other syndromes in which abnormal muscle tension raises suspicion for further diagnostic workup. These include forms of epilepsy, Psychogenic Nonepileptic Seizures (PNES), Amyotrophic Lateral Sclerosis (ALS), as well as Stiff Person Syndrome (baseline increased tone due to an autoimmune process in which antibodies are formed against glutamic acid decarboxylase (GAD)).

Pediatrics: Many genetic conditions with pediatric onset present with increased muscle tonicity that are detected in infancy or adolescence and worsen into adulthood. These are often associated with common clusters of symptoms. Myotonic dystrophy results in prolonged muscle contractions (myotonia) and patients are not able to relax certain muscles after use (e.g., grasping an object and not being able to let go). Patients also have cataracts, frontal balding, cardiac conduction defects, and testicular atrophy.

Clinical Evaluation of "Muscle Tension"

Patients complaining of muscle tension could have significant variance underlying the cause of this symptom and the differential diagnosis may be inappropriately prematurely narrowed due to the location (e.g., psychiatrist's office) in which the patient's complaint is heard. To quote, "When you're a hammer, everything looks like a nail." Thus, when a patient reports muscle tension, it is important to explore this further with a broad frame of mind. This can be accomplished using the mnemonic "OLD CARTS," which stands for **O**nset, **L**ocation, **D**uration, **C**haracter, **A**ggravation/**A**lleviation, **T**iming, and **S**everity (e.g., on a scale from 1 to 10).

A history of trauma or previous surgical operation in the affected anatomical area might yield further insight into the current symptom. Such a line of questioning may help accurately hone the differential diagnosis underlying muscle tension, which can be broad, since this symptom can represent disease from musculoskeletal, psychiatric, neuromuscular, autoimmune, genetic/syndromic, and metabolic/endocrine system origins. A patient's previous medical history is important, as some diseases lead to muscle tension as part of the normal illness progression. A patient's previous psychiatric history is equally important, as it may refine the differential away from solely systemic medical causes. However, ignoring/minimizing this symptom, or merely attributing it to solely psychiatric origins, can have potentially harmful consequences.

A Psychiatric Illness Differential for Muscle Tension

Muscle tension is primarily implicated in anxiety disorders but may be a significant component of other psychiatric illnesses as described in the DSM-5-TR.

Anxiety Disorders

Anxiety disorders include disorders that share features of excessive fear, anxiety, and other related behavioral disturbances. *Fear* can be thought of as an emotional *response* to either real or perceived imminent threat, whereas *anxiety* is *anticipation* of a future threat. While these two states overlap, there are some key differences. Fear is more associated with rushes of autonomic arousal necessary for fight or flight, thoughts of anger, and escape behaviors. This sensation may be challenging for patients to articulate, especially if it is chronic. Anxiety is more frequently associated with muscle tension, hypervigilance in preparation for future danger, and cautious/avoidant behaviors. Similarly, anxiety and these related symptoms can blend imperceptibly into the background noise for someone with chronically elevated anxiety levels. Another factor is that anxiety-related emotions can be primarily experienced as somatic symptoms like muscle tension. There may be trembling, twitching, feeling shaky, and muscle aches or soreness [19].

Generalized Anxiety Disorder (GAD)

GAD is the disorder in the DSM-5-TR in which the symptom of muscle tension is part of a diagnostic criteria. To be precise, "The anxiety and worry are accompanied by at least three of the following additional symptoms: restlessness or feeling keyed up or on edge, being easily fatigued, difficulty concentrating or mind going blank, irritability, **muscle tension**, and disturbed sleep, although only one additional symptom is required in children." The symptom of anxiety is present for at least 6 months duration, causes functional impairment, and is not better explained by another diagnosis or due to substance use [19]. Of important note is the symptom of "feeling keyed up or on edge," which was described in a previous study earlier. Perhaps *muscle tension* in this context may represent more of a *somatic* sensation, whereas feeling *keyed up or on edge* may represent more of a *mental* state. Regardless, this suggests that anxiety generates tension through these pathophysiological ways [20].

Another explanation for muscle tension in GAD patients is that excessive worry keeps the patient from sensing prolonged static tension in the muscles and this tension builds up. In contrast, people that are less chronically anxious may more easily sense that their muscles are getting tense during prolonged postures or repetitive motions and they will consequently act to relax and minimize muscle tension, pain, and exhaustion. Patients that suffer from chronic anxiety will thus accumulate repeated bouts of muscle tension that progresses to painful, semi-contracted, and stiff muscles that is manifested as one of the symptomatic criteria of generalized anxiety disorder [20].

Another explanation is that GAD patients experience a high degree of emotional stress during daily life and their muscle tension may thus primarily reflect their tonically increased stress levels. In fact, an association between daily stress and muscle tension has been demonstrated in female supermarket cashiers (measured objectively using electromyography (EMG)) and medical secretaries [21, 22]. Hence, muscle tension may be understood as a reaction to externally experienced stress in addition to intrinsically generated anxiety.

Pathological muscle tension is that muscle tension may be a way of coping with excessive arousal caused by anxiety. One study has shown that masseter (jaw muscle) tension increased anxiety in subjects who initially reported low anxiety, while it decreased anxiety in those who initially reported high anxiety. The shift in anxiety levels was quite dramatic; initially, low-anxiety subjects became noticeably irritable and withdrawn, whereas initially high-anxiety subjects tolerated the maneuver quite well, and even enjoyed it. Thus, voluntary, purposeful voluntary muscle tensing be explored as an anxiety-reducing technique for highly anxious subjects [23].

Incidence/Prevalence

According to Ruscio et al., the combined lifetime prevalence of GAD was 3.7%, 12-month prevalence was 1.8%, and 30-day prevalence was 0.8%. Lifetime prevalence estimates varied widely across countries, ranging from less than 1% of the populations of Nigeria and Shenzhen, China, to approximately 8% of the populations of Australia, New Zealand, and the United States [24].

Incidence/Prevalence of Diagnosis Presenting with Muscle Tension

According to Faravelli et al., muscle tension was the only symptom actually associated with a higher risk of having GAD. Out of 105 patients, 82 (78.1%) presented with muscle tension [25].

Typical Findings of the HPI

Patients will often report chronically increased anxious state characterized by excessive worrying, a tendency to catastrophize the likely outcomes of life circumstances, poor or irregular sleep, irritability, and risk of comorbid depressive disorder. The formal DSM-5-TR diagnostic criteria include excessive anxiety/worry, difficulty in control of worrying, three or more symptoms among restlessness, fatigue, poor concentration, irritability, muscle tension, and poor sleep, with clinically significant distress and/or social/occupational dysfunction.

Typical Findings on Physical and Mental Status Exam

- Mild tenderness over the affected muscles.
- A tense and/or anxious affect; may be dysphoric/tearful if comorbid depressive disorder.
- Motor restlessness.
- Patient may be easily startled by sounds.

Typical Laboratory/Radiological Findings

There are no specific diagnostic laboratory or radiological findings.

Generalized Anxiety disorder

The clinical presentation of adjustment disorder with anxiety may overlap phenomenologically and physically with GAD, but the social context will be different. The adjustment disorder patient will not have had a lifelong or at least 6-month pattern of anxiety symptoms but will be symptomatic in temporal response to a clear and discrete stressor (e.g., relationship problem, academic problem, occupational disruption). As with GAD, nervousness, worry, jitteriness, or separation anxiety is predominant. Although muscle tension per se is not part of the DSM-5-TR criteria for adjustment disorder with anxiety, the appearance of adjustment disorder with anxiety may overlap with the presentation of GAD, which makes the argument that anxiety allowed to run a chronic course leads to elevated states of muscle tension via pathways described before.

Delirium and Related Syndromes

Motor abnormalities of tone, movements, posturing, and agitation may be important elements in the clinical presentation and may need separate consideration from the cognitive and more "cortical" aspects of the delirium syndrome, which occurs frequently in the inpatient setting. While neuroleptic malignant syndrome, catatonia, and serotonin syndrome are not necessarily associated with delirium in all cases, they are included in this section due to their typical association with motor signs involving skeletal muscular activation. It is further a priori acknowledged and not all delirium presentations involved increased muscular tension/restlessness/agitation, but ascertainment and assessment of motor function is essential in all cases of delirium.

Delirium

Delirium is a neurocognitive disorder characterized by disturbances in arousal, attention, circadian rhythm, global cognition, and perception that is attributable to the physiological effects of CNS and/or systemic illness and/or effects of medications/substances. A major risk factor for delirium is comorbid neurocognitive disorder/dementia. Standard delirium workup includes CBC, BMP, liver-associated enzymes, ammonia, TSH, calcium, vitamin B12, vitamin D, folate, thiamine, urinalysis, urine toxicology, blood alcohol, acetaminophen, and CT head. EEG revealing bilateral slowing confirms delirium, but EEG can be negative. Standard delirium precautions for delirium include avoidance of opioids, anticholinergics, and benzodiazepines (unless delirium is due to benzodiazepine/alcohol withdrawal), promotion of normal sleep/wake cycle, correction of sensory disturbances, and provision of adequate fluid/electrolyte/nutritional status. Serial cognitive assessment is used as part of the clinical database to ascertain treatment response.

Psychotropic off-label medication options include antipsychotics, anticonvulsants, adrenergic agents, propofol, and benzodiazepines (which are the primary intervention for benzodiazepine/alcohol withdrawal). Environmental management to promote normal sleep/wake cycle (e.g., lights off at night, blinds open/lights on during day, PT/OT as tolerated, frequent reorientation and cognitive monitoring by nursing staff recommended). As delirium is, by definition, a "whole brain" disorder, any psychiatric and/or neurological finding can be attributed to delirium.

Pertinent to the finding of muscle tension, hyperactive or mixed delirium, characterized by periods of agitation, may manifest increased muscle tension. Three specific syndromes seen in psychiatry *commonly*, though not *necessarily*, associated with delirium are catatonia, neuroleptic malignant syndrome (NMS), and serotonin syndrome (SS) [26].

Incidence/Prevalence

Variable, estimated at less than 2% in outpatient clinical populations, 20% in ED presentations, up to 87% in hospitalized patients (highest risk is in ICU patients) [26].

Incidence/Prevalence of Diagnosis Presenting with Muscle Tension

This has not been studied explicitly. Fifty percent of delirium patients present with hyperactive type while 25% present with mixed hyperactive/hypoactive type. The 20% who present with hypoactive type will not exhibit motor signs/muscle tension. A small fraction of delirium patients cannot be classified clearly into one of these three subtypes [27].

Typical Findings of the HPI

Variable, to the degree that patients are cognitively capable of reporting an HPI. The presentation of the delirium syndrome including motor signs (muscle tension, restlessness, agitation) may be subacute to acute and be associated with cognitive symptoms such as confusion, disorientation, global cognitive impairment, altered LOC, and sleep-wake disturbances.

Typical Findings on Physical and Mental Status Exam

For hyperactive and mixed types, increased motor activity ranging from restlessness to agitation to combativeness (as quantified by RASS scale clinically), psychosis, cognitive impairment, mood disturbances, and altered LOC.

Typical Laboratory/Radiological Findings

There are neither classic nor specific neuroimaging findings, though neuroimaging revealing atrophy, white matter disease and other stigmata of premorbid/commingled dementia/MNCD are common. EEG is typically abnormal with bilateral diffuse slowing without seizure foci in 80% of delirium cases [28]. A myriad of laboratory abnormalities can be seen in delirium depending on the delirium risk factors associated with the delirium presentation, but there is no laboratory finding specific for the delirium syndrome.

Catatonia

Catatonia is a behavioral syndrome which can occur in the context of other underlying psychiatric and general medical disorders, with the hallmark feature being a motor disturbance in which patients are unable to move normally despite presumed full physical capacity in the limbs and trunk. The disturbance can range from marked reduction in movements to significant agitation. Catatonia is now considered a subtype or complication of another illness, e.g., "major depressive disorder with catatonic features." There are well-documented abnormal motor symptoms of catatonia including immobility (hypokinesis or akinesia), waxy flexibility, posturing, excessive and purposeless motor activity (excitement), and echopraxia (senseless repetition of another person's movements) [29].

Catatonia can present in the context of several psychiatric illnesses, including delirium, psychotic disorders, depressive disorders, and NMS. Catatonia symptoms are quantified by the Bush-Francis Catatonia Rating Scale. Treatment includes trial of IV lorazepam; treatment refractory cases may need evaluation for ECT. Precautions for DVT and other complications of low motor function are needed.

Abnormal and variable states of muscle tension/tonicity are implicated in these abnormal movements. One theory of the presumed mechanism of catatonia is acute GABA depletion, leading to loss of GABAergic inhibition causing increased muscle tone, which explains how acute GABA replacement with benzodiazepines promptly reverses the hypertonicity characteristic of catatonia [30]. Other theories describe mechanisms that involve dopamine depletion and conversely increased activity at *N*-methyl-D-aspartate receptors. The four components of the hypothesis are: (1) GABA-A agonists have been shown to alleviate catatonia and NMS; (2) D2 antagonism is proportional to the relative likelihood of NMS and catatonia; (3) 5-HT1A agonism with 5-HT2A antagonism is implicated in catatonia and NMS; and (4) NMDA receptor antagonists, such as phencyclidine and ketamine, reduce glutamate transmission. This hypothesis proposes that it is the interaction of these systems that predisposes, initiates, and maintains the twin syndromes of catatonia and NMS [31].

Incidence/Prevalence

According to a comprehensive meta-analysis conducted by Solmi et al., the overall pooled, mean prevalence of catatonia was 9.2% among subjects diagnosed with a variety of psychiatric or medical conditions [32].

Incidence/Prevalence of Diagnosis Presenting with Muscle Tension

By definition, all patients with catatonia will have abnormal motor findings but the report of muscle tension as a specific complaint is unknown.

Typical Findings of the HPI

Patients are typically minimally verbal at presentation. HPI may reflect antecedent commingled psychiatric illness. If it is a catatonic presentation of delirium, HPI will overlap with that of delirium.

Typical Findings on Physical and Mental Status Exam

Multiple signs of catatonia will include those on the Bush-Francis Catatonia Rating Scale; examples of catatonia signs reflecting increased muscle tension include rigidity, posturing, waxy flexibility, and *geggenhalten*.

Typical Laboratory/Radiological Findings

There are no specific laboratory/radiological findings for catatonia per se. Laboratory/radiological findings may represent those of commingled delirium in cases of delirium-associated catatonia.

Neuroleptic Malignant Syndrome (NMS)

NMS is a delirium syndrome associated with the use of antipsychotic medication. It is further characterized by hyperthermia, rigidity, increased CPK, low Fe^{2+}. All antipsychotics should be held and CPK followed serially until normalized; if sedation is needed, IV lorazepam is preferred. For persistent rigidity, dantrolene and bromocriptine can be considered. For treatment refractory cases, ECT can be utilized.

There are two main postulated hypotheses for the genesis of NMS, which are not necessarily mutually exclusive. Firstly, NMS is traditionally considered to be the result of dopaminergic D2 receptor antagonism in the CNS. This receptor antagonism triggers a series of homeostatic responses that raise core body temperature, provoke muscular rigidity, and impair mental status because of autonomic nervous system dysregulation. Secondly, it has recently been postulated that NMS is the result of a toxic effect of the pharmacological compounds on musculoskeletal fibers, leading secondarily to the full NMS syndrome [33].

Incidence/Prevalence

A meta-analysis conducted by Gurrera et al. estimated that the incidence ranges from 0.02% to3% among patients taking antipsychotic agents and there are 0.991 cases per thousand people [34].

Incidence/Prevalence of Diagnosis Presenting with Muscle Tension

Unknown.

Typical Findings of the HPI

Chronic psychotic, bipolar, or depressive disorder leading to intervention with antipsychotics, concomitant use of lithium, recent change in antipsychotic therapy such as an increased dose of antipsychotic agent, a switch to a relatively higher dopamine-blocking antipsychotic, augmentation with lithium, dehydration, and (rarely) a decrease in antiparkinsonian medication.

Typical Findings on Physical and Mental Status Exam

Tetrad of hyperpyrexia, muscle rigidity, autonomic dysfunction, and delirium.

Typical Laboratory/Radiological Findings

Dramatically elevated creatinine kinase level, elevated white blood count and low serum iron are common to NMS and malignant catatonia [33].

Serotonin Syndrome (SS)

Serotonin syndrome is a delirium syndrome following the use of serotonergic medications, due to the over-activation of both the central and peripheral serotonin receptors because of high levels of serotonin. Given the range of presentation from mild to life-threatening, serotonin syndrome is also referred to *serotonin toxicity*, where the level of toxicity correlates to its severity.

In *mild* cases, the predominating features are mild hypertension and tachycardia, mydriasis, diaphoresis, shivering, tremor, myoclonus, and hyperreflexia. Patients with a mild episode of serotonin syndrome are usually afebrile.

In moderate cases usually have the above symptoms plus hyperthermia (e.g., 40 °C), hyperactive bowel sounds, horizontal ocular clonus, mild agitation, hypervigilance, and pressured speech.

In *severe cases*, patients have all the above symptoms plus hyperthermia greater than 41.1 °C, dramatic swings in pulse rate and blood pressure, delirium, and muscle rigidity. Severe cases may result in significant systemic medical complications, e.g., seizures, rhabdomyolysis, myoglobinuria, metabolic acidosis, renal failure, acute respiratory distress syndrome, respiratory failure, diffuse intravascular clotting, coma, and death. The symptoms of hyperreflexia, rigidity, and clonus tend to be more prominent in the lower extremities [35].

Serotonin syndrome can result from 5-HT agonism (either from increased concentrations of 5-HT or medications that act directly as serotonin receptor agonists) and/or antagonism of varying combinations of the 5-HT receptor subtypes. Animal studies have demonstrated that the life-threatening effects of SS, in particular, severe hypertonicity and hyperthermia, are primarily mediated by the activation of 5-HT2A receptors at higher serotonin concentrations. The 5-HT1A receptors, which have a higher affinity for 5-HT and are therefore likely to be nearly fully occupied at much lower extracellular 5-HT concentrations, may contribute to some of the milder symptoms including anxiety and hyperactivity [36].

Incidence/Prevalence

The true incidence of SS is unknown, as is the number of cases that are mild, moderate, or severe. Observed across the full range of age groups, from neonates all the way through to the elderly. Relatively uncommon condition that cannot be easily picked up in randomized clinical control trials and the condition is under-recognized and under-reported by physicians [36].

Incidence/Prevalence of Diagnosis Presenting with Muscle Tension

Unknown.

Typical Findings of the HPI

Important components of the history include prescription drug use, over-the-counter medication and dietary supplement use, illicit substance use, any recent changes in dosing, or the addition of new drugs to a drug regimen. The most recent diagnostic criteria are the Hunter Serotonin Toxicity Criteria (HSTC) and must include the use of a serotonergic agent plus 1 of the 5 following criteria: spontaneous clonus, inducible clonus plus agitation or diaphoresis, ocular clonus plus agitation or diaphoresis, tremor and hyperreflexia, hypertonia and a temperature above 38°C. Clonus and hyperreflexia are most important for the diagnosis; however, severe muscle rigidity may mask these symptoms. Prominent features of life-threatening cases include hyperthermia (>38.5°C), peripheral hypertonicity, and truncal rigidity because of the high risk of progression to respiratory failure.

Typical Findings on Physical and Mental Status Exam

The clinical examination should focus on eliciting any signs of muscle rigidity, hyperreflexia, or the observation of clonus, as well as autonomic signs such as the presence of diaphoresis, increased bowel sounds, and mydriasis [35].

Typical Laboratory/Radiological Findings

A diagnosis of SS is entirely clinical and is based on the history and physical examination along with history of the patient's use of a serotonergic drug. Some nonspecific laboratory abnormalities may be seen in serotonin syndrome: leukocytosis, low bicarbonate level, elevated creatinine level, and elevated transaminases. Serum serotonin concentrations do not correlate with the severity of this syndrome [35, 36].

Stimulant (Including Cocaine, Methamphetamine) Intoxication

Here acute (presumed) dopamine and NE excess cause direct hyperadrenergia/dystonia. This may be manifest primarily as increased muscle tension accompanied by an anxious/paranoid mood state, but will typically occur in concert with numerous other CNS and peripheral signs of increased arousal such as tachycardia, hypertension, psychomotor agitation, dyskinesias, or dystonias. The clinician should be vigilant for comorbid perceptual disturbances (delusions, hallucinations) occurring during stimulant intoxication, which may be the primary focus of clinical attention, especially if associated with behavioral regression or acting out. More severe stimulant intoxication is associated with cognitive impairment verging on delirium, seizures, and even coma.

The clinician seeing milder states of stimulant intoxication may see muscle tension and other evidence of mild hyperadrenergia in the setting of recent exposure to stimulants. The intoxication with stimulants will typically abate within 1 or 2 days, though the patient may continue to experience increased muscle tension throughout the withdrawal period. Given the context of presentation, it is unlikely that stimulant intoxication will present as an isolated complaint of increased muscle tension, although this complaint in the proper clinical context of recent substance exposure and other clinical signs should lead to the attribution of increased muscle tension to stimulant intoxication [37].

Incidence/Prevalence

Stimulant intoxication is not studied as a distinct entity. Stimulant use disorder prevalence is reported as 0.2–0.5% in the US [38].

Incidence/Prevalence of Diagnosis Presenting with Muscle Tension

Unknown.

Typical Findings of the HPI

Recent stimulant use, muscle tension, and other associated hyperadrenergic signs.

Typical Findings on Physical and Mental Status Exam

Increased muscle tone/tremors/dystonia/dyskinesia, psychosis, increased pulse and BP, pupillary dilatation, flushing, and cognitive impairment.

Typical Laboratory/Radiological Findings

Urine toxicology reveals stimulant (e.g., cocaine, methamphetamine). Stimulants when combined with increased motor activity and dehydration are at risk of inducing rhabdomyolysis (discussed below)—evidence of such would include an elevated creatine kinase.

Anti-*N*-methyl-D-aspartate (NMDA) Receptor Encephalitis (ANMDARE)

Anti-*N*-methyl-D-aspartate (NMDA) receptor encephalitis (ANMDARE) is a presumably autoimmune illness with various neuropsychiatric symptoms which may progress through three phases. A prodromal phase may present with nonspecific constitutional, "flu-like" symptoms accompanied by subtle psychiatric symptoms such as anxiety, agitation, and memory loss. This may be followed by more severe and debilitating psychiatric symptoms (including psychosis), with third phase including neurological symptoms including dyskinesia, seizures, and dysautonomia. Muscle tension could be part of the presentation [38–40].

Incidence/Prevalence

Rare, prevalence unknown.

Incidence/Prevalence of Diagnosis Presenting with Muscle Tension

Unknown.

Typical Findings of the HPI

Atypical presentation of psychotic illness, either concurrent or subsequent neurological signs.

Typical Findings on Physical and Mental Status Exam

Psychosis, dyskinesias, dystonia.

Typical Laboratory/Radiological Findings

CSF+ for IgG for NMDA receptor, increased protein, pleocytosis, oligoclonal bands [41].

A Systemic Medical Differential for Muscle Tension

Medication Induced

There are many medications that either directly or indirectly result in increased muscle tension and cause involuntary spasm or even dystonia. Some medications, like statin medications that lower cholesterol and antimalarial drugs are notorious for causing painful, cramped, and sore muscles. Muscle cramps from statin medications are often referred to as **statin-induced myopathy**. In randomized control trials, the incidence is approximately 1.5–5% [42].

Acute dystonic reactions are most commonly caused by antipsychotics, especially high-potency antipsychotic agents like haloperidol, but also antiemetics that block dopamine receptors such as metoclopramide can also cause these reactions. The pathophysiology is most often linked with the blockage of dopamine receptors. When acute dystonic reactions affect the neck region, difficulty swallowing, speaking, and even breathing can ensue—representing a medical emergency. Important risk factors for acute dystonia in this setting include young age, male sex, and muscular body habitus.

Another commonly seen side effect of antipsychotics is **akathisia**, which is an internal sense of restlessness that often results in an inability to sit still, pacing, and moving one's extremities in an effort to relieve the feeling of restlessness. Such a symptom is commonly treated with β-blockers such as propranolol.

Lastly, **diuretics** such as hydrochlorothiazide and furosemide may cause muscle spasm through dehydration or an electrolyte imbalance, especially hypokalemia, hypocalcemia, or hypomagnesemia [43].

When suspecting and evaluating medication-induced muscle tension and related pathologies, it is important to check [43]:

- Potassium, calcium, and magnesium levels.
- Creatine phosphokinase (CPK) to evaluate for any evidence of muscle breakdown.
- Electromyogram (EMG) if myopathy or ALS is being considered.
- Liver function tests (LFTs) for evidence of hepatotoxicity.

Tension Headache

Incidence/Prevalence

Tension-type headache (TTH) is the most common primary headache disorder, with a worldwide lifetime prevalence of 46–78% [44].

Incidence/Prevalence of Diagnosis Presenting with Muscle Tension

Estimated to be high, as a common presenting symptom of a tension headache is feeling a band of tension and pressure around one's head.

Typical Findings of the HPI/Exam

Tension-type headache are recurrent episodes of headache lasting minutes to weeks. The pain is typically pressing or tightening in quality, of mild to moderate intensity, and bilateral in location. Nausea and vomiting are usually absent, but photophobia or phonophobia may be present. These headaches were previously known by many terms such as psychogenic headache, stress headache, psychomyogenic headache, and muscle contraction headache [45]. Among psychiatric illness, anxiety and depression are more frequently associated with tension headaches [46].

Typical Laboratory/Radiological Findings

Clinical diagnosis only.

Myositis

The idiopathic inflammatory myopathies (IIMs), known collectively as myositis, constitute a large spectrum of clinical phenotypes. As indicated by the name, the classical clinical manifestations of IIMs, such as muscle weakness, relate to chronic inflammation in skeletal muscle. Such conditions include polymyositis, dermatomyositis, and inclusion body myositis. The classical clinical manifestations of IIMs, such as muscle weakness, relate to chronic inflammation in skeletal muscle. This inflammation frequently affects other organs, including the skin, joints, lungs, gastrointestinal tract, and heart, indicating the systemic nature of this disease [47].

Incidence/Prevalence of Diagnosis Presenting with Muscle Tension

Unknown.

Typical Findings on Physical and Mental Status Exam

Patients with amyopathic dermatomyositis and classic dermatomyositis have cutaneous manifestations which frequently include heliotrope erythema, erythema over joints (Gottron sign), and papules over joints (Gottron papules) [47].

Typical Laboratory/Radiological Findings

In addition to clinical history, they are often diagnosed and subclassified based upon specific antibody testing.

Rhabdomyolysis

Incidence/Prevalence

Approximately 25,000 cases of rhabdomyolysis are reported each year in the USA [48].

Typical Findings of the HPI

Rhabdomyolysis is a complex medical condition involving the rapid dissolution of damaged or injured skeletal muscle. This disruption of skeletal muscle integrity leads to the direct release of intracellular muscle components, including myoglobin, creatine kinase (CK), aldolase, and lactate dehydrogenase, as well as electrolytes, into the bloodstream and extracellular space. Rhabdomyolysis ranges from an asymptomatic illness with elevation in the CK level to a life-threatening condition associated with extreme elevations in CK, electrolyte imbalances, acute renal failure (ARF), and disseminated intravascular coagulation [48].

Although rhabdomyolysis is most often caused by direct traumatic injury, the condition can also be the result of drugs, toxins, infections, muscle ischemia, electrolyte and metabolic disorders, genetic disorders, exertion or prolonged bed rest, and temperature-induced states such as NMS and malignant hyperthermia [49].

Incidence/Prevalence of Diagnosis Presenting with Muscle Tension

Muscle pain is the most common presenting symptom and is presented in about 50% of adults with rhabdomyolysis, and dark-colored urine is seen in about 30–40% [48].

Typical Findings on Physical and Mental Status Exam

Muscle pain, weakness, and tea-colored urine are the characteristic triad of rhabdomyolysis, but this is not always seen. Malaise, abdominal pain, nausea, palpitations, and fever might be present. Depending on the cause of rhabdomyolysis, patients may provide a history of illicit drugs (stimulants like methamphetamines or cocaine), insect bites, heat exertion, recent surgical procedure, accidents, recent increasing dosages of regularly used medications, antibiotic use, and over-the-counter body enhancing supplements. Patients may have atrophic or hypertrophic muscles [48, 49].

Typical Laboratory/Radiological Findings

The hallmark of acute rhabdomyolysis is elevated creatine kinase (CK)/creatine phosphokinase (CPK) levels. Reddish-brown urine from myoglobinuria is present in ~50% of cases. Normal CPK levels are 20–200 IU/L. Elevated levels usually at least five times the upper limit of normal is considered rhabdomyolysis [48].

Of note, in a study of 89 subjects with single stimulant exposure, the prevalence of rhabdomyolysis was as follows: synthetic cathinone, 12/19 (63%); methamphetamine, 22/55 (40%); cocaine, 3/9 (33%) [50].

Spasticity

Spasticity is defined as disordered sensory motor control, resulting from an upper motor neuron lesion, presenting as intermittent or sustained involuntary activation of muscles. The pathophysiologic basis of spasticity is incompletely understood. The changes in muscle tone probably result from alterations in the balance of inputs from reticulospinal and other descending pathways to the motor and interneuronal circuits of the spinal cord, and the absence of an intact corticospinal system. Loss of descending tonic or phasic excitatory and inhibitory inputs to the spinal motor apparatus, alterations in the segmental balance of excitatory and inhibitory control, denervation supersensitivity, and neuronal sprouting may be observed [51].

Incidence/Prevalence

The epidemiology depends upon the cause of the spasticity. For example, post-stroke spasticity vs. spasticity due to a specific genetic disorder.

Incidence/Prevalence of Diagnosis Presenting with Muscle Tension

Increase muscle tone is expected to be part of the natural disease course of most diseases and resultant spastic disorders.

Typical Findings of the HPI, Physical, and Mental Status Exam

When the injury is acute, such as in the hours after a cerebral infarction, muscle tone is flaccid with hyporeflexia before the appearance of spasticity. The interval between injury and the appearance of spasticity varies from days to months according to the level of the lesion. After neuronal injury and loss of tonic inhibition sets in after several years, the affected muscles (e.g., of the arm or leg) remain in a state of increased tone. Symptoms can range from mild muscle stiffness to severe, painful, and uncontrollable muscle spasm. It is associated with some common neurological disorders: multiple sclerosis, long-term sequelae of stroke, cerebral palsy, spinal cord and brain injuries, and neurodegenerative diseases affecting the upper motor neuron, pyramidal and extrapyramidal pathways. Left untreated, it gives rise to many problems, such as pain, spasms, limb contracture, and deformity [51].

Typical Laboratory/Radiological Findings

Monitored clinically.

Parkinson's Disease (PD)

PD is the most common neurodegenerative movement disorder. It is also a neurocognitive disorder characterized physically by tremor, bradykinesia, and postural instability attributed to the loss of dopaminergic neurons in the substantia nigra and accumulation of misfolded α-synuclein, which is found in intra-cytoplasmic inclusions called Lewy bodies. When patients are first diagnosed, a substantial proportion of dopaminergic neurons have already been lost and neurodegeneration has spread to other brain areas [52].

Incidence/Prevalence

Parkinson's disease (PD) affects 1–2 per 1000 of the population at any time. PD prevalence is increasing with age and PD affects 1% of the population above 60 years [52].

In Europe, prevalence and incidence rates for PD are estimated at approximately 108–257/100,000 and 11–19/100,000 per year, respectively [52].

Incidence/Prevalence of Diagnosis Presenting with Muscle Tension

Rigidity/increased muscle tone is almost always seen later rather than sooner in the disease course.

Typical Findings of the HPI, Physical, and Mental Status Exams

The cardinal symptoms of Parkinson's disease are shaking, stiffness, slowness, and poverty of movement. The condition leads to physical signs including tremors at rest, rigidity on passive movement, slowness of movement (bradykinesia), and poverty of movement (hypokinesia). These features are unilateral at the onset but become bilateral as the condition progresses. Postural instability refers to imbalance and loss of righting reflexes (increased risk of falls). Mental status exam findings might include what is known as masked facies, with a blunted or even flat facial expression [52]. Other notable characteristics include decreased blinking, dysphagia, sialorrhoea, dysarthria, hypophonia, hypomimia, disturbances of sleep and wakefulness, micrographia, and cardiovascular symptoms of blood pressure variations (postural, postprandial) and dysrhythmias [53].

Typical Laboratory/Radiological Findings

The diagnosis is clinical, although specific investigations can help the differential diagnosis from other forms of parkinsonism.

Huntington's Disease (HD)

HD is a devastating autosomal dominant genetic illness leading to caudate nucleus degeneration within the basal ganglia. The characteristic motor changes are involuntary, unwanted movements for instance within the distal extremities such as fingers and toes, but also in small facial muscles. Initially, these muscle twitches are often overlooked or can be explained as nervousness [54].

Incidence/Prevalence

Huntington's disease (HD) is a fully penetrant neurodegenerative disease caused by a dominantly inherited CAG trinucleotide repeat expansion in the huntingtin gene on chromosome 4. In Western populations HD has a prevalence of 10.6–13.7 individuals per 100,000 [55].

Incidence/Prevalence of Diagnosis Presenting with Muscle Tension

No official studies. Dystonia (for instance, torticollis) or tics can be the first motor sign in Huntington's disease [55].

Typical Findings of the HPI

Typically presents in males in their late 30s with a positive family history or positive genetic test and the onset of motor disturbance as defined by the Unified HD Rating Scale (UHDRS) total motor score (TMS) diagnostic confidence score.

Typical Findings on Physical and Mental Status Exam

Characterized by motor (as described above), psychiatric (apathy, anxiety, irritability, depression, obsessive-compulsive behavior, and psychosis), and cognitive disturbances (impaired emotion recognition, processing speed, visuospatial, and executive function).

Movement disturbance in HD can be split into a hyperkinetic phase with prominent chorea in the early stages of the disease, which then tends to plateau. The hypokinetic phase is characterized by bradykinesia, dystonia, balance, and gait disturbance.

Gradually the unwanted movements spread from distal to proximal until choreatic movements are present anytime the patient is awake. Walking becomes unstable and the person might appear to be ambulating in a drunken manner. No single pattern exists, but facial choreatic movements can lead to a continuous movement of facial muscles where for instance an eyebrow is lifted, an eye closed, the head is bent or turned while the tongue is protruded with the lips pouting. Dysarthria and dysphagia become very prominent during the course of the disease with high risk of aspiration. All patients develop hypokinesia, akinesia, and rigidity [55].

Typical Laboratory/Radiological Findings

Macroscopic degeneration of the caudate on brain imaging.

Amyotrophic Lateral Sclerosis ALS

ALS is a devastating neurological illness affecting both upper and lower motor neurons and patients experience localized muscle weakness that begins distally in either the upper or lower extremities. Usually, the onset symptoms are asymmetric and develop in progressive generalized weakness and wasting of the muscles. Most of the patients develop bulbar and respiratory symptoms and spasticity which affects manual dexterity and gait. Muscle atrophy, including muscles of the hands, forearms or shoulders, and proximal thigh or distal foot muscle in lower limbs, is usually discovered early in the development of limb-onset ALS. In the later stages of ALS, some patients develop flexor spasms or involuntary spams due to excess activation of the flexor arc in spastic limbs [56].

Incidence/Prevalence

Estimated to be ~1.59% for North America [57].

Incidence/Prevalence of Diagnosis Presenting with Muscle Tension

Not studied, the first stage presents with fasciculations followed by muscle weakness [58].

Typical Findings of the HPI

Amyotrophic lateral sclerosis is a devastating neurodegenerative disease with a median survival of just 3 years from symptom onset. Fasciculations represent an early pathophysiological hallmark of amyotrophic lateral sclerosis. As ALS is a motor neuron disease, the sensory tracts are spared in the spinal cord.

Typical Findings on Physical and Mental Status Exam

Depending upon the stage, a mixture of upper and lower motor neuron findings are striking: hyperreflexia, fasciculations, spasticity.

Typical Laboratory/Radiological Findings

While the diagnosis of ALS has historically been primarily clinical, electromyography (EMG) is useful in detecting the findings of acute denervation, chronic denervation, and chronic reinnervation. As observed clinically, nerve conduction studies will also show normal sensory action potentials [59].

Stiff Person Syndrome (SPS)

SPS is a rare neuroimmunological disorder characterized by progressive rigidity and painful muscle spasms affecting axial and lower extremity musculature. EEG and MRI of the brain may be unremarkable; however, the condition is often diagnosed with LP and CSF studies that are positive for antiglutamic acid decarboxylase (GAD) antibodies. The episodes of muscle spasms can be triggered by sudden movement, noise, or emotional stress, which may present as a psychiatric condition [60].

Incidence/Prevalence

Unknown/poorly studied.

Incidence/Prevalence of Diagnosis Presenting with Muscle Tension

Estimated to be high given that the disease presents with fluctuating muscle rigidity and spasm.

Typical Findings of the HPI

A rare disorder, characterized by fluctuating rigidity and stiffness of the axial and proximal lower limb muscles, with superimposed painful spasms [61].

Typical Findings on Physical and Mental Status Exam

Body stiffness is associated with painful muscle spasms, and varies in location and severity. It is subdivided into stiff trunk versus stiff limb presentation and progressive encephalomyelitis. Stiff person-type syndrome also reflects a paraneoplastic picture.

Typical Laboratory/Radiological Findings

Roughly 60% of patients have antiglutamic acid decarboxylase antibodies in the blood and the cerebrospinal fluid. Continuous motor unit activity on electromyography [61, 62].

References

1. Bhimani R, Gaugler JE, Felts J. Consensus definition of muscle tightness from multidisciplinary perspectives. Nurs Res. 2020;69(2):109–15. https://doi.org/10.1097/NNR.0000000000000404. PMID: 31702702
2. Bhimani R, Soomar D. Understanding symptoms of muscle tightness, weakness, and rigidity from a nursing perspective. Rehabil Nurs J. 2019;44:271–81. https://doi.org/10.1097/rnj.0000000000000151.
3. Cram JR. The history of surface electromyography. Appl Psychophysiol Biofeedback. 2003;28(2):81–91. https://doi.org/10.1023/a:1023802407132. PMID: 12827987
4. Sainsbury P, Gibson JG. Symptoms of anxiety and tension and the accompanying physiological changes in the muscular system. J Neurol Neurosurg Psychiatry. 1954;17(1954):216–24.
5. Biga LM, et al. Anatomy & physiology. https://open.oregonstate.education/aandp/chapter/10-4-nervous-system-control-of-muscle-tension/. Publication date unknown.
6. Adeyinka A, Kondamudi NP. Cholinergic crisis. In: StatPearls [Internet]. Treasure Island, FL: StatPearls Publishing; 2021. PMID: 29494040.
7. van't Groenewout JL, Stone MR, Vo VN, Truong DD, Matsumoto RR. Evidence for the involvement of histamine in the antidystonic effects of diphenhydramine. Exp Neurol. 1995;134(2):253–60. https://doi.org/10.1006/exnr.1995.1055. PMID: 7556545
8. Schwarz PB, Yee N, Mir S, Peever JH. Noradrenaline triggers muscle tone by amplifying glutamate-driven excitation of somatic motoneurones in anaesthetized rats. J Physiol. 2008;586(23):5787–802. https://doi.org/10.1113/jphysiol.2008.159392.
9. Mir S, Yee N, Brooks PL, Peever JH. Noradrenergic control of motoneurons during natural sleep in rats. Sleep. 2006;29:A27.
10. Guilleminault C, Wilson RA, Dement WC. A study on cataplexy. Arch Neurol. 1974;31:255–61.
11. Onofrj M, Luciano AL, Thomas A, Iacono D, D'Andreamatteo G. Mirtazapine induces REM sleep behavior disorder (RBD) in parkinsonism. Neurology. 2003;60:113–5.
12. Dvir Y, Smallwood P. Serotonin syndrome: a complex but easily avoidable condition. Gen Hosp Psychiatry. 2008;30(3):284–7. https://doi.org/10.1016/j.genhosppsych.2007.09.007. PMID: 18433663
13. Sakai M, Matsunaga M, Kubota A, Yamanishi Y, Nishizawa Y. Reduction in excessive muscle tone by selective depletion of serotonin in intercollicularly decerebrated rats. Brain Res. 2000;860(1–2):104–11. https://doi.org/10.1016/s0006-8993(00)02022-9. PMID: 10727628

14. Hanna T. Load pattern and pressure pain threshold in the upper trapezius muscle and psychosocial factors in medical secretaries with and without shoulder/neck disorders. Int Arch Occup Environ Health. 1988;69:423–32.
15. Joormann J, Stöber J. Somatic symptoms of generalized anxiety disorder from the DSM-IV: associations with pathological worry and depression symptoms in a nonclinical sample. J Anxiety Disord. 1999;13(5):491–503. https://doi.org/10.1016/s0887-6185(99)00017-1. PMID: 10600050
16. Bordoni B, Sugumar K, Varacallo M. Muscle cramps. [Updated 2020 Nov 20]. In: StatPearls [Internet]. Treasure Island, FL: StatPearls Publishing; 2020. https://www.ncbi.nlm.nih.gov/books/NBK499895/.
17. Batla A. Dystonia: a review. Neurol India. 2018;66(Suppl):S48–58. https://doi.org/10.4103/0028-3886.226439. PMID: 29503327
18. Schmidt J. Current classification and management of inflammatory myopathies. J Neuromusc Dis. 2018;5(2):109–29. https://doi.org/10.3233/JND-180308.
19. American Psychiatric Association Content Provider. Anxiety disorders: DSM-5 selections; 2016. Web.
20. Pluess M, Conrad A, Wilhelm FH. Muscle tension in generalized anxiety disorder: a critical review of the literature. J Anxiety Disord. 2009;23(1):1–11. https://doi.org/10.1016/j.janxdis.2008.03.016. Epub 2008 Apr 7. PMID: 18472245
21. Lundberg U, Dohns IE, Melin B, Sandsjö L, Palmerud G, Kadefors R, Ekström M, Parr D. Psychophysiological stress responses, muscle tension, and neck and shoulder pain among supermarket cashiers. J Occup Health Psychol. 1999;4(3):245–55. https://doi.org/10.1037//1076-8998.4.3.245. PMID: 10431284
22. Hägg GM, Aström A. Load pattern and pressure pain threshold in the upper trapezius muscle and psychosocial factors in medical secretaries with and without shoulder/neck disorders. Int Arch Occup Environ Health. 1997;69(6):423–32. https://doi.org/10.1007/s004200050170. PMID: 9215929
23. Grim PF. Anxiety change produced by self-induced muscle tension and by relaxation with respiration feedback. Behav Ther. 1971;2(1):11–7., ISSN 0005-7894. https://doi.org/10.1016/S0005-7894(71)80141-7.
24. Ruscio AM, Hallion LS, Lim CCW, et al. Cross-sectional comparison of the epidemiology of DSM-5 generalized anxiety disorder across the globe. JAMA Psychiat. 2017;74(5):465–75. https://doi.org/10.1001/jamapsychiatry.2017.0056.
25. Faravelli C, Castellini G, Benni L, Brugnera A, Landi M, Lo Sauro C, Pietrini F, Rotella F, Ricca V. Generalized anxiety disorder: is there any specific symptom? Compr Psychiatry. 2012;53(8):1056–62. https://doi.org/10.1016/j.comppsych.2012.04.002. Epub 2012 May 11. PMID: 22578985
26. Maldonado JR. Acute brain failure: pathophysiology, diagnosis, management, and sequelae of delirium. Crit Care Clin. 2017;33(3):461–519. https://doi.org/10.1016/j.ccc.2017.03.013. PMID: 28601132
27. Grover S, Sharma A, Aggarwal M, Mattoo SK, Chakrabarti S, Malhotra S, Avasthi A, Kulhara P, Basu D. Comparison of symptoms of delirium across various motoric subtypes. Psychiatry Clin Neurosci. 2014;68(4):283–91. https://doi.org/10.1111/pcn.12131. Epub 2013 Dec 25. PMID: 24372977
28. Naeije G, Bachir I, Gaspard N, Legros B, Pepersack T. Epileptic activities are common in older people with delirium. Geriatr Gerontol Int. 2014;14(2):447–51. https://doi.org/10.1111/ggi.12128. Epub 2013 Aug 4. PMID: 23910220
29. Fink M. Catatonia from its creation to DSM-V: considerations for ICD. Indian J Psychiatry. 2011;53(3):214–7. https://doi.org/10.4103/0019-5545.86810. PMID: 22135438; PMCID: PMC3221176
30. Unal A, Bulbul F, Alpak G, Virit O, Copoglu US, Savas HA. Effective treatment of catatonia by combination of benzodiazepine and electroconvulsive therapy. J ECT. 2013;29(3):206–9. https://doi.org/10.1097/YCT.0b013e3182887a1a. PMID: 23965606

31. Carroll BT. The universal field hypothesis of catatonia and neuroleptic malignant syndrome. CNS Spectr. 2000;5(7):26–33. https://doi.org/10.1017/s1092852900013365. PMID: 18197153
32. Solmi M, Pigato GG, Roiter B, Guaglianone A, Martini L, Fornaro M, Monaco F, Carvalho AF, Stubbs B, Veronese N, Correll CU. Prevalence of catatonia and its moderators in clinical samples: results from a meta-analysis and meta-regression analysis. Schizophr Bull. 2018;44(5):1133–50. https://doi.org/10.1093/schbul/sbx157.
33. Tse L, Barr AM, Scarapicchia V, Vila-Rodriguez F. Neuroleptic malignant syndrome: a review from a clinically oriented perspective. Curr Neuropharmacol. 2015;13(3):395–406. https://doi.org/10.2174/1570159x13999150424113345. PMID: 26411967; PMCID: PMC4812801
34. Gurrera RJ, Simpson JC, Tsuang MT. Meta-analytic evidence of systematic bias in estimates of neuroleptic malignant syndrome incidence. Compr Psychiatry. 2007;48(2):205–11. https://doi.org/10.1016/j.comppsych.2006.10.004. Epub 2007 Jan 2. PMID: 17292713
35. Volpi-Abadie J, Kaye AM, Kaye AD. Serotonin syndrome. Ochsner J. 2013;13(4):533–40.
36. Scotton WJ, Hill LJ, Williams AC, Barnes NM. Serotonin syndrome: pathophysiology, clinical features, management, and potential future directions. Int J Tryptophan Res. 2019;12:1178646919873925. https://doi.org/10.1177/1178646919873925.
37. American Psychiatric Association. Diagnostic and statistical manual of mental disorders. 5th ed., text rev. Washington, DC: American Psychiatric Association; 2022.
38. Reddy MSS, Thippeswamy H, Ganjekar S, et al. Anti-NMDA receptor encephalitis presenting as postpartum psychosis-a clinical description and review. Arch Womens Ment Health. 2018;21(4):465–9.
39. Kayser MS, Dalmau J. Anti-NMDA receptor encephalitis in psychiatry. Curr Psychiatr Rev. 2011;7(3):189–93.
40. Dalmau J, Gleichman AJ, Hughes EG, et al. Anti-NMDA-receptor encephalitis: case series and analysis of the effects of antibodies. Lancet Neurol. 2008;7(12):1091–8.
41. Blinder T, Lewerenz J. Cerebrospinal fluid findings in patients with autoimmune encephalitis-a systematic analysis. Front Neurol. 2019; 10(804).
42. Tomaszewski M, Stępień KM, Tomaszewska J, Czuczwar SJ. Statin-induced myopathies. Pharmacol Rep. 2011;63(4):859–66. https://doi.org/10.1016/s1734-1140(11)70601-6. PMID: 22001973
43. Le Quintrec JS, Le Quintrec JL. Drug-induced myopathies. Baillieres Clin Rheumatol. 1991;5(1):21–38. https://doi.org/10.1016/s0950-3579(05)80294-8. PMID: 2070426
44. Scripter C. Headache: tension-type headache. FP Essent. 2018;473:17–20. PMID: 30346680
45. Chowdhury D. Tension type headache. Ann Indian Acad Neurol. 2012;15(Suppl 1):S83–8. https://doi.org/10.4103/0972-2327.100023.
46. Song TJ, Cho SJ, Kim WJ, Yang KI, Yun CH, et al. Anxiety and depression in tension-type headache: a population-based study. PLoS One. 2016;11(10):e0165316. https://doi.org/10.1371/journal.pone.0165316.
47. Lundberg I, de Visser M, Werth V. Classification of myositis. Nat Rev Rheumatol. 2018;14:269–78. https://doi.org/10.1038/nrrheum.2018.41.
48. Stanley M, Chippa V, Aeddula NR, et al. Rhabdomyolysis. [Updated 2021 Jul 10]. In: StatPearls [Internet]. Treasure Island, FL: StatPearls Publishing; 2021. https://www.ncbi.nlm.nih.gov/books/NBK448168/.
49. Zimmerman JL, Shen MC. Rhabdomyolysis. Chest. 2013;144(3):1058–65. https://doi.org/10.1378/chest.12-2016. PMID: 24008958
50. O'Connor AD, Padilla-Jones A, Gerkin RD, Levine M. Prevalence of rhabdomyolysis in sympathomimetic toxicity: a comparison of stimulants. J Med Toxicol. 2015;11(2):195–200. https://doi.org/10.1007/s13181-014-0451-y.
51. Ghai A, Garg N, Hooda S, Gupta T. Spasticity - pathogenesis, prevention and treatment strategies. Saudi J Anaesth. 2013;7(4):453–60. https://doi.org/10.4103/1658-354X.121087.
52. Tysnes OB, Storstein A. Epidemiology of Parkinson's disease. J Neural Transm (Vienna). 2017;124(8):901–5. https://doi.org/10.1007/s00702-017-1686-y. Epub 2017 Feb 1. PMID: 28150045

53. Balestrino R, Schapira AHV. Parkinson disease. Eur J Neurol. 2020;27(1):27–42. https://doi.org/10.1111/ene.14108. Epub 2019 Nov 27. PMID: 31631455
54. Roos RA. Huntington's disease: a clinical review. Orphanet J Rare Dis. 2010;5:40. https://doi.org/10.1186/1750-1172-5-40.
55. McColgan P, Tabrizi SJ. Huntington's disease: a clinical review. Eur J Neurol. 2018;25:24–34. https://doi.org/10.1111/ene.13413. Epub 2017 Sep 22. PMID: 28817209
56. Zarei S, Carr K, Reiley L, Diaz K, Guerra O, Altamirano PF, Pagani W, Lodin D, Orozco G, Chinea A. A comprehensive review of amyotrophic lateral sclerosis. Surg Neurol Int. 2015;6:171. https://doi.org/10.4103/2152-7806.169561.
57. Marin B, Boumédiene F, Logroscino G, et al. Variation in worldwide incidence of amyotrophic lateral sclerosis: a meta-analysis. Int J Epidemiol. 2017;46(1):57–74. https://doi.org/10.1093/ije/dyw061.
58. Bashford JA, Wickham A, Iniesta R, et al. The rise and fall of fasciculations in amyotrophic lateral sclerosis. Brain Commun. 2020;2(1):fcaa018. Published 2020 Feb 20. https://doi.org/10.1093/braincomms/fcaa018.
59. Brotman RG, Moreno-Escobar MC, Joseph J, et al. Amyotrophic lateral sclerosis. [Updated 2021 Jun 8]. In: StatPearls [Internet]. Treasure Island, FL: StatPearls Publishing; 2021. https://www.ncbi.nlm.nih.gov/books/NBK556151/.
60. Cervantes CE, Lee Lau H, Binazir TA, O'Brien KO, Cross JS. Why it is not always anxiety: a tough diagnosis of stiff person syndrome. Case Rep Neurol Med. 2017;2017:7431092. https://doi.org/10.1155/2017/7431092.
61. Hadavi S, Noyce AJ, Leslie RD, Giovannoni G. Stiff person syndrome. Pract Neurol. 2011;11(5):272–82. https://doi.org/10.1136/practneurol-2011-000071. PMID: 21921002
62. Ciccotto G, Blaya M, Kelley RE. Stiff person syndrome. Neurol Clin. 2013;31(1):319–28. https://doi.org/10.1016/j.ncl.2012.09.005. PMID: 23186907

Visual Hallucinations

9

Peter J. Ureste, Matthew Gunther, Jonathan Artz,
and Kara Wang

Definition of Visual Hallucinations

Visual hallucinations are the perceived presence of a visual image, without the actual presence of an external stimulus. They can range from static objects to fully articulated faces and people. In contrast to visual hallucinations, visual *illusions* are distortions of visual stimuli, including color, shape, and size and are precipitated by an actual external stimulus [1].

One of the most succinct and comprehensible definitions of a visual hallucination was provided by Waters et al.: "a visual percept, experienced when awake, which is not elicited by an external stimulus." In defining the symptom this way, visual hallucinations are immediately separated from other perceptual disturbances in terms of time and trigger [2]. Waters' definition of visual hallucinations draws clarity between hallucinations experienced when awake versus those that occur at the onset or cessation of sleep. *Hypnagogic* and *hypnopompic* hallucinations are two examples of this, where auditory or visual perceptions are experienced just prior to falling asleep or just upon awakening, respectively. This distinction is

P. J. Ureste (✉)
Department of Psychiatry and Behavioral Sciences, University of California, San Francisco, San Francisco, CA, USA
e-mail: Peter.Ureste@ucsf.edu

M. Gunther
Department of Psychiatry and Behavioral Sciences, Stanford University, Stanford, CA, USA

J. Artz
Department of Psychiatry, Baylor Scott & White Health, Temple, TX, USA
e-mail: Jonathan.Artz@bswhealth.org

K. Wang
Department of Psychiatry, San Mateo County Behavioral Health and Recovery Services, San Mateo, CA, USA
e-mail: kwang@smcgov.org

E. G. Meyer et al. (eds.), *The Medical Evaluation of Psychiatric Symptoms*,
https://doi.org/10.1007/978-3-031-14372-4_9

important because visual hallucinations occurring while falling asleep or waking up are considered to be within the range of normal experience.

Historical Definitions of Visual Hallucinations

Visual hallucinations were once commonly thought to be visions and apparitions due to a divine revelation [3]. In two groundbreaking papers by neurologist Georges de Morsier and psychiatrists Julian de Ajuriaguerra and Jean L'Hermitte published in 1936 and 1938, respectively; they established that visual hallucinations were a separate entity from other types of hallucinations [4]. Given these physicians' different backgrounds, these papers focused on different etiologies of visual hallucinations. de Ajuriaguerra and L'Hermitte looked at visual hallucinations within the scope of a general hallucinatory state and its psychological implications [4]. de Morsier on the other hand looked at the neurological correlation and named specific pathways as causes for visual hallucinations, while also giving eponyms to these syndromes [4]. For example, the Charles Bonnet syndrome was hypothesized to be caused by the degeneration of pulvino-cortical pathways. He also named the Zingerle syndrome, symptoms of which included visual hallucinations, forced movements, and vestibular disturbances. It was hypothesized that visual hallucinations were caused by damage to the vestibular, motor, and pulvino-cortical pathways [4].

The 1930s were also when visual hallucinations were classified into simple and complex. Simple hallucinations were thought to be caused by lesions in the visual sensory cortex, whereas complex hallucinations were thought to arise from lesions in the visual association cortex. However, it was soon discovered that these locations were not solely responsible for each type of hallucination. The definitions of simple and complex hallucinations have evolved over time, leading to our current definitions, with simple hallucinations to mean colors, lines, and shapes and complex hallucinations to mean fully formed objects, animals, people, or events [5].

Clinical Evaluation of Visual Hallucinations

When a clinician first learns of a patient with visual hallucinations, both the literature and medical training focus first on the more common underlying structural pathology. Two categories stand out in this regard: neurodegenerative diseases and ophthalmologic diseases. When looking at populations with neurodegenerative disorders, between 60% and 90% of those with Lewy body dementia (LBD) report visual hallucinations with lower, but still appreciable, rates observed in those with Parkinson's disease (PD) and Parkinson's disease dementia, 15–40% and 30–90%, respectively [6]. In terms of ophthalmologic disease, up to 10% of people with diagnoses such as macular degeneration can experience visual hallucinations [7]. A psychiatrist or other mental health clinician should always consider these etiologies when coming up with a differential diagnosis, especially if a visual disturbance is the primary focus or complaint of the patient.

Psychiatric research on visual hallucinations is limited. This is likely due to how psychiatrists and other mental health clinicians categorize and view hallucinations as a symptom class. In the Diagnostic and Statistical Manual of Mental Disorders, Fifth Edition (DSM-5-TR), a set of heterogeneous symptoms make up a particular diagnosis. At times, symptoms can overlap among diagnoses, such as delusions, which can be found in bipolar I disorder and schizophrenia. This makes conducting research on particular symptom aspects of a diagnosis difficult. The National Institute of Mental Health's Research Domain Criteria (RDoC) aims to alleviate this problem by focusing instead on behavior and function in psychiatric illness through identifying domains and, subsequently, constructs to help better link symptoms with neurobiological measures [8]. For example, with visual hallucinations, the cognitive domain is an area of focus given its inclusion in the memory construct. Hallucinations in those with schizophrenia are often reported to have qualities from specific memories of the patient—for example, a family member's voice or appearance.

While visual hallucinations can also be farther away from reality in a fantastic way, understanding how the content of the symptom is shaped by a person's recollections can be helpful. The negative valence domain is another area of interest given the often-persecutory nature of hallucinations in patients with psychotic disorders. By breaking down a patient's symptoms into these "units of analysis," research is better able to focus on which area of the CNS is disrupted and with that information, better develop effective treatments [8]. This is still an area of development in the psychiatric literature. However, the available research highlights well how we can conceptualize a patient's individual experience when they present with perceptual disturbance.

In psychiatric disorders, hallucinations, in general, are one of the predominant symptoms mentioned in some of the psychotic, depressive, and bipolar spectrum illnesses. In the literature and psychiatric training programs, however, more attention is paid to auditory hallucinations as a classic symptom of a psychotic disorder. This is likely due to the higher prevalence of visual hallucinations in nonpsychiatric pathology, in addition to the symptom itself being less common in major psychiatric illnesses. In individuals with psychosis, McCarthy-Jones et al. found that the lifetime prevalence of visual hallucinations was between 23% and 30%, while the range for auditory hallucinations was 64–80% [9]. Interestingly, visual hallucinations should not be viewed as a discrete entity. When visual hallucinations are present in a patient with psychosis, 84% of the time the symptom is accompanied by a co-occurring auditory hallucination [10]. This introduces the concept that hallucinations should be treated as involving multiple modalities, rather than a perception involving a single sense.

When evaluating a patient with a perceptual disturbance, it is key to obtain as much descriptive data as possible as well as to distinguish what modality (or combination) is typically involved. Visual hallucinations can vary widely in their presentation to the patient. For example, in those with ophthalmologic disease, unformed perceptions, such as floaters, flashes, or lines, tend to be more common [11]. Migraines are similar in that the perception is typically unformed but can involve a perceived flickering of light or color called a scintillating scotoma. In psychiatric disorders however the hallucinations are typically formed and complex [11]. As opposed to flashes of color across one's visual field, patients can experience seeing a family member talking to them, animals in their room, or catch glimpses of faces in inanimate objects. The hallucination can be of a stationary being or can be more involved, with the individual observing a scene unfolding before them, such as an angelic being interacting with the patient. While specific details of visual hallucinations in the literature are sparse, the disturbance is said to be realistic enough that the patient frequently attempts to interact with it in some way such as through conversation or direct physical interaction.

There is also a key differentiation between levels of distress induced by visual hallucination when looking at etiologies. In those with visual hallucinations due to neurodegenerative disease, patients are typically unbothered by the perceptual disturbance and perhaps may even find it comforting [2]. However, in patients with schizophrenia, the visual disturbance can be distressing and anxiety-producing. In particular, if the content of the hallucination has a negative emotional valence (such as involving death, persecutory religious themes, or threatening images), patients can be frightened to the point of acting on the hallucination with the intent to stop or reduce the symptom. Therefore, obtaining this history is critical to differentiate between etiologies of these symptoms, both for patient safety and targeted treatment.

Literature on the different characteristics of visual hallucination across psychiatric disorders is scarce. As mentioned above, in schizophrenia spectrum and other psychotic disorders, patients often experience persecutory, threatening, or frightening hallucinations involving multiple modalities. In individuals with symptoms of depressive disorder triggered by grief, patients can hallucinate that their deceased loved one is in the room with them. Negative emotions in depressive disorders often precede these perceptual disturbances and it is thought that multiple sensory disturbances are less likely in depressive disorders than in psychotic disorders [2]. In bipolar spectrum disorders, little is written on the content variation of visual hallucinations as compared to psychotic disorders. However, if hallucinations do occur during a manic or depressive phase, a patient's hospitalization typically lasts longer, and the disorder is viewed as more severe [2]. More research is required to better distinguish characteristics of visual hallucinations between psychiatric disorders, as most data includes distinctions between psychotic and neurologic disorders, as well as other etiologies such as substance withdrawal and advanced ophthalmologic disease.

Psychiatric Differential for Visual Hallucinations

Schizophrenia Spectrum and Other Psychotic Disorders

Schizophrenia spectrum and other psychotic disorders include schizophrenia, schizoaffective disorder, brief psychotic disorder, schizophreniform, and schizotypal personality disorder, which are all primary psychotic disorders.

Incidence/Prevalence

The lifetime prevalence of schizophrenia is between 0.3% and 0.7%, although reports have varied between race and ethnicity, for immigrants, children of immigrants, and across countries [12]. The prevalence of schizoaffective disorder is estimated to be about one-third as common as schizophrenia. Brief psychotic disorder may account for 9% of first-onset psychosis [12]. In the US and other developed countries, the incidence of schizophreniform disorder is low, possibly fivefold less than that of schizophrenia. The prevalence of schizotypal personality disorder is 1.9% in clinical settings and 4.6% in a US community sample [12]. Epidemiologic studies show a prevalence of visual hallucinations 16–72% and 25% in patients with schizophrenia and schizoaffective disorder, respectively [10, 12, 13].

Typical Findings of the HPI

Psychotic symptoms include hallucinations, delusions, disorganized thinking or speech, grossly disorganized or abnormal motor behavior, and negative symptoms. For a diagnosis of schizophrenia, the patient must have two or more psychotic symptoms, at least one being from the first three symptoms, present for a significant portion of 1 month, and cause at least a 6-month disturbance in occupational or social functioning. For a diagnosis of schizoaffective disorder, the patient meets criteria for schizophrenia, but also has an uninterpreted period of illness with a major depressive or manic episode; however, the mood symptoms must be absent for at least 2 weeks while hallucinations or delusions remain present. In brief psychotic disorder, there is the presence of at least one psychotic symptom for at least 1 day but less than 1 month, whereas in schizophreniform there are at least two symptoms for at least 1 month but less than 6.

Unusual perceptual experiences can also be present in schizotypal personality disorder. Other symptoms present in this condition include ideas of reference, odd beliefs, or magical thinking inconsistent with subcultural norms, odd thinking and speech, suspiciousness or paranoid ideations, inappropriate or reduced affect, eccentric behavior, lack of close friends, or excessive social anxiety associated with paranoid fears. For a diagnosis of schizotypal personality disorder, a patient must have five or more of these symptoms.

PPV information related to visual hallucinations and schizophrenia spectrum and other psychotic disorders was not found in a review of relevant literature.

Typical Findings on Physical Exam and Mental Status Exam

The patient may appear to be responding to unseen stimuli, such as looking at and talking to unseen others. They may also have fixed false beliefs that could be grandiose, persecutory, erotomanic, somatic, or bizarre in nature, which may affect behavior. For example, they may appear frightened while believing ghosts are out to harm them. Their speech or thinking may be disorganized. The patient may behave in a disorganized manner or appear catatonic. Lastly, they may have negative symptoms consisting of diminished emotional expression and a decrease in self-motivated initiated purposeful activities (avolition), pleasure (anhedonia), speech production (alogia), and social interactions (asociality).

Typical Laboratory/Radiological Findings

Substance-induced psychotic disorders should be ruled out with a urine toxicology test. A psychotic disorder due to another medical condition can be ruled out with CMP (electrolyte disturbances, hepatic encephalopathy), CBC (infectious causes), TSH (hyperthyroidism), RPR (neurosyphilis), and HIV. Neuroimaging may show an underlying structural abnormality.

Bipolar and Related Disorders

The hallmark of bipolar disorders is a fluctuation between mania or hypomania and major depression. Bipolar I disorder fluctuates between manic and major depressive episodes, whereas bipolar II disorder moves between hypomania and major depression. Visual hallucinations and other psychotic symptoms have been reported in cases of bipolar I disorder. Psychosis can occur during major depressive episodes in bipolar I or II disorder. Since hypomania is not severe enough to cause significant impairment in social or occupational functioning, psychosis cannot occur in hypomanic states [12]. If psychotic features are present, then the episode is considered manic. However, visual hallucinations can occur in patients with bipolar disorder including type II during major depressive episodes.

Incidence/Prevalence

The estimated prevalence is 0.6% for bipolar I disorder and 0.8% for bipolar II disorder in the US [12]. In a study with 990 patients diagnosed with bipolar I disorder, visual hallucinations were reported in 28.6% of the sample [14]. Among those with psychotic features (92.5% of the sample), hallucinations occurred in 58% of patients, of which 39% reported visual hallucinations [14]. In another study of patients with bipolar disorder, visual hallucinations occurred predominately during a manic episode, whereas auditory hallucinations most often occurred when patients were in a depressive episode [15]. It is important to note that this study included a small sample of only 40 subjects.

Typical Findings of the HPI

For a diagnosis of bipolar I disorder, the patient must meet the following criteria for a manic episode: elevated, expansive, or irritable mood with increased energy lasting 1 week, present every day for most of the day. In addition to the mood and increased energy, the patient must also have four of the following symptoms: inflated sense of self, decreased need for sleep, talkative than usual or pressured speech, flight of ideas or racing thoughts, distractibility, increase in goal-directed activity, or involvement in high-risk activities.

For a diagnosis of bipolar II disorder, the patient must meet the following criteria for a hypomanic episode: elevated, expansive, or irritable mood with increased energy lasting at least 4 consecutive days, present every day for most of the day. They must also have three or more of the symptoms noted above, four if one of them is irritability.

If a patient with bipolar disorder is in a major depressive episode, they will meet the criteria for major depression, as described below.

PPV information related to visual hallucinations and bipolar disorders was not found in a review of relevant literature.

Typical Findings on Physical Exam and Mental Status Exam

During the interview, the patient may appear irritable or euphoric, with mood lability. Their speech may be pressured and loud. They may be extremely talkative, to the point that it is difficult to ask questions. If questions can be asked, the patient may respond with answers loosely related or unconnected. They may also be easily distracted by external stimuli such as often looking around the room due to loud ambient noise. The patient may exhibit impulsivity in their behavior, such as abruptly leaving the interview without notice or psychomotor agitation. If they are in a major depressive episode, the typical findings on examination will be similar to major depression as described below.

Typical Laboratory/Radiological Findings

Substance induced bipolar disorder should be ruled out with a urine toxicology test. Rule out bipolar disorder due to another medical condition with CBC (infectious causes), TSH (hyperthyroidism), RPR (neurosyphilis), and HIV. MRI Brain or CT scan of the head may show an underlying structural abnormality.

Major Depressive Disorder

Incidence/Prevalence

The prevalence of major depressive disorder in the US is 7% [12].

Typical Findings of the HPI

Patients with major depressive disorder will report five or more of the following symptoms, one of which must be either depressed mood or anhedonia, occurring for at least 2 weeks or more: depressed mood most of the day and nearly every day; loss of interest or pleasure; changes in appetite, either reduced or increased intake; changes in sleep, either insomnia or hypersomnia; loss of energy; feelings of worthlessness or excessive guilt; difficulties in concentration; psychomotor agitation or slowing; or suicidal thoughts, intent, or plan. In addition, these symptoms result in functional impairment.

PPV information related to visual hallucinations and major depressive disorder was not found in a review of relevant literature.

Typical Findings on Physical Exam and Mental Status Exam

The patient with major depressive disorder may appear sad or tearful. Their movement or speech may be slowed. They may also appear agitated, perhaps yelling. In severe cases, their cognition may be poor due to difficulties with concentration. Their thought content contains suicidal ideas, intent, or a plan.

Typical Laboratory/Radiological Findings

Rule out substance-induced depressive disorder with toxicology and a blood alcohol level. Rule out depressive disorder due to another medical condition with CMP (electrolyte disturbance or hypoglycemia) or TSH (hypothyroidism). Neuroimaging may show an underlying structural abnormality, such as a tumor.

Posttraumatic Stress Disorder

Incidence/Prevalence

The estimated prevalence of posttraumatic stress disorder (PTSD) is 3.5% among US adults [12].

Typical Findings of the HPI

For a diagnosis of PTSD, the patient must have exposure to serious injury, sexual violence, or actual or threatened death. As a result of the trauma, there is a disturbance in function for more than 1 month characterized by intrusive symptoms such as reexperiencing in the form of nightmares or flashbacks, persistent avoidance of stimuli associated with the trauma, hyperreactivity, and negative alterations in cognition or mood. Flashbacks can resemble visual hallucinations and other perceptual disturbances. The PPV of visual hallucinations-like flashbacks in PTSD was not found in a review of relevant literature.

Typical Findings on Physical Exam and Mental Status Exam

The patient may be hypervigilant or easily startled. They may avoid discussing memories, thoughts, or feelings about their traumatic event or events. The patient may also have dissociative reactions such as a flashback in which the patient feels as if the trauma is recurring.

Typical Laboratory/Radiological Findings

Check a urine drug screen or alcohol blood level, as substance intoxication or withdrawal can present with symptoms like PTSD.

Substance-Related Disorders

Incidence/Prevalence

The prevalence of a substance-induced psychotic disorder in the general population is unknown. However, it has been reported that between 7% and 25% of patients with first episode psychosis have substance-induced psychotic disorder [12]. Development of psychosis may vary depending on the substance, amount used, duration, and may occur during intoxication or withdrawal. Hallucinogens such as mescaline, psilocybin, and lysergic acid diethylamide (LSD), and dissociative drugs such as phencyclidine and ketamine have been associated with psychosis [13]. Other drugs such as stimulants and cannabis have been reported to induce visual hallucinations in 40% and 20% of users, respectively [16, 17]. Opioid-induced visual hallucinations are rare but have been reported in case reports [18]. Visual hallucinations have also been observed in 2% of alcohol drinkers withdrawing from alcohol intoxication [19]. The prevalence of visual hallucinations due to prescription medication is unknown. However, numerous case reports have indicated baclofen, benzodiazepines, corticosteroids, and dopamine agonists, among others, to be associated with visual hallucinations.

Typical Findings of the HPI

Visual hallucinations developed during intoxication or during withdrawal from a substance, but not prior. They may also have other types of hallucinations or delusions with the same temporal pattern. If due to prescription medication, the patient may have a recent change in their medication regimen. PPV information related to visual hallucinations and substance-related disorders was not found upon a review of relevant literature.

Typical Findings on Physical Exam and Mental Status Exam

Examination findings vary depending on the type of substance involved and whether the patient has acute intoxication or withdrawal. For example, a patient with stimulant intoxication may have diaphoresis, hypertension, tachycardia, and severe agitation. They may also have skin excoriations or "track marks" over a vein if the drug was used intravenously. A patient withdrawing from alcohol or benzodiazepines may be tremulous with diaphoresis and autonomic instability. There may also be hallucinosis (if the last alcoholic drink was 12–24 h previously), generalized tonic-clonic seizures (12–48 h after last alcohol), or delirium tremens (48–96 h after last alcohol).

Typical Laboratory/Radiological Findings

A urine drug screen can be used to determine the presence of illicit drugs. A blood alcohol level can be obtained to determine the presence of ethanol. It is important to note that withdrawal can still occur when the blood alcohol level is still elevated.

Delirium

Delirium is a syndrome of acute onset of disturbance in awareness and attention and is the direct consequence of another medical condition or a substance. This disturbance must not be better explained by worsening neurodegeneration or occur in the context of severely reduced arousal state such as during a coma.

Incidence/Prevalence

The prevalence of delirium ranges from 14% to 24% among hospitalized individuals. Older hospitalized patients are at greater risk than their younger counterparts, occurring in rates as high as 53% postoperatively and 87% of those in intensive care. Psychotic symptoms occur in 43% of delirium cases, of which 27% had visual hallucinations [20].

Typical Findings of the HPI

The individual has an acute onset of fluctuations in their attention or awareness. History may suggest that this abrupt disturbance is a direct physiological consequence of another medical condition or multiple etiologies. For example, a new medication may have recently been introduced to the patient's regimen. Or the patient was recently diagnosed with a urinary tract infection and has poor adherence with their antibiotic therapy.

On review of relevant literature, the PPV of visual hallucinations in delirium was not found.

Typical Findings on Physical Exam and Mental Status Exam

Fluctuation in consciousness or inattention is observed. Motor activity may be hyperactive, such as the patient attempting to pull out their intravenous lines and/or climb out of their hospital bed. Or they may be hypoactive, such as staring in space with minimal to no motoric response. Patients could also present with a mixture of motoric activity.

Typical Laboratory/Radiological Findings

Typical EEG findings in delirium include theta-delta slowing. To evaluate the underlying cause of delirium, laboratory tests include urine drug screen (drug intoxication) and alcohol blood level (withdrawal). Check CMP (electrolyte disturbances, hepatic encephalopathy), CBC (infectious causes), TSH, RPR, and HIV. Infectious etiologies can be evaluated with a urine analysis (urinary tract infection), blood culture (bacteremia), and chest X-ray (pneumonia). If this infectious work-up is unrevealing and the patient has signs of infection and an abnormal neurological examination, then a lumbar puncture may be considered. Neuroimaging may show an underlying structural abnormality.

Major Neurocognitive Disorders

Incidence/Prevalence

Tauopathies and alpha-synucleinopathies are two major groups of neurodegenerative diseases characterized by aggregation of abnormal protein in the brain. Two examples of tauopathies are Alzheimer's disease (AD) and frontotemporal dementia (FTD). The reported prevalence of AD is 11.3% in people 65 years and older. Visual hallucinations are the most common hallucination associated with AD and have been reported in 21–49% of clinic populations [21]. FTD is a common cause of early onset (midlife) major neurocognitive disorder and is estimated to occur at similar rates to AD in patients younger than 65 years old. Visual hallucinations may occur in less than 10% of FTD cases [21]. In alpha-synucleinopathies, two examples are LBD and Parkinson's disease (PD) dementia. Visual hallucinations have been reported in 60–80% of LBD cases and between 25% and 50% of PD cases [22].

Typical Findings of the HPI

Visual hallucinations in AD and FTD are not detailed as found in LBD or PD. The patient may have cooccurring delusions. In AD, these delusions are often paranoid, simple, and non-bizarre [21]. A patient with AD may also have progressive impairment in memory, diminished executive function, semantic fluency, increased wandering, falls, aggressive behavior, or difficulties with basic or instrumental activities of daily living. A patient with FTD may also have progressive changes in behavior and personality, hyperorality, and impulsivity, possibly resulting in violations of the law. Visuospatial, psychomotor, and memory are generally preserved. In AD and FTD, family history may be significant for the same condition.

LBD and PD both typically have detailed hallucinations of people or animals. They are typically a presenting symptom in LBD and occur an average of 12 years after presentation of motor symptoms in PD [23]. The presence of visual hallucinations at initial presentation is one of the strongest clinical indicators of LBD, with a reported PPV of 83% when differentiating from AD early in the disease course [13, 24]. In both, LBD and PD, patients will also have symptoms of parkinsonism consisting of muscle rigidity, tremor, or bradykinesia. Symptoms of Parkinsonism are often mild enough in earlier stages of LBD that their presence is not a reliable way to differentiate from AD, with a reported PPV of only 26% [24]. Additionally, patients with LBD may have cognitive fluctuations and rapid eye movement sleep behavior disorder, which are not core features in PD. The PPV of these features in distinguishing LBD from PD is currently unclear, although there have been attempts to gather such information using structured assessments and questionnaires.

Typical Findings on Physical Exam and Mental Status Exam

Patients with AD typically have no motor or sensory deficits early in the course of illness. Mental status exam may show apathy or poor orientation due to progressive memory decline. Cognitive screening tools or neuropsychological testing may show mild deficits in memory, visuospatial, language, and attention early in the course, and more severe as the disease progresses. In FTD, there may be no focal findings on physical examination early in the disease course. Mental status exam may show disinhibition, impaired judgment, and insight in an individual with FTD. Cognitive screening or neuropsychological testing in patients with FTD may show pronounced executive impairment, cognitive inflexibility, and perseveration, while memory is less impaired early in the course.

In alpha-synucleinopathies, a motor exam may find impaired amplitude or frequency in finger tapping or other rapid motor movements (i.e., bradykinesia), muscular rigidity with passive flexion of joints, impaired gait, retropulsion, and postural tremor. Mental status exam may show reduced facial expression or "masked faces" and decreased volume of speech or other disruptions. Impaired memory, attention, or other aspects of cognition may be found as well. Orthostatic vitals may be positive due to autonomic dysfunction.

Typical Laboratory/Radiological Findings

Laboratory assessment for major neurocognitive disorder includes CBC, CMP, TSH, B12, HIV, and syphilis test. Neuroimaging such as MRI or CT may be used to support clinical diagnosis. In AD, imaging may show reduced hippocampal volume or medial temporal lobe atrophy. Amyloid PET imaging may be helpful in differentiating AD from other causes of major neurocognitive disorders. In FTD, neuroimaging shows frontal or temporal lobe atrophy. Functional imaging for FTD may reveal hypometabolism or hypoperfusion in these brain regions. If there is a strong family history of FTD then genetic testing for microtubule-associated protein tau, progranulin, and C9orf72 may be useful in confirming the diagnosis. In PD dementia, the Movement Disorder Society-Sponsored Revision of the Unified Parkinson's Disease Rating Scale may also be used [25].

General Medical Differential for Visual Hallucination

Migraine Headaches

Incidence/Prevalence

Upto 31% of migraines are associated with an aura, with 99% of those being visual [13].

Typical Findings of the HPI

Visual hallucinations in migraine headaches are rarely complex hallucinations and are classically described as monochromatic jagged lines or flashing lights beginning in the central portion of the field of vision and progressing to the periphery. Hallucinations may be perceived as occurring in one eye as the visual phenomenon frequently occurs within a hemifield of vision. Visual symptoms typically develop gradually over at least 5 min, resolve within an hour, and proceed or are accompanied by a unilateral, throbbing, or pulsatile headache [26]. PPV information related to these findings was not found upon a review of relevant literature.

Typical Findings on Physical Exam

Typically, there will be no associated abnormal neurological or physical exam findings. Migraine subtypes with associated findings, such as hemiplegic migraines, are extremely rare in their incidence. They also present with symptoms consistent with the International Classification of Headache Disorders criteria [23].

Typical Laboratory/Radiological Findings

Neuroimaging is not necessary unless the headache is severe and sudden.

Seizure Disorders

Incidence/Prevalence

Visual hallucinations occur in 60% of occipital lobe seizures and 16–18% of temporal lobe seizures [13].

Typical Findings of the HPI

Visual hallucinations are typically simple, described as flashing shapes or colors which may change in characterization, and are generally brief in duration. They occur in both eyes with hallucinations localized within one visual field suggesting a contralateral seizure focus. Generally associated with stereotyped movements with blinking and eye deviation being most common in occipital seizures and a broader range of focal motor activity occurring in temporal lobe seizures [13]. PPV information related to these findings was not found upon a review of relevant literature.

Typical Findings on Physical Exam and Mental Status Exam

Although there are no commonly associated findings on exam, the presence of lateraling neurological deficits can be indicative of a contralateral brain lesion. Although oral lacerations are also associated with syncope, biting of the lateral aspect of the tongue is highly specific for seizure disorders.

Typical Laboratory/Radiological Findings

Neuroimaging may show an underlying structural abnormality. An electroencephalogram (EEG) is essential in the evaluation of seizures, although a normal EEG does not definitively rule them out. Interictal EEG has a variable rate of findings, between 25% and 50%, depending on the type of seizure.

Cerebrovascular Accident

Incidence/Prevalence

Psychosis occurs in 1–2% of stroke cases [27]. Patients have developed visual hallucinations after a cerebrovascular accident (CVA) anywhere between the retina and occipital cortex, as well as in the midbrain [1, 28]. The incidence or prevalence of visual hallucinations post-stroke is unknown.

Typical Findings of the HPI

Patients with a CVA between their retina and occipital cortex may report seeing abnormal brightness or flashing lights [28]. Midbrain CVAs may present with vivid, well-formed, colorful hallucinations of people, animals, and complex scenes [1]. The visual hallucinations may last minutes to hours, are less prominent during the day and more vivid in the evening, and frequently occur during sedation [1]. Patients often have insight into their hallucinations and may find it amusing or interesting [28]. On review of relevant literature, the PPV of visual hallucinations in CVAs was not found.

Typical Findings on Physical Exam and Mental Status Exam

Physical examination may show focal neurologic deficits that are unilateral. Eye movements or visual fields may be abnormal.

Typical Laboratory/Radiological Findings

Neuroimaging may show an infarct in the occipital lobe or brainstem.

Rare medical conditions with cooccurring visual hallucinations are listed in Table 9.1.

Table 9.1 Rare medical conditions with visual hallucinations

Disorder	Distinctive features	VH Description
Anton's syndrome	• Combination of anosognosia and confabulation • Patients with cortical blindness deny that they have visual loss	• Prevalence unknown, but 3 out of 50 patients with cortical blindness denied having blindness
Autoimmune encephalitis	• Subacute onset, systemic markers of autoimmune processes, history of concurrent malignancy • CSF studies generally show elevated WBC, protein, IgG index, and oligoclonal bands • Can be targeted towards intracellular antigens (Amphiphysin, CASPR2, or CRMP-5) or Surface Antigens (AMPAR, NMDAR)	• Unknown
Creutzfeldt-Jakob disease	• Fatal progressive neurodegenerative prion disease • More advanced Creutzfeldt-Jakob disease presents with ataxia and myoclonus • Heidenhain variant has non-generalizing complexes over the occipital	• Associated with the Heidenhain illness variant due to the occipitoparietal distribution of pathology • VH includes color changes, visual field defects, visual agnosia, cortical blindness, and metamorphosia
Narcolepsy	• Occur in 30% of narcolepsy patients • Hallucinations occur while entering sleep (hypnagogic) or awakening (hypnopompic)	• Characterized as colorful images and may include people, animals, and panoramic scenes • VH last several minutes
Neurosyphilis	• 10–15% of primary syphilis cases progress to tertiary syphilis, and of these cases, less than 20% present with psychosis	• Unknown
Occipital lobe tumor/mass	• Space occupying lesion found in the occipital lobe of the brain	• Characterized as spots of light or shapes similar to occipital seizures
Retinal pathologies	• Retinal detachment or various retinopathy	• Unknown
Reversible posterior leukoencephalopathy syndrome	• A neurological disorder characterized by subacute or acute presentation of neurological symptoms such as headache, altered consciousness, and visual deficits • Typically presents with significantly elevated blood pressure and findings of vasogenic edema on MRI in parieto-occipital distribution	• VH reported in up to 67% of cases

(continued)

Table 9.1 (continued)

Disorder	Distinctive features	VH Description
Temporal lobe tumor/mass	• Unlike occipital masses, tumors compressing the optic tract produce more complex hallucinations	• In one case study, prevalence of 22% among 59 individuals with temporal lobe tumors • Many of these hallucinations may be secondary to seizure activity secondary to the tumor
Visual release hallucinations (Charles Bonnet Syndrome)	• VH in the visually impaired	• VH is described as clear, detailed, and often involves people, faces, animals, and inanimate objects • Hallmark of the disorder is development of insight into hallucinations

AMPAR α-amino-3-hydroxy-5-methyl-4-isoxazolepropionic acid receptor, *CASPR2* contactin-associated protein-like 2, *CRMP-5* collapsin response-mediator protein-5, *CSF* cerebral spinal fluid, *IgG* immunoglobulin G, *MRI* magnetic resonance imaging, *NMDAR* *N*-methyl-D-aspartate receptor, *VH* visual hallucinations, *WBC* white blood count
Source: [1, 5, 13, 29–31]

Conclusion

Visual hallucination is a perceptual disturbance that occurs in the absence of an actual external stimulus. It has a broad differential diagnosis that includes psychiatric and medical etiologies. It is important for the clinician to identify the underlying cause because the treatments are different. This chapter attempted to help the clinician better understand visual hallucinations and assist in its evaluation and assessment. It is essential to keep in mind the psychiatric and medical differential diagnoses for visual hallucinations. We attempted to outline common disorders and briefly list rare conditions that present with visual hallucinations.

References

1. Norton JW, Corbett JJ. Visual perceptual abnormalities: hallucinations and illusions. Semin Neurol. 2000;20(1):111–21.
2. Waters F, Collerton D, Ffytche DH, Jardri R, Pins D, Dudley R, et al. Visual hallucinations in the psychosis spectrum and comparative information from neurodegenerative disorders and eye disease. Schizophr Bull. 2014;40(Suppl 4):S233–45. https://doi.org/10.1093/schbul/sbu036.
3. Berrios GE, Markova IS. Visual hallucinations: history and context of current research. In: Collerton D, Mosimann UP, Perry E, editors. The neuroscience of visual hallucinations. Oxford: Wiley Blackwell; 2015. p. 5.
4. Ffytche DH. Visual hallucinatory syndromes: past, present, and future. Dialogues Clin Neurosci. 2007;9(2):173–89. https://doi.org/10.31887/DCNS.2007.9.2/dffytche.

5. O'Brien J, Taylor JP, Ballard C, Barker RA, Bradley C, Burns A, et al. Visual hallucinations in neurological and ophthalmological disease: pathophysiology and management. J Neurol Neurosurg Psychiatry. 2020;91(5):512–9. https://doi.org/10.1136/jnnp-2019-322702.
6. Waters F, Fernyhough C. Hallucinations: a systematic review of points of similarity and difference across diagnostic classes. Schizophr Bull. 2017;43(1):32–43. https://doi.org/10.1093/schbul/sbw132.
7. Carter R, Ffytche DH. On visual hallucinations and cortical networks: a transdiagnostic review. J Neurol. 2015;262(7):1780–90. https://doi.org/10.1007/s00415-015-7687-6.
8. Ford JM, Morris SE, Hoffman RE, Sommer I, Waters F, Mccarthy-Jones S, et al. Schizophr Bull. 2014. https://doi.org/10.1093/schbul/sbu011.
9. McCarthy-Jones S, Smailes D, Corvin A, Gill M, Morris DW, Dinan TG, et al. Occurrence and co-occurrence of hallucinations by modality in schizophrenia-spectrum disorders. Psychiatry Res. 2017;252:154–60. https://doi.org/10.1016/j.psychres.2017.01.102.
10. Mueser KT, Bellack AS, Brady EU. Hallucinations in schizophrenia. Acta Psychiatr Scand. 1990;82(1):26–9. https://doi.org/10.1111/j.1600-0447.1990.tb01350.x. PMID: 2399817
11. Hamedani AG, Pelak VS. Correction to: The Charles Bonnet syndrome: a systematic review of diagnostic criteria. Curr Treat Options Neurol. 2019;21(10). https://doi.org/10.1007/s11940-019-0594-x.
12. American Psychiatric Association. Diagnostic and statistical manual of mental disorders. 5th ed., text rev. Washington, DC: American Psychiatric Association; 2022.
13. Teeple RC, Caplan JP, Stern TA. Visual hallucinations: differential diagnosis and treatment. Prim Care Companion J Clin Psychiatry. 2009;11(1):26–32. https://doi.org/10.4088/pcc.08r00673.
14. van Bergen AH, Verkooijen S, Vreeker A, Abramovic L, Hillegers MH, Spijker AT, Hoencamp E, Regeer EJ, Knapen SE, Riemersma-van der Lek RF, Schoevers R, Stevens AW, Schulte PFJ, Vonk R, Hoekstra R, van Beveren NJ, Kupka RW, Sommer IEC, Ophoff RA, Kahn RS, Boks MPM. The characteristics of psychotic features in bipolar disorder. Psychol Med. 2019;49(12):2036–48. https://doi.org/10.1017/S0033291718002854.
15. Hammersley P, Taylor K, McGovern J, Kinderman P. Attributions for hallucinations in bipolar affective disorder. Behav Cogn Psychother. 2010;38(2):221–6. https://doi.org/10.1017/S1352465809990592. Epub 2010 Jan 5. PMID: 20047708
16. Glasner-Edwards S, Mooney LJ. Methamphetamine psychosis: epidemiology and management. CNS Drugs. 2014;28(12):1115–26. https://doi.org/10.1007/s40263-014-0209-8.
17. Pearson NT, Berry JH. Cannabis and psychosis through the lens of DSM-5. Int J Environ Res Public Health. 2019;16(21):4149. https://doi.org/10.3390/ijerph16214149.
18. Sivanesan E, Gitlin MC, Candiotti KA. Opioid-induced hallucinations: a review of the literature, pathophysiology, diagnosis, and treatment. Anesth Analg. 2016;123(4):836–43. https://doi.org/10.1213/ANE.0000000000001417.
19. Stephane M, Arnaout B, Yoon G. Alcohol withdrawal hallucinations in the general population, an epidemiological study. Psychiatry Res. 2018;262:129–34. https://doi.org/10.1016/j.psychres.2018.02.021.
20. Webster R, Holroyd S. Prevalence of psychotic symptoms in delirium. Psychosomatics. 2000;41(6):519–22. https://linkinghub.elsevier.com/retrieve/pii/S0033318200705706
21. Burghaus L, Eggers C, Timmermann L, Fink GR, Diederich NJ. Hallucinations in neurodegenerative diseases. CNS Neurosci Ther. 2012;18(2):149–59. https://doi.org/10.1111/j.1755-5949.
22. Bertram K, Williams DR. Visual hallucinations in the differential diagnosis of parkinsonism. J Neurol Neurosurg Psychiatry. 2012;83(4):448–52.
23. Headache Classification Committee of the International Headache Society (IHS). The international classification of headache disorders, 3rd edition. Cephalalgia. 2018;38(1):1–211. http://journals.sagepub.com/doi/10.1177/0333102417738202
24. Tiraboschi P, Salmon DP, Hansen LA, Hofstetter RC, Thal LJ, Corey-Bloom J. What best differentiates Lewy body from Alzheimer's disease in early-stage dementia? Brain. 2006;129(Pt 3):729–35. https://doi.org/10.1093/brain/awh725.

25. Goetz CG, Tilley BC, Shaftman SR, Stebbins GT, Fahn S, Martinez-Martin P, et al. Movement Disorder Society-sponsored revision of the Unified Parkinson's Disease Rating Scale (MDS-UPDRS): scale presentation and clinimetric testing results. Mov Disord. 2008;23(15):2129–70. https://doi.org/10.1002/mds.22340.
26. Liu GT, Volpe NJ, Galetta SL. Visual hallucinations and illusions. In: Liu GT, Volpe NJ, Galetta SL, editors. Liu, Volpe, and Galetta's neuro-ophthalmology. 3rd ed. Amsterdam: Elsevier Inc.; 2019. p. 395–413. https://doi.org/10.1016/B978-0-323-34044-1.00012-2.
27. Stern TA, Freudenreich O, Smith FA, Fricchione GL, Rosenbaum JF. Massachusetts General Hospital handbook of general hospital psychiatry. 7th ed. Amsterdam: Elsevier Inc.; 2017. p. 246.
28. Beckson M, Cummings JL. Neuropsychiatric aspects of stroke. Int J Psychiatry Med. 1991;21(1):1–15. https://doi.org/10.2190/EUMY-3MGP-MWB2-CWG9.
29. Fischer M, Schmutzhard E. Posterior reversible encephalopathy syndrome. J Neurol. 2017;264(8):1608–16. http://www.ncbi.nlm.nih.gov/pubmed/28054130
30. Jackson ML, Ferencz J. Cases - Charles Bonnet syndrome: visual loss and hallucinations. CMAJ. 2009;181(3–4):175–6.
31. Nutile LM. Neurosyphilis with psychosis as the primary presentation. Am J Psychiatry Residents J. 2021;16(3):6–8. https://doi.org/10.1176/appi.ajp-rj.2021.160304.

Conclusions

10

Eric G. Meyer, Kelly L. Cozza, and James A. Bourgeois

The Pros and Cons of Specificity

In the Introduction, we frankly stated that each chapter in this book would focus on a singular symptom. *This is easier said than done.* The complexity of psychiatric symptoms, the dangers of oversimplification, the often synergistic and even reciprocal relationships among symptoms, and the limitations of the constructs available to fully comprehend human behavior all complicate the goal of treating psychiatric symptoms as *unique symptom entities*. Indeed, patients live their lives in an integrated, not discrete, symptom-driven fashion. These challenges are *not* a result of clarifying psychiatric symptoms. These are the *inherent* challenges of psychiatry—of attempting to describe and clinically classify pathologic human behavior. Defining and differentiating psychiatric symptoms illuminates this challenge and is a necessary step in improving our ability to understand our patients.

For some symptoms, clearly defining and differentiating them from other symptoms was relatively straightforward, achieving our goals without much fuss. Decreased appetite is *not* equivalent to weight loss—and it may *not* result in weight loss. Concentration is *not* simply momentary attention, and each cannot be assessed using the same set of questions or tools. Muscle tension is *not* muscle pain, even though it is reasonable to expect a patient to report pain, they may be wholly unaware of their muscle tension.

E. G. Meyer (✉) · K. L. Cozza
Department of Psychiatry, Uniformed Services University of the Health Sciences, Bethesda, MD, USA
e-mail: eric.meyer@usuhs.edu; kelly.cozza@usuhs.edu

J. A. Bourgeois
Department of Psychiatry and Behavioral Sciences, University of California, Davis, Sacramento, CA, USA
e-mail: jbourgeois@ucdavis.edu

E. G. Meyer et al. (eds.), *The Medical Evaluation of Psychiatric Symptoms*,
https://doi.org/10.1007/978-3-031-14372-4_10

Once such straightforward symptoms are clearly understood and differentiated, the task of developing a differential is simplified and, as a result, the following steps of determining the most accurate explanatory diagnosis and treatment approach are markedly easier. Instead of exploring a vast list of all possible symptoms as if they are all equally important, the process of considering other signs and symptoms in relation to the primary symptom is more focused.

Irritability also has a clear definition and can be differentiated from other symptoms. However, this clarity does *not* provide the same diagnostic efficiencies seen with the previous three symptoms. While there are many diagnoses that include irritability as a *symptom*, there are many *more* diagnoses where irritability occurs in *response* to the *other symptoms*. While we elected to primarily explore a differential where irritability was a direct result of the pathophysiology of a disease process, it remains important to consider irritability as a response to other symptoms and/or social stressors related to other symptoms and treatments.

Anxiety, a symptom ubiquitous in psychiatry, becomes remarkably *narrow* when robbed of its commonly associated comorbid symptoms (e.g., decreased concentration, muscle tension, insomnia). Indeed, in its reductionistic, non-contextual simplicity, anxiety may become purely an element of universal human experience. While focusing on this singular symptom may facilitate a better understanding of the person seeking help, it is also quite limiting diagnostically. It is here that the DSM-5-TR's ontology and the need to evaluate for a syndrome-defining *constellation* of associated symptoms becomes apparent.

Insomnia and *dizziness* chapters (Chaps. 4 and 5) stand together as markedly different approaches to the problem of reductionism. For insomnia, we elected to provide tools to differentiate insomnia into three discrete symptoms and explored each with a separate differential. Dizziness, on the other hand, revealed itself to be an almost *meaninglessly nonspecific* word, even as it is commonly reported by patients and frequently noncritically accepted by clinicians. Dizziness, though nonspecific, is certainly not meaningless to the patient—indeed, the patient's words must be respected as having the *utmost meaning and importance* to the patient. However, this import did not absolve us from attempting to understand what dizziness actually means. Any attempt to reduce "dizziness" to some parsimoniously specific core construct was fruitless—as was developing a differential for such a vast experience. Dividing dizziness directly into diagnostic subtypes was also folly—as syncope and vertigo are only possibilities for the same symptom if one is comfortable allowing that symptom to be ambiguous.

The solution was instead to clarify dizziness as one of *three* meaningful symptoms (vertigo, syncope, and disequilibrium) *before* attempting a differential. For space, we only explored vertigo, as it has more elaborated pathophysiology and somewhat more specific meaning. While it was tempting to retitle the chapter as "vertigo," this would have undermined the process of clarifying "dizziness." This is an important point for all clinicians—while we might know the right official, medically validated "title" for a patient's experience, it is important not to discount the "titles" our patients use to capture their lived experience. We hope a future edition might explore all three symptoms more fully.

In the *memory loss* and *visual hallucinations* chapters (Chaps. 6 and 9), the desire to hone down to a specific symptom was especially challenging—and potentially misleading. While a clinician *can* differentiate *working memory* from *semantic memory*, it is unlikely that a patient will have just one of these subtypes or report their experience in sufficient detail to reliably make this distinction on their own. Instead, the clinician needs to look for the preponderance of *both* of these types of memory difficulties and parse out the differences with careful history-taking and clinical evaluation, as this is what helps clarify the diagnostic picture.

Similarly, while visual hallucinations are clearly different from auditory hallucinations, the cooccurrence of the two modalities of hallucinations is *common*. Again, the clinician's task is to assess for *both* types of hallucinations, differentiate them, and determine the relationship between them and the frequency of each. In sum, while it is important to define and differentiate each individual psychiatric symptom, clinicians should *not* expect to necessarily find only one symptom. Instead, after all symptoms have been clearly identified, clinicians must consider them *in concert* to develop an appropriate differential and determine the most unifying diagnosis.

The Urge to Jump to Differentials

Throughout this book, we were consistently reminded of the clinical urge to leave symptoms as ambiguous constructs and accept them at face value while moving directly into the development of a differential diagnosis and treatment plan. While this practice may ultimately result in a *defensible* differential, it is wholly insufficient. Returning to our introductory example, if chest pain is not first clarified as epigastric, a clinician is left asking a plethora of review of systems questions for every potentially related organ system. While the clinician may eventually arrive at a diagnosis of gastroesophageal reflux disease (GERD), it will only be after exhaustively ruling out many other diagnoses, an unnecessary process, as GERD can be characterized and discovered directly—it is not a diagnosis of exclusion.

The temptation to radically accept a symptom without clarification is further compounded for psychiatric symptoms, as the review of symptoms (interestingly and not clearly interchangeably, sometimes called "review of systems") often does not result in a focused review of related symptoms. Instead, it splays out, widely looking for a combination of symptoms that may be conflated to indicate a diagnosis. For example, a patient who presents with "depression" that is never fully characterized may also report difficulty concentrating, insomnia, decreased energy, and psychomotor agitation. While this constellation of symptoms appears to be describing a major depressive episode, if the primary symptom is clarified to be anxiety (a commonly confused experience), the diagnosis quickly coalesces as a generalized anxiety disorder. So, for psychiatric symptoms, the practice of jumping to related symptoms in the defense of a differential is not usually efficient or effective.

The Falsity of Dichotomizing Psychiatric and Medical Differentials

An important conceptual point in this book is the distinction between "psychiatric" and "systemic medical" illness. This distinction, artificial and to a degree arbitrary at best, continues to be the source of active debate. To be consistent, we elected to limit the psychiatric differential to disorders found in the DSM-5-TR—but then obviously ignored all disorders described as primarily due to a general medical condition. The largely anachronistic cartesian dualism of "brain" vs. "mind" as an anatomic vs. functional distinction "between" neurologic (and by inference, general medical) and psychiatric illness, *though rendered obsolete by recent scientific progress*, persists in common language. To illustrate, the concept of "organic" disease as pertains to psychiatric illness has been officially obsolete since the publication of the DSM-IV in 1994. Despite this, some still refer to "neurologic" disease as "due to organic lesions," while "psychiatric" disease is due to "functional" (implicitly "nonanatomic") causes.

Such distinctions regrettably persist among clinicians themselves, many of whom attribute psychiatric illness as solely the result of "social" problems, such as the experience of distressing events, victimization of abuse, or interpersonal problems, while neurologic illness is the consequence of "real disease." This regrettable distinction persists despite decades of research that repeatedly demonstrates that schizophrenia, bipolar disorder, major depressive disorder, and panic disorder have substantially heritable components. To further illustrate this, the only psychiatric illnesses that *a priori* require the experience of traumatic personal events are acute stress disorder and PTSD.

In light of this, it is far preferable to conceptualize psychiatric illness by its symptomatic manifestations, not its implicit "nonanatomic, functional" causation. This is well illustrated by many examples of syndromes with classic "psychiatric" presentations that are substantially, if not solely, clearly attributable to temporally corresponding CNS or systemic disturbances. A brief list of such illnesses includes postpartum depressive disorder (caused by acute hormonal fluctuations), post-stroke depressive disorder (caused by cortical injury), and corticosteroid-associated manic episode (caused by medication exposure).

Fundamental Gaps in the Literature

Throughout this book, basic knowledge gaps in the current literature also became apparent. While the field of neuroscience is exploding with fascinating findings related to a wide variety of complex systems, there is still a limited exploration of medical disorders presenting with primarily psychiatric symptoms. Incidence and prevalence of conditions presenting with specific neuropsychiatric symptoms, the timeline that neuropsychiatric symptoms precede or follow constitutional symptoms, or the associated morbidity and mortality of presenting with a neuropsychiatric symptom are all together wanting for most of the conditions we explored in this text.

What is especially worrisome is that we know that this basic information *matters*. Comorbid depressive disorder increases the risk of diabetes mellitus by 37% [1]. Limited understanding of the incidence and prevalence of such psychiatric comorbidities *perpetuates* (and even *potentiates*) concerns mentioned in the Introduction: hypothyroidism presenting as depression appears to be remarkably rare, even if it is considered a "classic" presentation. How many other conditions are prioritized as part of a workup when they are, in fact, highly unlikely? To put it bluntly, why are not fasting blood glucose and neuroimaging *routine* parts of the evaluation of depressive disorder? Abnormalities in these areas are clearly more likely and clinically significant than thyroid dysfunction.

Another concerning gap in the literature is the limited description of the accuracy of signs, symptoms, laboratory values, and screening tests as they relate to psychiatric symptoms. Psychiatric disorders are often considered to be diagnoses of exclusion. To effectively rule them out we need to know the accuracy of our assessment tools.

Future Work

We hope this text has been as informative and exciting for you to read as it has been for us to design and produce. While we assumed that we could anticipate the result of each chapter's description of its assigned symptom, this could not be further from the truth. Even as seasoned clinicians, we still found our eyebrows raised as the nuance of each symptom was revealed to us. The process of delineating each symptom has reinvigorated our respect for the human condition and humanity's ongoing efforts to understand it. We have only scratched the surface with nine symptoms—continued clarification and delineation of psychiatric symptoms are needed. We further hope that as symptoms are further ascertained, research of these symptoms and their related disorders might gain additional focus, improving treatment, and, ultimately, our patients' lives.

Reference

1. Knol MJ, Twisk JW, Beekman AT, Heine RJ, Snoek FJ, Pouwer F. Depression as a risk factor for the onset of type 2 diabetes mellitus. A meta-analysis. Diabetologia. 2006;49(5):837–45.

Index

E. G. Meyer et al. (eds.), *The Medical Evaluation of Psychiatric Symptoms*,
https://doi.org/10.1007/978-3-031-14372-4

MIX
Papier aus verantwortungsvollen Quellen
Paper from responsible sources
FSC® C105338

If you have any concerns about our products,
you can contact us on
ProductSafety@springernature.com

In case Publisher is established outside the EU,
the EU authorized representative is:
Springer Nature Customer Service Center GmbH
Europaplatz 3, 69115 Heidelberg, Germany

Printed by Libri Plureos GmbH
in Hamburg, Germany